TEXTBOOK ON PSYCHOLOGY
for BSc Nursing Students

TEXTBOOK ON PSYCHOLOGY
for BSc Nursing Students
(As Per INC Syllabus)

I Clement
MSc (N) MSc (Psy) MA (Sociol)
MA (Childcare and Edu) PhD (N) PGDHA
Professor and Principal
VSS College of Nursing
Bengaluru, Karnataka, India

Professional Life Member
PhD Society of India, Chennai, Tamil Nadu
Nursing Research Society of India, New Delhi
Trained Nurses' Association of India, New Delhi
Christian Medical Association of India, New Delhi
Indian Society of Psychiatric Nurses, Bengaluru, Karnataka
Medical Surgical Nursing Society of India, Chennai
Indian Society of Neuroscience Nursing, New Delhi
Asian Association of Cardiac Nurses, Kolkata, West Bengal
Health Organization Member
Indian Red Cross Society
St John's Ambulance Association
General Secretary, Indian Society of Medical Surgical Nurses
Bengaluru, Karnataka, India

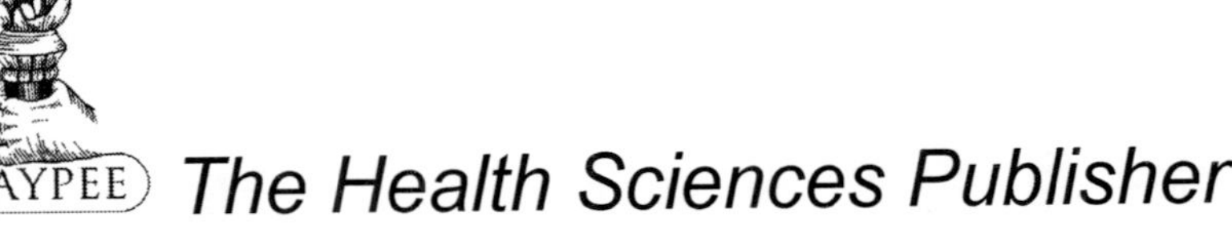

The Health Sciences Publisher
New Delhi | London | Philadelphia | Panama

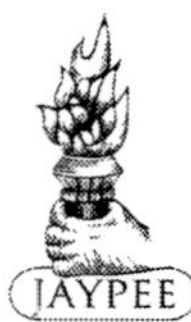

Jaypee Brothers Medical Publishers (P) Ltd

Headquarters

Jaypee Brothers Medical Publishers (P) Ltd
4838/24, Ansari Road, Daryaganj
New Delhi 110 002, India
Phone: +91-11-43574357
Fax: +91-11-43574314
Email: jaypee@jaypeebrothers.com

Overseas Offices

J.P. Medical Ltd
83 Victoria Street, London
SW1H 0HW (UK)
Phone: +44 20 3170 8910
Fax: +44 (0)20 3008 6180
Email: info@jpmedpub.com

Jaypee-Highlights Medical Publishers Inc
City of Knowledge, Bld. 235, 2nd floor Clayton
Panama City, Panama
Phone: +1 507-301-0496
Fax: +1 507-301-0499
Email: cservice@jphmedical.com

Jaypee Medical Inc
325 Chestnut Street
Suite 412, Philadelphia, PA 19106, USA
Phone: +1 267-519-9789
Email: support@jpmedus.com

Jaypee Brothers Medical Publishers (P) Ltd
17/1-B Babar Road, Block-B, Shaymali
Mohammadpur, Dhaka-1207
Bangladesh
Mobile: +08801912003485
Email: jaypeedhaka@gmail.com

Jaypee Brothers Medical Publishers (P) Ltd
Bhotahity, Kathmandu
Nepal
Phone: +977-9741283608
Email: kathmandu@jaypeebrothers.com

Website: www.jaypeebrothers.com
Website: www.jaypeedigital.com

Inquiries for bulk sales may be solicited at: jaypee@jaypeebrothers.com

Textbook on Psychology for BSc Nursing Students

First Edition: **2016, Reprint 2025**

ISBN 978-93-85891-00-7

Printed in India

Preface

Nursing is a dynamic profession where the nurse takes up the multiple roles such as caregiver, health advocate, health counselor, communicator, and comforter; hence, the nurse is able to empathize the problems better by understanding the psychology of the patient to provide better nursing care.

Understanding basic psychology of human will help every nurse plan better nursing care; basically, mental health is the main source of energy to attain a complete health. All the diseases take up the sick-role behavior and every patient will have unique behavior; therefore, it will be challenging for the nurses to understand the specific behavior and handle patients at any setting.

In collaboration with the psychologist, every nurse should work as a team in health care to learn psychological problems in the patients and to tackle them by solving the emotional and psychological issues. Therefore, to develop the knowledge of psychology, this book is a good source of valid information where the students can learn better as per their requirements.

This book on psychology will definitely help every BSc (Nursing) student understand the basic psychology and its application in nursing care. This book has 27 chapters and 6 sections framed carefully in simple language with adequate tables and diagrams for easy understanding of the basic psychology.

The book has appendices with glossary to attain good clarity on the content, and previous years question papers (from 2015 to 1999) to help the students understand the subject better. All the topics are chosen in accordance with Indian Nursing Council (INC) syllabus and their requirements.

This book will be a student-friendly guide for BSc (Nursing) students and a refreshing book for teachers.

I wish all the best for all nursing students!

I Clement

Acknowledgments

I am thankful to the Lord Almighty who strengthens me with his abundant blessing through innumerable means, helping me in all my accomplishments.

My heartfelt thanks to Shri Sommana, Former Minister of Karnataka and Chairman of VSS Group of Institutions, Bengaluru, Karnataka, India, for his constant support and encouragement.

My sincere thanks to my guru Dr BT Basavanthappa (Principal, Rajarajeswari College of Nursing, Bengaluru) and Professor PV Ramachandran (Chairman, College of Nursing, Sri Ramachandra University, Chennai, Tamil Nadu, India), a great philosopher and internationally renowned teacher of nursing, who helped me in discovering the world of knowledge. I am thankful to Ms Shylaja Sommana (Managing Director), Dr BS Naveen, Dr BS Arun and Ms Divya, from VSS Group of Institutions for their support and encouragement.

I am also grateful to Dr BC Bhagavan (Syndicate Member of RGUHS, Bengaluru and Professor, Department of Surgery, Kempegowda Institute of Medical Sciences, Bengaluru) and Dr Ashwathnarayanan (MLA, Chairman, Padmashree Group of Institutions, Bengaluru). Special thanks to Dr TV Ramakrishnan (Professor of Anesthesiology and Head of Clinical Services, Department of Accident and Emergency Medicine, Sri Ramachandra University), Dr Jeyaseelan Manickam Devadasan (Syndicate Member, The Tamil Nadu Dr MGR Medical University, Chennai, and Dean and Professor, Annai JKK Sampoorani Ammal College of Nursing, Namakkal, Tamil Nadu), Dr Tamilmani (Principal) and Professor (Mrs) Jessie Sudarsanum (Head of Department of Medical Surgical Nursing), Annai JKK Sampoorani Ammal College of Nursing, and all my teachers and students.

I convey my sincere thanks to my beloved parents, brothers and sisters, and my wife Nisha Clement, for her continuous support and constant encouragement in each step of my life. I take this opportunity to thank my little ones, Cibin, Cynthia and Cavin. I extend thanks to my beloved friend and brother Mr Regi T Kurien, USA.

Special thanks to Shri Jitendar P Vij (Group Chairman), Mr Ankit Vij (Group President), Mr Tarun Duneja (Director–Publishing), Mr KK Raman (Production Manager) and Mr Rajesh Sharma (Production Coordinator) of M/s Jaypee Brothers Medical Publishers (P) Ltd, New Delhi, India, and also Mr Venugopal Vishnumurthy [Associate Director-South (Sales and Marketing)], Mr Santhosh Kumar (Author Coordinator), Ms Sajini SV (Team Head) and other staff members of M/s Jaypee Brothers Medical Publishers (P) Ltd, Bengaluru branch.

Contents

Section III

Cognitive Process

Section IV

Motivational/Emotional Process and Personality

Section V

Developmental/Educational/Social Psychology

Section VI

Mental Health Process

Appendices

Section I

Introduction to Psychology

CHAPTER 1

History and Origin of Science of Psychology

■ INTRODUCTION

The word 'psychology' is derived from two Greek words, 'psyche' and logos'. 'Psyche' means 'soul' and 'logos' means 'the study of'. Psychology, as a scientific discipline is an extremely exciting field of knowledge. It continuous to grow at an accelerating field pace each year and continues to provide answer to basic question about the human behavior. Psychology has enormous potential. It offers us the hope of both understanding and improving the quality of life. Psychological knowledge has been used in measuring intelligence, designing school curricula, helping troubled marriages, controlling aggression, selling products and treating both the young and old with greater sensitivity and humaneness.

Psychology is the academic and applied scientific study of mental processes and behavior. Psychology also involves the application of knowledge to various spheres of human activity from daily life, work and family to the treatment of severe mental health problems. Psychology revolves around such broad areas as emotions, perception, individuality and personality, relationships, social dynamics and functions, and also many other subjects. Psychology also attempts to identify the physical and biological processes that underlie mental functioning.

■ EARLY ORIGIN OF PSYCHOLOGY

The earliest origins of psychology are, unsurprisingly, found in the ancient civilizations of Greece, Egypt, China and India. The early psychology involved theories on the mind, body and soul and how they all operate together, so they were not really what we would call psychology today. However, these great early psychological philosophers identified things such as the brain and speculation of its functions, basics of human nature and the 'self'. The Medieval Times saw more psychological progress. As early as the 700s, Medieval Muslim had built insane asylums and practices to help patients with diseases of the mind. Ahmed ibn Sahl al-Balkhi was the first to suggest that if the mind gets sick, the body may eventually develop a physical illness. He recognized and analyzed what we modernly call depression.

Several other modern psychological phenomena and neuropsychiatric conditions were emerging—hallucination, mania, dreams, nightmares, epilepsy, paralysis, stroke, vertigo, psychotherapy and musical therapy, social psychology, neurophysiology, and the subconsciously western psychology emerging. The ancient writings were preserved, thanks to Islamic translators, and together with their theories and experiments became the basis for modern psychology, which started to emerge during the Renaissance. While early psychology involved the study of the soul, modern psychology focused more on brain functions. During the Enlightenment period, thinkers Descartes, Thomas Willis and John Locke discussed the nature of mind and soul, but also supported the development of clinical psychology as a discipline of medicine. Those times also saw the rise of popular yet false psychological developments. This included the science of hypnotism, developed by Anton Mesmer as a way to cure diseases using the 'magnetism of the mind.'

Prehistoric Views

As far back as the Stone Age (7,000 years ago and maybe even as long as 50,000 years ago), humans tried to cure one another of various mental problems. Most prehistoric cultures had 'medicine men or women,' known as shamans, who would treat the possessed by driving out the demons with elaborate rituals such as exorcisms, incantations and prayers. Occasionally, some of these shamans appeared to practice the oldest of all known surgical procedures, trephination.

Trephination involves drilling a small hole in a person's skull, usually less than an inch in diameter (Alt et al 1997; Weber and Wahl, 2006). Some of these surgeries may have been for medical reasons such as an attempt to heal a brain injury. Some may also have been performed for psychological reasons to release the spirits and demons that possessed the afflicted person. Anthropological evidence suggests that a surprisingly large percentage of people survived such surgeries, which today's scientists can confirm by identifying bone growth after the procedure and the surgeons must have had moderately sophisticated knowledge and understanding of the brain.

Ancient Views

Around 2600 BCE (before the common era), the ancient Chinese moved away from supernatural explanations toward natural and physiological explanations of psychological disorders (Tseng, 1973). Specifically, they made connections between a person's bodily organs and emotions. The heart housed the mind; the liver, the spiritual soul; the lung, the animal soul; the spleen, ideas and intelligence; and the kidneys, will and vitality. The ancient Egyptians and Greeks also sought natural explanations for psychological disorders. For example, in the second century BCE, the ancient Egyptians apparently used narcotics to treat pain (Finger, 1994). The Greek physician Hippocrates (460–377 BCE) was the first to write about a man suffering from a phobia of heights—what we now call acrophobia.

■ HISTORY OF PSYCHOLOGY

The subject psychology has a long past, but a short history. The meaning of this statement is simply that human kind has given thought to psychological questions for many centuries. The ancient philosophers wrote at length about psychology. However, psychology as an established and recognized science in universities and colleges is less than 100 years old. The date, when psychology became a field of study formally detached from philosophy is generally taken as 1879, the date when Wilhelm Wundt, the Principal Founder of experimental psychology established the first psychological laboratory in Leipzig, Germany. Main contributors and their contribution in history of psychology are detailed in Table 1.1.

Table 1.1: History of psychology and important contributors

Sl No.	Contributors	Description
1.	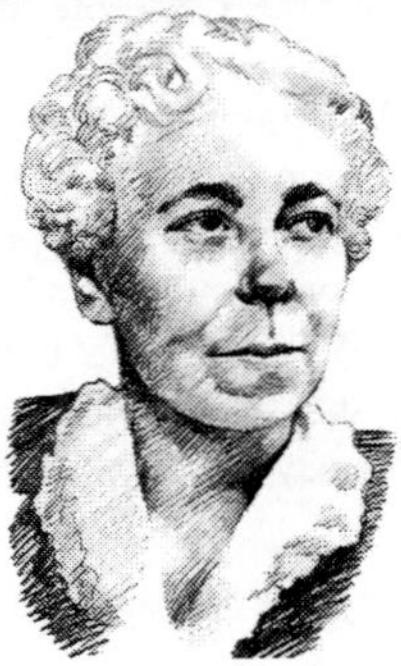 Karen Horney (1885–1952)	**Karen Horney** made significant contributions to humanism, self-psychology, psychoanalysis and feminine psychology. Her refutation of Freud's theories about women generated more interest in the psychology of women. Horney also believed that people were able to act as their own therapists, emphasizing the personal role each person has in their own mental health and encouraging self-analysis and self-help. Holistic psychology personality attributes are the result of the interaction between the person and environment.
2.	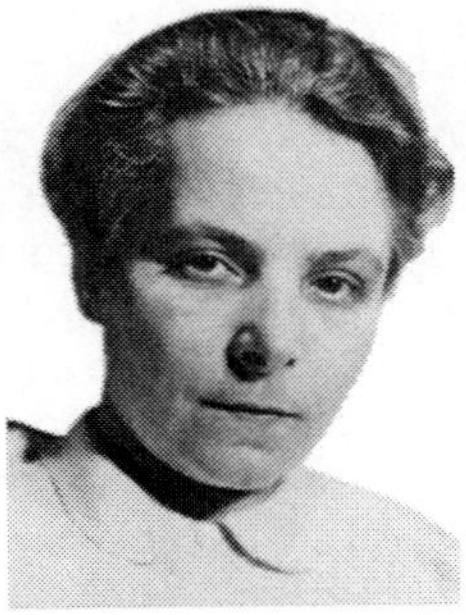 Edith Jacobson (1897–1978)	**Edith Jacobson** (September 10, 1897 to December 8, 1978) was a German psychoanalyst. Her major contributions to psychoanalytic thinking dealt with the development of the sense of identity and self-esteem, and with an understanding of depression and psychosis. She was able to integrate the tripartite structural model of classic psychoanalysis with the theory of object relations into a revised drive theory. Thereby, she increased the treatment possibilities of the more disturbed preoedipal patients.
3.	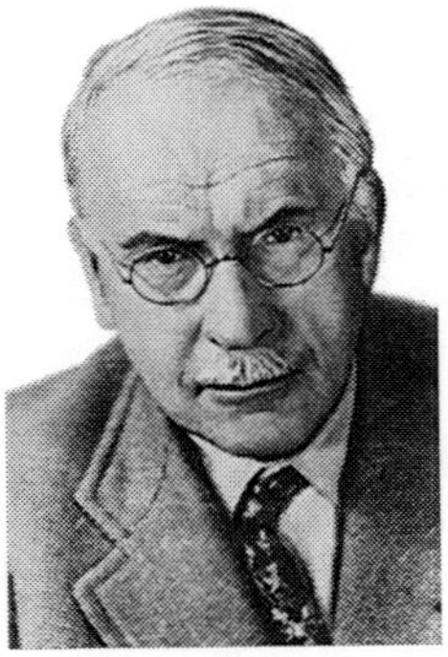 Carl Gustav Jung (1875–1961)	**Carl Gustav Jung** was a Swiss psychiatrist and Founder of the school of analytical psychology. He proposed and developed the concepts of the extroverted and introverted personality, archetypes and the collective unconscious. The issues that he dealt with arose from his personal experiences. For many years Jung felt as if he had two separate personalities. One introverted and other extroverted. This interplay resulted in his study of integration and wholeness. His work has been influential not only in psychology but also in religion and literature as well.
4.		**Maslow** [April 1, 1908 (Brooklyn) to June 8, 1970 (California)] took this idea and created his now famous hierarchy of needs. Beyond the details of air, water, food and sex, he laid out five broader layers—the physiological needs, the need for safety and security, the need for love and belonging, the need for esteem and the need to actualize the self, in that order. At a time

Contd...

Contd...

Sl No.	Contributors	Description
	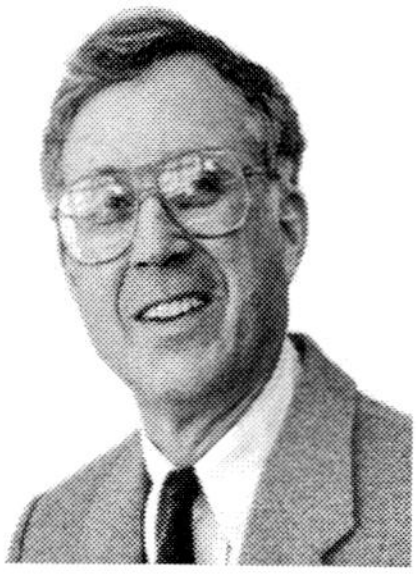 Abraham Maslow (1908–1970)	when most psychologists focused aspects of human nature that were considered abnormal, Abraham Maslow shifted to focus to look at the positive sides of mental health. His interest in human potential, seeking peak experiences and improving mental health by seeking personal growth had a lasting influence on psychology. While Maslow's work fell out of favor with many academic psychologists, his theories are enjoying resurgence due to the rising interesting in positive psychology.
5.	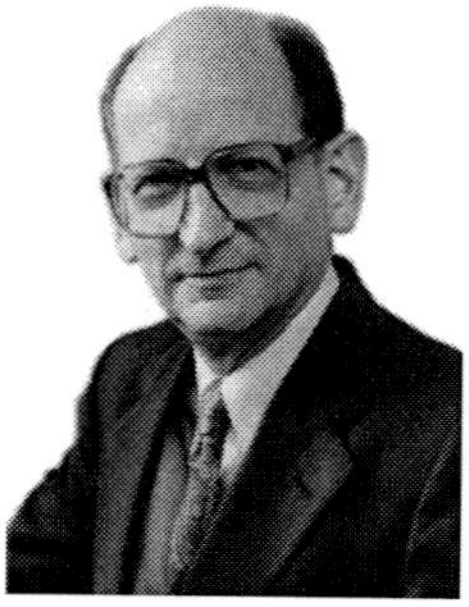 Kernberg (1928)	**Otto Friedmann Kernberg** (born September 10, 1928) is a psychoanalyst and Professor of Psychiatry at Weill Cornell Medical College. He is most widely known for his psychoanalytic theories on borderline personality organization and narcissistic pathology. In addition, his work has been central in integrating postwar ego psychology (which was primarily developed in the United States and the United Kingdom) with Kleinian and other object relations perspectives (which was developed primarily in the United Kingdom and South America). His integrative writings were central to the development of modern object relations, a theory of mind that is perhaps the theory most widely accepted among modern psychoanalysts.
6.	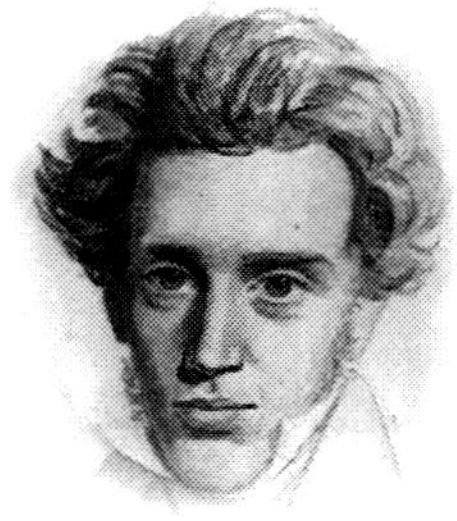 Søren Aabye Kierkegaard (1813–1855)	**Kierkegaard** explains a feeling in his book, *The Concept of Anxiety.* As an example, he asks us to consider a man standing on a cliff or tall building. If this man looks over the edge, he experiences two different kinds of fear—the fear of falling and fear brought on by the impulse to throw him off the edge. This second type of fear or anxiety arises from the realization that he has absolute freedom to choose whether to jump or not and this fear is as dizzying as his vertigo. Kierkegaard suggests that we experience the same anxiety in all our moral choices, when we realize that we have the freedom to make even the most terrifying decisions.
7.		**Murphy** was among the first researchers to conduct scientific experiments on telepathy, clairvoyance and other extrasensory powers. Murphy was also directly responsible for the creation of the Psychology Department and the Parapsychology Laboratory at Duck University. Murphy argued that a collective consciousness might support the theory of reincarnation. According to Murphy, a person's mind or soul could survive in an 'interpersonal field'. He further contended that this field might explain some paranormal phenomena, but that an individual consciousness or

Contd...

Contd...

Sl No.	Contributors	Description
	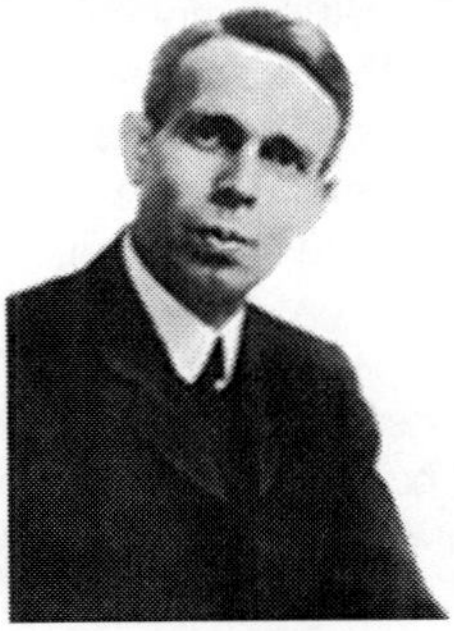 Gardner Murphy (1895–1979)	personality would not continue to exist in this field. Instead, a person's mind would be assimilated into the collective consciousness. Murphy paranormal phenomena were as scientific as any other psychological phenomena and he argued that there were scientific benefits to recreating contexts in which paranormal events were likely to occur. He also argued that personality could play a role in an individual's experience of paranormal events. Murphy was a prolific author and contributed publication of many psychology books. Much of what he wrote is still considered/cited as valuable research and essential to teaching in the field of parapsychology. Murphy also wrote articles highlighting his theories on social and clinical psychology, personality, parapsychology and humanistic psychology.
8.	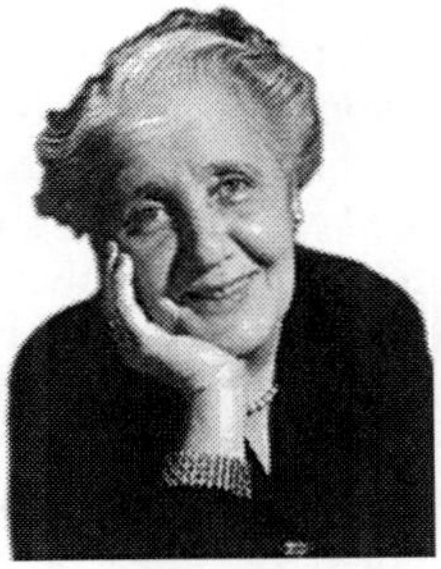 Melanie Klein (1882–1960)	**Melanie Reizes Klein** (March 30, 1882 to September 22, 1960) was an Austrian-born British psychoanalyst, who devised novel therapeutic techniques for children that had an impact on child psychology and contemporary psychoanalysis. She was a leading innovator in theorizing object relation theory. Melanie Klein is perhaps the most important woman psychoanalyst, who ever lived and yet is probably the least well known to American psychologists.
9.	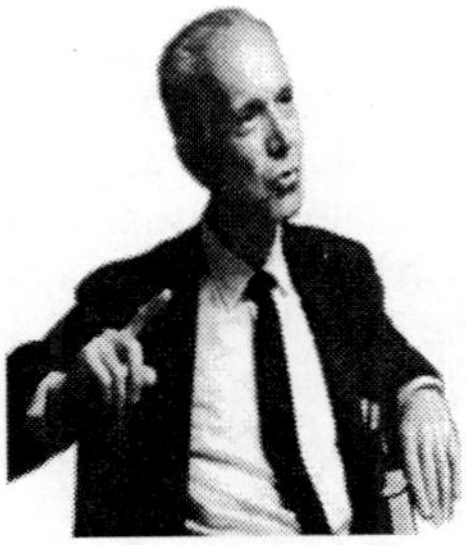 Heinz Kohut (1913–1981)	**Kohut** defined empathy as a key element of analysis, a viewpoint he maintained and extended throughout his life (1990–1991a). Patients become aware of their excessive needs for approval and self-gratification. *'Forms and Transformations of Narcissism'* (1966) and *'The Psychoanalytic Treatment of Narcissistic Personality Disorders'* (1990–1991b) introduced a new way of analyzing narcissism that culminated in the publication of *The Analysis of the Self* (1971) and *How Does Analysis Cure?* (1984), which was published posthumously in 1984.
10.	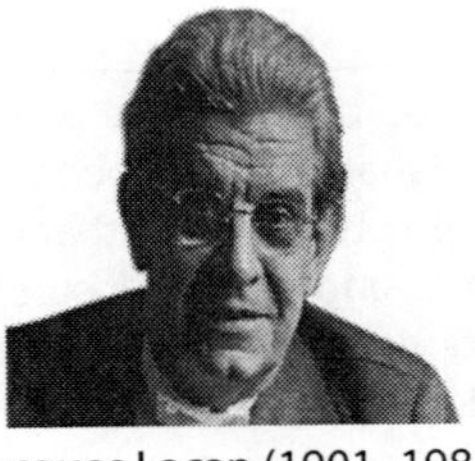 Jacques Lacan (1901–1981)	**Jacques Marie Émile Lacan** (French; April 13, 1901 to September 9, 1981) was a French psychoanalyst and psychiatrist, who have been called 'the most controversial psychoanalyst since Freud'. Giving yearly seminars in Paris from 1953 to 1981, Lacan influenced many leading French intellectuals in the 1960s and the 1970s, especially those associated with poststructuralism. Primary process of thought is actually uncontrolled free-flowing sequences of meaning.

Contd...

Contd...

Sl No.	Contributors	Description
11.	Kurt Lewin (1890–1947)	**Kurt Lewin** contributed to Gestalt psychology by expanding on Gestalt theories and applying them to human behavior. He was also one of the first psychologists to systematically test human behavior, influencing experimental psychology, social psychology and personality psychology. He was a prolific writer, publishing more than 80 articles and eight books on various psychology topics. Many of his unfinished papers were published by his colleagues after his sudden death at age 56. Lewin is known as the Father of modern social psychology because of his pioneering work that utilized scientific methods and experimentation to look as social behavior.
12.	Adolf Meyer (1866–1950)	**Adolf Meyer** (September 13, 1866 to March 17, 1950) was a psychiatrist who rose to prominence as the President of the American Psychiatric Association and was one of the most influential figures in psychiatry in the first half of the 20th century. His focus on collecting detailed case histories on patients is the most prominent of his contributions; along with his insistence that patients could best be understood through consideration of their 'psychobiological' life situations. He is most remembered for reframing mental disease as biopsychosocial 'reaction types' rather than as biologically specifiable natural disease entities. In 1906, he reframed dementia precox as a 'reaction type'; a discordant bundle of maladaptive habits that arose as a response to biopsychosocial stressors.
13.	Henry Murray (1893–1988)	**Henry A Murray** (Harry), organizer and primary author of *Explorations in Personality* = = *w* (Murray et al, 1938) and with his long-time partner and collaborator Christiana Morgan, deviser of the Thematic Apperception Test (TAT), was a humanistic psychologist on the grand scale. Since he felt alienated from the irrationalistic, antiscientific aspects of the humanistic psychology movement, when it became substantially captured by the counterculture of the 1960s and therefore limited his participation, probably rather few Henry A Murray participants in humanistic psychology.
14.		**Carl Rogers** was a humanistic psychologist, who agreed with the main assumptions of Abraham Maslow, but added that for a person to 'grow', they need an environment that provides them with genuineness (openness and self-disclosure), acceptance (being seen with unconditional positive regard) and empathy (being listened to and understood). Rogers identified five characteristics of the fully functioning person:

Contd...

Contd...

Sl No.	Contributors	Description
	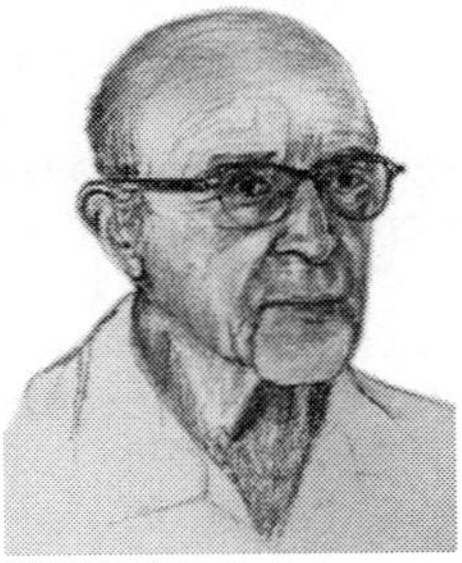 Carl Rogers (1902–1987)	*Open to experience:* Both positive and negative emotions accepted. Negative feelings are not denied, but worked through (rather than resort to ego defense mechanisms). *Existential living:* In touch with different experiences as they occur in life, avoiding prejudging and preconceptions. Being able to live and fully appreciate the present, not always looking back to the past or forward to the future (i.e. living for the moment). *Trust feelings:* Feeling, instincts and gut reactions are paid attention to and trusted. People's own decisions are the right ones and we should trust ourselves to make the right choices. *Creativity:* Creative thinking and risk taking are features of a person's life. Person does not play safe all the time. This involves the ability to adjust and change and seek new experiences. *Fulfilled life:* Person is happy and satisfied with life and always looking for new challenges and experiences.
15.	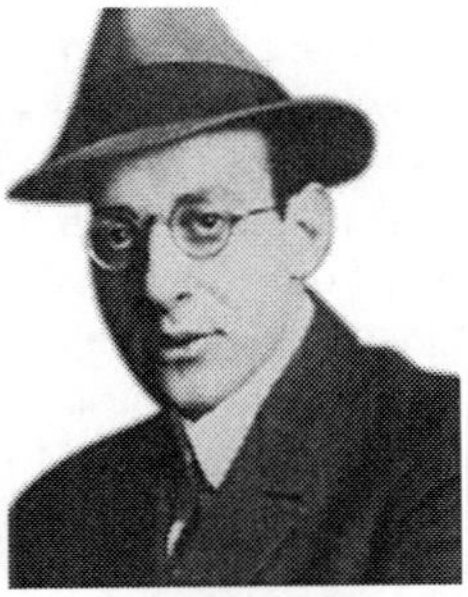 Frederick S Perls (1893–1970)	**Perls** was a German-American psychotherapist, who co-founded Gestalt therapy. Perls was born in Berlin in 1893 into a middle class family. He was a bright student, but his interest in science did not emerge until after he enrolled in college in 1913. Before that he had been interested in the theater. He toyed briefly with the idea of studying law, but settled on medicine. Frederick S Perls, known to his friends and colleagues as Fritz, was the Co-Founder with his wife Laura (1905–1990) of the Gestalt School of Psychotherapy. Trained as a Freudian, Perls felt that Freud's ideas had limitations, in part, because they focused on past experiences. One of the key elements of Gestalt therapy is its focus on what Perls called the 'here and now.'
16.	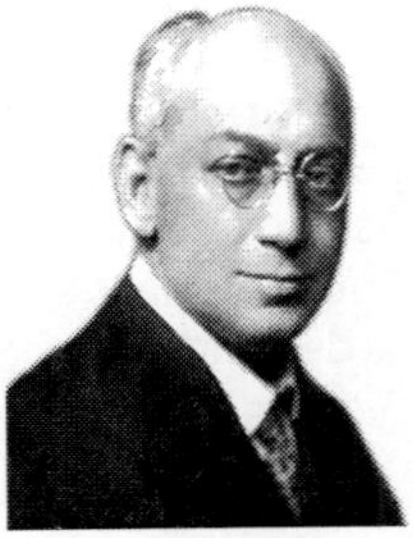 Sándor Radó (1890–1972)	**Sándor Radó,** [1890 (Kisvarda) May 14, 1972 New York City] was a Hungarian psychoanalyst and physician. Radó's work culminates in his writings on *'Adaptational Psychodynamics',* a concise reformulation of what has come to be known as ego analysis. In them he presciently criticizes the exclusive preoccupation of the therapist with the patient's past and the neglect of his present, among other matters—on all these points Radó was way ahead of his time.
17.		**Skinner** described his Pennsylvania childhood as 'warm and stable'. As a boy, he enjoyed building and inventing things; a skill he would later use in his own psychological experiments. In 1945, Skinner moved to Bloomington, Indiana and became Psychology Department Chair at the University of Indiana. In 1948, he joined the Psychology Department at Harvard University,

Contd...

Contd...

Sl No.	Contributors	Description
	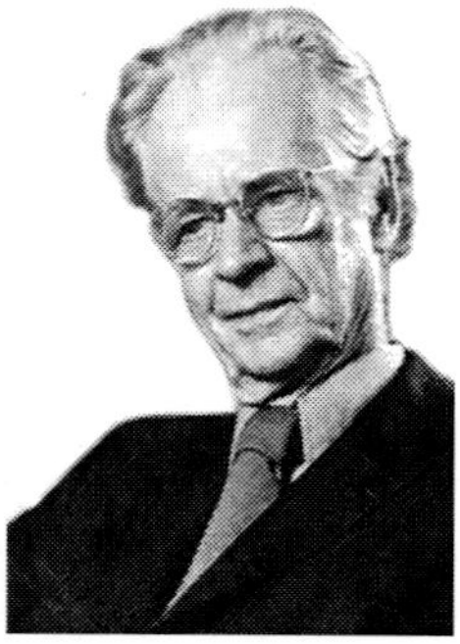 Skinner BF (1904–1990)	where he remained for the rest of his life. He became one of the leaders of behaviorism and his work contributed immensely to experimental psychology. He also invented the 'Skinner box' in which a rat learns to obtain food by pressing a lever. BF Skinner is famous for his research on operant conditioning and negative reinforcement. He developed a device called 'cumulative recorder', which showed rates of responding as a sloped line. Using this device, he found that behavior did not depend on the preceding stimulus as Watson and Pavlov maintained. Instead, Skinner found that behaviors were dependent upon what happens after the response. Skinner called this operant behavior.
18.	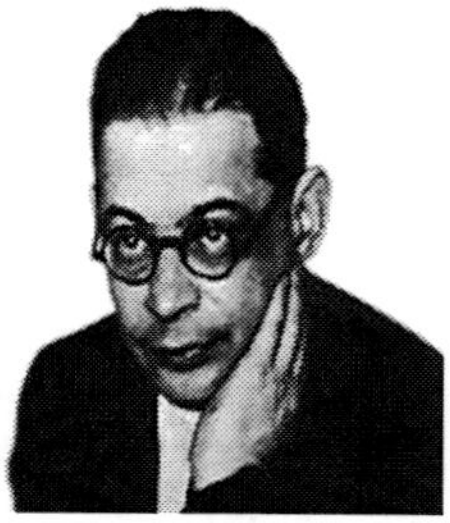 Otto Rank (1884–1939)	**Otto Rank** (April 22, 1884 to October 31, 1939) was an Austrian psychoanalyst, writer and teacher. Born in Vienna as Otto Rosenfeld, he was one of Sigmund Freud's closest colleagues for 20 years, a prolific writer on psychoanalytic themes, an editor of the two most important analytic journals, Managing Director of Freud's publishing house and a creative theorist and therapist. He remains famous for his 'trauma-of-birth theory' and 'will therapy'. Rank's work diverged from Freud's, when he became interested in the way the infant experiences separating from the mother at the time of birth. He developed the idea that freedom, namely independence from others, is essential to the development of our creativity. For Rank, how we deal with the independence from our mother that is thrust on us at birth determines the type of personality we develop.
19.	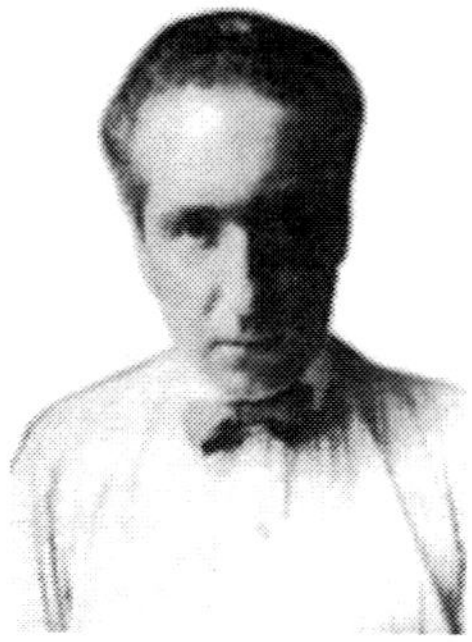 Wilhelm Reich (1897–1957)	**Reich** born in Austria, obtained his medical degree in 1922 and after graduate studies in neurology and psychiatry, became the first Clinical Assistant at Sigmund Freud's Psychoanalytic Polyclinic in 1922 and the clinic's first Director in 1928. In 1930, he moved to Berlin, where he helped establish a program for sexual education for young people. During his early days as a psychoanalytic, Reich made important observations about the nature of human character and how to deal with character structure in therapy.
20.		**Harry Stack Sullivan,** American psychiatrist, who conceived of psychiatry as the study of interpersonal relations, was born in Norwich. Sullivan was strongly influenced by psychoanalytic studies of schizophrenic patients, but always related psychoanalytic interpretations to the broader concepts

Contd...

Contd...

Sl No.	Contributors	Description
	Harry Stack Sullivan (1892–1949)	developed by non-psychoanalytic psychiatrists. Harry Stack Sullivan is known primarily for his theory of interpersonal relations, though he is also well known for his system of psychotherapy to which it is closely related. Essentially, Sullivan's theory holds that human experience primarily consists of interactions or transactions between people, whether the people are real, imaginary (as in many dreams and psychotic experiences), or a blend of both the real and imaginary.

■ SCHOOLS OF PSYCHOLOGY

When psychology was first established as a science separate from biology and philosophy, the debate over how to describe and explain the human mind and behavior began. The different schools of psychology represent the major theories within psychology. The first school of thought, structuralism, was advocated by the Founder of the first psychology laboratory, Wilhelm Wundt. Almost immediately, other theories began to emerge and vie for dominance in psychology. In the past, psychologists often identified themselves exclusively with one single school of thought. Today, most psychologists have an eclectic outlook on psychology. They often draw on ideas and theories from different schools rather than holding to any singular outlook. The following are some of the major schools of thought that have influenced our knowledge and understanding of psychology.

Structuralism

Structuralism emerged as the first school of thought and some of the ideas associated with the structuralist school were advocated by Wilhelm Wundt (Fig. 1.1). Structuralism was the first school of psychology and focused on breaking down mental processes into the most basic components. Researchers tried to understand the basic elements of consciousness using a method known as introspection.

Wilhelm Wundt, is often associated with this school of thought despite the fact that it was his student Edward B Titchener, who first coined the term to describe this school of thought. While Wundt's work helped to establish psychology as a separate science and contributed methods to experimental psychology, Wundt himself referred to his view of psychology as volunteerism and his theories tended to be much more holistic than the ideas that Titchener later introduced in the United States. Titchener's development of structuralism helped establish the very first 'school' of psychology, but structuralism itself did not last long beyond Titchener's death.

Strengths of Structuralism

1. Structuralism is important because it is the first major school of thought in psychology.
2. Structuralism also influenced experimental psychology.

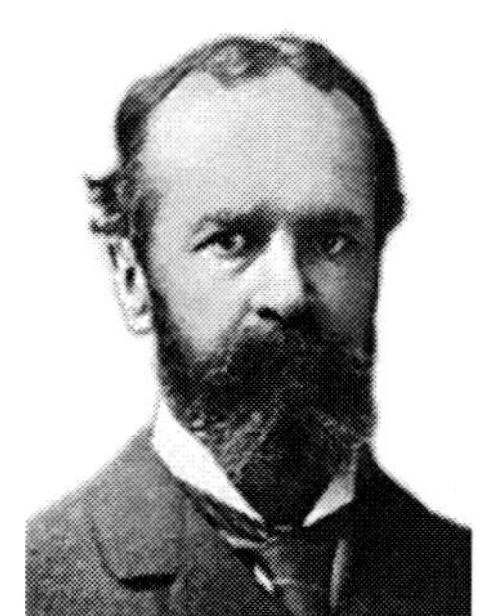

Figure 1.1: Wilhelm Wundt

Functionalism

Functionalism formed as a reaction to the structuralism and was heavily influenced by the work of William James and the evolutionary theory of Charles Darwin. Functionalists sought to explain the mental processes in a more systematic and accurate manner. Rather than focusing on the elements of consciousness, functionalists focused on the purpose of consciousness and behavior. Functionalism also emphasized individual differences, which had a profound impact on education:

1. Functionalism is contrast to structuralism, emphasized the changing and dynamic quality of consciousness.
2. The Father of functionalism William James (1890) compared the human mind to a river always flowing and changing.
3. Functionalism as its name implies, asserts that consciousness has a function and aim. Functionalism provided an impetus for psychologists, who are interested in applying psychology to industry and education.

Strengths of Functionalism

1. Influenced behaviorism and applied psychology.
2. Influenced the educational system, especially with regards to John Dewey's belief that children should learn at the level for which they are developmentally prepared.

Behaviorism

Behaviorism suggests that all behavior can be explained by environmental causes rather than by internal forces. Behaviorism is focused on observable behavior. Theories of learning including classical conditioning and operant conditioning were the focus of a great deal of research. The behavioral school of psychology had a major influence on the course of psychology and many of the ideas and techniques that emerged from this school of thought are still widely used today. Behavioral training, token economies, aversion therapy and other techniques are frequently used in psychotherapy and behavior modification programs:

1. Behaviorism came into being in the 1910s with the writings of John B Watson (Fig. 1.2).
2. Watson (1919) claimed that the concept of consciousness was unnecessary for psychology. He thus attacked at once both structuralism and functionalism.
3. The essential idea in behaviorism is that consciousness cannot be observed. It is completely private and personnel.
4. Watson suggested using more specific concepts such as habits or Pavlov's conditioning reflexes. Watson's aim has to transform psychology from quasi philosophical study of the mind into valid 'science of behavior.'

There are two major types of conditioning:

1. **Classical conditioning:** It is a technique used in behavioral training in which a naturally occurring stimulus is paired with a response. Next, a previously neutral stimulus is paired with the naturally occurring stimulus. Eventually, the previously neutral stimulus comes to evoke the response without the presence of

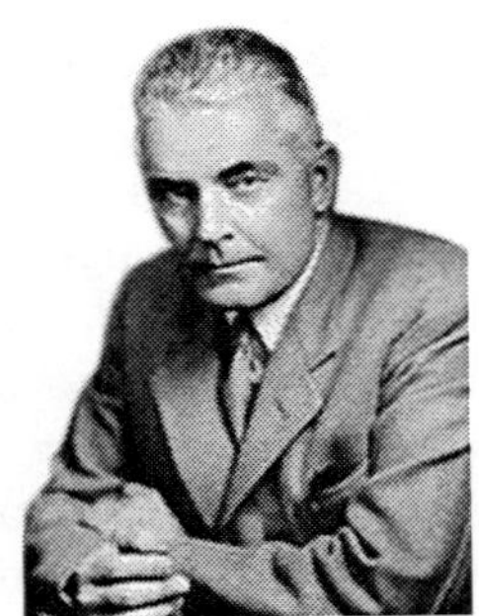

Figure 1.2: John B Watson

the naturally occurring stimulus. The two elements are then known as the condition stimulus and conditioned response.

2. **Operant conditioning:** Sometimes referred to as instrumental conditioning. This is a method of learning that occurs through rewards and punishments for behavior. Through operant conditioning, an association is made between a behavior and a consequence for that behavior.

Strengths of Behaviorism

1. Behaviorism is based upon observable behaviors, so it is easier to quantify and collect data and information, when conducting research.
2. Effective therapeutic techniques such as intensive behavioral intervention, behavior analysis, token economies and discrete trial training are all rooted in behaviorism. These approaches are often very useful in changing maladaptive or harmful behaviors in both children and adults.

Gestalt Psychology

Gestalt psychology is a school of psychology based upon the idea that we experience things as unified wholes. This approach to psychology began in Germany and Austria during the late 19th century in response to the molecular approach of structuralism. Instead of breaking down thoughts and behavior to their smallest elements, the Gestalt psychologists believed that you must look at the whole of experience. According to the Gestalt thinkers, the whole is greater than the sum of its parts:

1. Gestalt psychology came into being as a reaction against Wundt's structuralism. It came into prominence in Germany simultaneously when behaviorism was gaining attention in America.
2. During 1910s without being aware of one another's development. The Father of Gestalt psychology is Max Wertheimer.
3. The essential point of Gestalt psychology is that it is important to explain everything by analyzing it downward, by always reducing it something that is presumably on a more basic level.

The fundamental 'formula' of Gestalt theory might be expressed in this way', Max Wertheimer wrote "There are wholes, the behavior of which is not determined by that of their individual elements, but where the part-processes are themselves determined by the intrinsic nature of the whole. It is the hope of Gestalt theory to determine the nature of such wholes (1924)."

Psychoanalysis

Psychoanalysis is a school of psychology founded by Sigmund Freud (Fig. 1.3). This school of thought emphasized the influence of the unconscious mind on behavior. Freud believed that the human mind was composed of three elements—the id, the ego and the superego.

The id is composed of primal urges, while the ego is the component of personality charged with dealing with reality. The superego is the part of personality that holds all of the ideals and values we internalize from our parents and culture. Freud believed

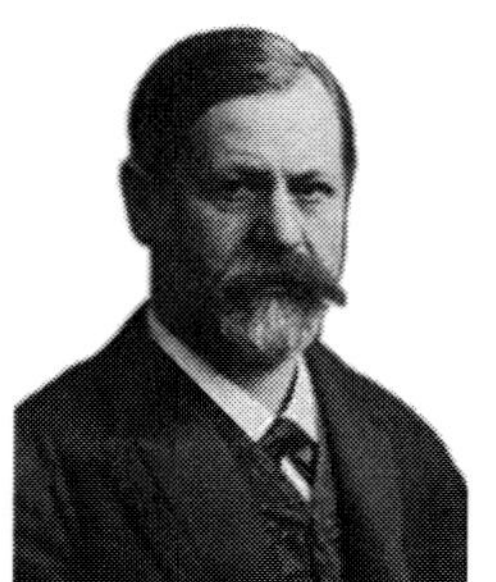

Figure 1.3: Sigmund Freud

that the interaction of these three elements was what led to all of the complex human behaviors. Freud's school of thought was enormously influential, but also generated a great deal of controversy. This controversy existed not only in his time but also in modern discussions of Freud's theories:

1. The Father of psychoanalysis is Sigmund Freud. His personal influence in psychology made itself known over a long period of time beginning in the later part of the 19th century and ending in the 1930s.
2. Freud argued that motives, ideas and memories often exist in human personality outside of consciousness (awareness).
3. The human mind is similar to iceberg. The exposed tip represents consciousness. The large region below water level represents the unconscious domain of the mind. Freud argued that the unpleasant or painful ideas are repressed or pushed down into the unconscious.
4. Freud devised a technique called free association for making repressed material available to consciousness. Freud believed that if a neurotic patient could see into the nature of his conflicts, then those conflicts would lose most of their power to make the patient suffer.

Strengths of Psychoanalysis

1. While most psychodynamic theories did not rely on experimental research, the methods and theories of psychoanalytic thinking contributed to experimental psychology.
2. Many of the theories of personality developed by psychodynamic thinkers are still influential today including Erikson's theory of psychosocial stages and Freud's psychosexual stage theory.
3. Psychoanalysis opened up a new view on mental illness, suggesting that talking about problems with a professional could help relieve symptoms of psychological distress.

Criticisms of Psychoanalysis

1. Freud's theories overemphasized the unconscious mind, sex and aggression, and childhood experiences.
2. Many of the concepts proposed by psychoanalytic theorists are difficult to measure and quantify.

Neo-Freudian Theories

Neo-Freudian psychologists were thinkers, who agreed with the basis of Freud's psychoanalytic theory, but changed and adapted the theory to incorporate their own beliefs, ideas and theories. Psychologist Sigmund Freud proposed a number of ideas that were highly controversial, but also attracted a number of followers. Many of these thinkers agreed with Freud's concept of the unconscious mind and the importance of early childhood. There were, however, a number of points that other thinkers disagreed with or directly rejected. Because of this, these individuals went on to propose their own unique theories of personality:

1. Several contemporary psychoanalysts such as Karen Horney, Erich Fromm and Harry Stack Sullivan are all referred to as Neo-Freudians.
2. Their theories of personality are essentially revisions of Freud's while they differ from each other in many specific

details and they are similar in that they all emphasized the role of culture in the development of personality rather than biological drives or instincts.

3. According to Harry Stack Sullivan (Fig. 1.4), personality does not exist apart from interpersonal relations. In other words, there is no personality, unless one is interacting with others.

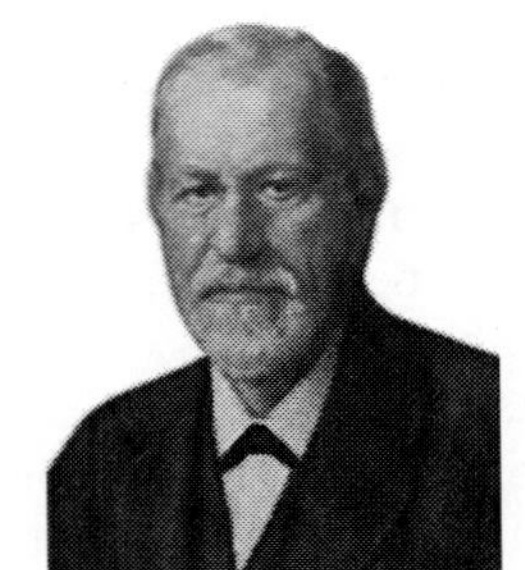

Figure 1.4: Harry Stack Sullivan

Neo-Freudian Disagreements with Freud

There are a few different reasons why these Neo-Freudian thinkers disagreed with Freud. For example, Erik Erikson believed that Freud was incorrect to believe that personality is shaped almost entirely by childhood events. Other issues that motivated Neo-Freudian thinkers included:

1. Freud's emphasis on sexual urges as a primary motivator.
2. Freud's negative view of human nature.
3. Freud's belief that personality is entirely shaped by early childhood experiences.
4. Freud's lack of emphasis on social and cultural influences on behavior and personality.

While the Neo-Freudian may have been influenced by Freud, they developed their own unique theories and perspectives on human development, personality and behavior.

Humanistic Psychology

Humanistic psychology emerged during the 1950s as a reaction to psychoanalysis and behaviorism, which dominated psychology at the time. Psychoanalysis was focused on understanding the unconscious motivations that drive behavior, while behaviorism studied the conditioning processes that produce behavior. Humanist thinkers felt that both psychoanalysis and behaviorism were too pessimistic, either focusing on the most tragic of emotions or failing to take into accounts the role of personal choice.

Humanistic psychology was instead focused on each individual's potential and stressed the importance of growth and self-actualization. The fundamental belief of humanistic psychology is that people are innately good and that mental and social problems result from deviations from this natural tendency:

1. A single individual cannot be named as the Father of humanistic psychology. The movement known as humanistic psychology did not become a powerful force in psychology until the 1960s.
2. Humanistic psychology is characterized by the belief that man is always struggling to become. Humanistic psychology sees the individual's task in life as the making of a series of conscious choices between constructive and destructive alternatives.
3. The humanistic psychology is also termed existential psychology or existential humanistic psychology.

Strengths of Humanistic Psychology

1. One of the major strengths of humanistic psychology is that it emphasizes the role of the individual. This school of psychology gives people more credit in controlling and determining their state of mental health.
2. It also takes environmental influences into account. Rather than focusing solely on our internal thoughts and desires,

humanistic psychology also credits the environment's influence on our experiences.

3. Humanistic psychology continues to influence therapy, education, healthcare and other areas.
4. Humanistic psychology helped remove some of the stigma attached to therapy and made it more acceptable for normal, healthy individuals to explore their abilities and potential through therapy.

Criticisms of Humanistic Psychology

1. Humanistic psychology is often seen as too subjective; the importance of individual experience makes it difficult to objectively study and measure humanistic phenomena. How can we objectively tell if someone is self-actualized? The answer, of course, is that we cannot. We can only rely upon the individual's own assessment of their experience.
2. Another major criticism is that observations are unverifiable; there is no accurate way to measure or quantify these qualities.

Cognitive Psychology

The term 'cognitive psychology' was first used in 1967 by American psychologist Ulric Neisser (Fig. 1.5) in his book *Cognitive Psychology*. According to Neisser, cognition involves all processes by which the sensory input is transformed, reduced, elaborated, stored, recovered and used.

It is concerned with these processes even when they operate in the absence of relevant stimulation, as in images and hallucinations. Given such a sweeping definition, it is apparent that cognition is involved in everything a human being might possibly do; that every psychological phenomenon is a cognitive phenomenon.

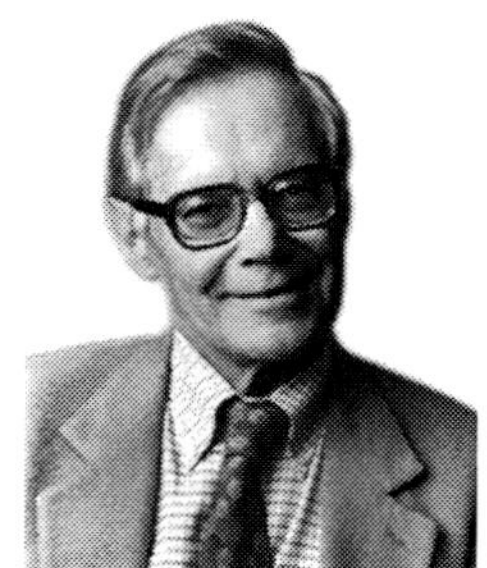

Figure 1.5: Ulric Neisser

Cognitive psychology is the school of psychology that studies mental processes including how people think, perceive, remember and learn. As part of the larger field of cognitive science, this branch of psychology is related to other disciplines including neuroscience, philosophy and linguistics. Cognitive psychology began to emerge during the 1950s, partly as a response to behaviorism. Critics of behaviorism noted that it failed to account for how internal processes impacted behavior. This period of time is sometimes referred to as the 'cognitive revolution' as a wealth of research on topics such as information processing, language, memory and perception began to emerge.

▪ CONCLUSION

The development of psychology as a science has followed a long and somewhat an uncertain course through the centuries. Psychology is a body of systematized knowledge that is gathered by carefully observing and measuring the events. Psychologist does experiments and makes observations, which others can repeat and verify. It has vast scope with its numerous sub-branches. The present world of psychology is dominated by a mixed trend involving so many schools of thought. Some schools worth mentoring are behaviorism, psychoanalysis, humanist psychology, transpersonal psychology and cognitive psychology.

■ REVIEW QUESTIONS

Long Essays

1. Explain the early origin of psychology in detail.
2. Describe in detail about history of psychology and its contributors.

Short Essays

3. Discuss in brief about the schools of psychology.
4. Gestalt psychology.
5. Psychoanalysis.
6. Neo-Freudian theories.
7. Humanistic psychology.

Short Answers

8. Strengths of structuralism.
9. Functionalism.
10. Sigmund Freud.
11. Cognitive psychology.

CHAPTER 2

Nature and Scope of Psychology

■ INTRODUCTION

A sound mind is a sound body; man's mind should be healthy. Brain and its functions are so complex, still there are many unrevealed facts about brain. Each person is unique; we cannot read the mind from outside, but can understand only through their activities and behaviors. As a nurse, we come across different kinds of people with divergent culture, taboos, ideas, customs, belief, religion, race, creed, caste, etc. It will differ for the nurse to give care, communicate, unless until she understand the mind of people, thoughts, ideas, psychological concepts, once he/she learns, empathizes, understand and behave accordingly to gain the cooperation from the patient.

■ DEFINITION

1. Psychology is defined as a science of human and animal behavior.
2. Psychology is a science, which aims to give us better understanding and control of the behavior of the organism as a whole.
3. Psychology as the scientific study of behavior does not exclude mind and other internal process from the field of psychology; what a person does his/her behavior is the outcome of the internal mental process.
4. Psychology is the science of human and animal behavior; it includes the applications of this science to human problems.
5. Psychology is the study of processes or activities of man in relation to his environment. —*Woodworth*
6. Psychology related to reaction to any and every situation of life. —*Skinner*
7. Psychology is the science or study of the mind and how it functions. —*Oxford dictionary*
8. Psychology is the scientific study of behavior and mental processes. Behavior includes all of our outward or overt actions and reactions, such as talking, facial expressions and movements. Mental processes refer to all the internal covert activity of our minds, such as thinking, feeling and remembering. —*Ciccarelli and Meyer, 2006*

■ NATURE OF PSYCHOLOGY

1. Psychology deals with the mind and its working, and that the knowledge of psychology helps in reading other people's mind.
2. Psychology is concerned with behavior and while dealing with behavior it extends to animal behavior.

3. Psychology possesses a well-organized theory, which is supported by the relevant psychological laws and principles.
4. Psychology has its applied aspects in the form of various branches of applied psychology such as industrial, legal, clinical and educational psychology.
5. Psychology has established facts, principles and laws of the behavior in the subject. Psychology enjoys universal applicability in practical life, other bodies of the knowledge and future researches in its own field.
6. Psychology as a science deals systematically with human behavior, with the motives, feelings, emotions, thoughts and actions of men and women.

Psychology as a Science

1. A science is a body of systematized knowledge that is gathered through careful observations and measurements of events in experiments set up by the scientist to produce the events being studied. Of course, all events studied by a scientist are not necessarily produced experimentally. At times, scientist has to observe the spontaneous events.
2. The psychologist do experiments and make observations, which others can repeat. They obtain data often in the form of quantitative measurements, which others can verify.
3. As a science, psychology is a systematic data from experiments and observations are essential, but from them to make some sense in helping us understand events, they must be organized in some way. Scientific theories are important tools for the organization of observed facts.
4. The most three essential requirements for a field of knowledge to be called 'science' are:
    a. It deals with observable facts.
    b. Science is not a mere collection or description of facts; it aims at the explanation of facts.
    c. Every science has its own methods, accordingly to these a scientist has to choose a problem for investigation.
5. Measurement in psychology is often more difficult than it is in science such as physics and chemistry because many of the psychological studies cannot be measured directly by physical scales, e.g. emotion, intelligence and attitudes.
6. Psychology is related to many other sciences such as biological sciences, sociology, philosophy and psychiatry. Its scope is very wide, it has many branches such as general psychology, animal psychology, child psychology, abnormal psychology, clinical psychology and applied psychology.

Psychology as a Behavioral Science

1. Psychology deals with certain aspects of behavior as does anthropology, sociology, economics or political science. All these sciences concern themselves with a specific aspect of behavior.
2. Psychology deals with the general nature of behavior. It does not select a single aspect of behavior like the rest of the behavioral sciences. It pervades the entire range of behavior and the basic principles underlying it.
3. Psychology includes not only the conscious behavior and activities of human mind but also the subconscious and unconscious. Consequently it covers not only the overt behavior but also the covert behavior involving all the inner experiences and mental processes.
4. An organism, e.g. a human being constantly behaves, so also the animals.

Psychology as a science of behavior deals with these acts of the organism. The environment means the surroundings objects and circumstances. It may be physical or social in nature.

5. Overt behavior is the most obvious and outwardly expressed form of behavior. It is easily observable. Covert behavior is not so easily observable. The initial activities of feeling, thinking and the 'like' are the examples of covert behavior, while the activities such as walking, smiling, hitting, etc. are those overt behaviors.
6. Behavioral sciences are concerned with the observation and explanation of human behavior either in single individuals or in groups. Psychology also interrelated with many other biological sciences.

■ RELATION OF PSYCHOLOGY WITH OTHER FIELDS OF STUDY

Relation of psychology with other sciences is shown in Figure 2.1:

1. **Psychology and biological sciences:** These studies gives light on their behavior and are closely related to the study of mental functions.
2. **Psychology and sociology:** It deals with the activities of a group of people taken as a whole. It studies tradition, customs, intuitions and other group of behaviors.
3. **Psychology and philosophy:** There is a close relationship between the two as both philosophy and psychology attempt to interpret human behavior.

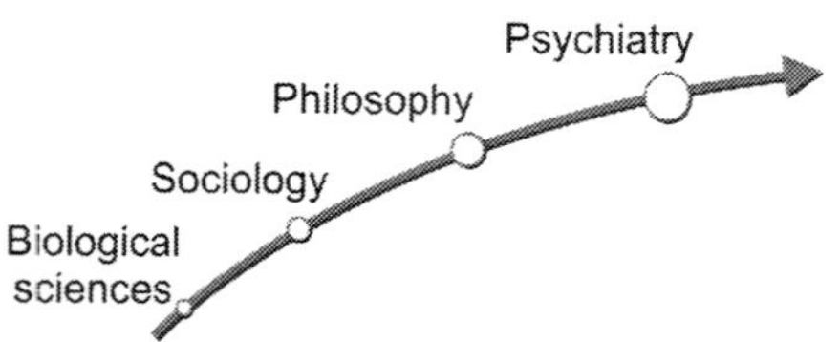

Figure 2.1: Relation of psychology with other sciences

4. **Psychology and psychiatry:** Psychiatry deals with study, diagnosis and treatment of the mentally ill.

■ SCOPE OF PSYCHOLOGY

Psychology deals with all types of experience in society or private such as those all phases that emerge in the realism of human life. Psychology discusses the inner dynamics of behavior such as motives and emotions. It concerns itself with individual differences in behavior and tries to find out the factors that explain these differences. It also deals with the study of abilities and aptitudes. Psychologists have also devised appropriate tests for measuring these abilities and aptitudes in people. Psychology also considers the working of the sensory and response mechanism.

It discusses the impact of the physical stimuli on sense organs. It also discusses and investigates the working of the senses organs, nervous system, muscles and glands. Social and community psychology deals with individual, family and group for the prevention of illness and promotion of health. It includes various types of group phenomena such as public opinion, propaganda, attitudes, beliefs and crowd behavior.

■ BRANCHES OF PSYCHOLOGY

The science of psychology, since its foundation, has grown into different levels. Its application is widely used. Among the other branches of pure psychology may be included experimental psychology, comparative psychology and physiological psychology. The branch of applied psychology includes clinical psychology, individual psychology, human psychology and educational psychology, etc.

Subfields of Psychology

Physiological Psychology

Physiological psychology is a branch, which experimentally investigates the physiological bases of behavior including the anatomical structure and physiological processes, which are related to psychological events, psychological processes and mental functions. It often uses operative technique, investigating the functions of brain for instance, by removing portions of the brain tissue and noting the effect upon behavior.

Experimental Psychology

1. Experimental psychology that studies the process of sensing, perceiving, learning and thinking about the mind.
2. It is the observation of concomitant variations and interpretation of the concomitance as cause and effects. In this method, a systematic controlled scientific methodology in the investigation of psychological phenomena is used.
3. The systematic presentation of the methodology and the results are usually within the context of a laboratory. The work of experimental psychology overlaps with that of the focus of biopsychology as well as that done by other types of psychologist.

Developmental Psychology

1. Developmental psychology deals with the changes in behavior that accompanies change in age from conception to death.
2. Since behavior and abilities change most rapidly during the early years, child psychology has traditionally received the most attention from developmental psychologist.
3. Development psychology has both pure and applied aspects.

Social and Personality Psychology

1. Social psychology is the study of the individuals in the growth and relationship of group to one another. Thus social psychology considers the psychological interrelations of people forming families, crowds, societies and mobs, and of the leader with his followers.
2. It includes the study of the formation of group attitudes and opinions. It is thus forced into a consideration of social and national conflict, or race prejudice and similar manifestation of the interrelations of the conflicting needs of many individuals.
3. Personality psychology is concerned with individual people and administration of psychological tests extensively. The personality psychologist is interested in understanding the non-deviant or normal cases.

Clinical Psychology

1. Clinical psychology is the practical application of dynamic and normal psychology to the problem of human adjustments.
2. Clinical psychology is devoted to study, diagnosis and treat behavior disorders. It is the largest subfield of psychology.
3. A clinical psychology is well-trained in the etiology of causes of the various forms of abnormal behavior such as psychoneurosis, psychoses, etc. and also trained in various methods of diagnosis of abnormal behavior through psychological testing.

Counseling Psychology

1. Counseling psychology is related to clinical psychology, but different in that the problem it deals with is generally of less serious in nature.

2. Personal, vocational and educational guidance are provided. Psychologist, who is well versed in the different diagnosis and treatment of such minor behavior problems are known as psychological counselors.
3. The counseling psychologist deals with individuals if milder emotional and personal problems exist. Also practices psychotherapy as well as depending upon the severity of the problems.

School Psychology

1. The counseling psychologist, who administers tests and guides individual students, is generally called school psychologists.
2. The school psychologist is on specializing in problems associated with elementary and secondary educational system. Also utilizes psychological concepts and methods in programs or reactions, which attempt to improve learning conditions for students.

Industrial-organizational Psychology

1. Industrial-organizational psychology is concerned with the psychology of the workplace. Specifically, it considers issues such as productivity, job satisfaction and decision-making.
2. The first application of psychology to the problems of industries and organizations was the use of intelligence and aptitude tests in selecting employees.
3. Now private and public organizations also apply psychology to problems of management and employee training, to supervise the personnel, to improve communication within the organizations, to do the counseling of employees and to alleviate the industrial conflict.

Consumer Psychology

1. Consumer psychology considers people's buying habits and the effects of advertising on behavior.
2. Consumer psychologist to research on consumer attitude toward the company's product.
3. As a subfield of psychology, in this the psychology principles are applied to practical problems of consumer products.

Health Psychology

1. Health psychology explores the relationships between psychological factors and physical ailments or disease.
2. For instance, health psychologist are interested in long-term stress can affect physical health.
3. They are also concerned with identifying ways of promoting behavior related to good health or discouraging unhealthy behavior such as smoking.

Cross-cultural Psychology

1. Cross-cultural psychology investigates the similarities and differences in psychological functioning in various cultural and ethnic groups.
2. Psychologist specializing in cross-cultural issues investigates the ways in which people in different culture attribute their academic successes or failures leading to differences in scholastic performance.

Forensic Psychology

1. Forensic psychology is another emerging specialty for the works handled with the legal, court and connectional system.
2. Forensic psychologist assists police in the variety of ways, from developing

personality profiles of criminal offenders to helping law enforcement personnel understand problems such as family conflict and substance abuse.

3. They may also assist judges and parole officers in making decisions about the disposition of convicted offenders.

■ CONCLUSION

Psychology is a scientific discipline in an extremely exciting field of knowledge as it continuous to grow at an accelerating field pace each year and continues to provide answer to basic question about the human behavior. Psychology has enormous potential; it offers us, the hope of both understanding and improving the quality of life. Psychological knowledge has been used in measuring intelligence, designing school curricula, helping troubled marriages, controlling aggression, selling products and treating both the young and old with greater sensitivity and humanness.

■ REVIEW QUESTIONS

Long Essays

1. Define psychology. Explain the nature of psychology in detail.
2. Discuss in detail about the branches of psychology.

Short Essays

3. Describe psychology as a science.
4. Relationship of psychology with other subjects.
5. Enumerate the scope of psychology.
6. Forensic psychology.
7. Subfields of psychology.

Short Answers

8. Experimental psychology.
9. Clinical psychology.
10. Developmental psychology.
11. School psychology.
12. Health psychology.

CHAPTER 3

Psychology and Nursing

■ INTRODUCTION

Psychology is a young science. A study of psychology can help to understand the self in better, understand other people, improve situations by helping others to solve problems and understand the close relationship of body, mind and spirit.

Literary meaning of psychology is the science of mind. Some others have accepted it, as the science of consciousness. Both of these meanings are not appropriate for psychology, as the modern psychology does not recognize mind and gives more importance to the mental processes or modes. According to modern concept, psychology is the study of human behavior. It includes stimulated behavior and internal mechanism. Psychology deals with the mind and its working and that the knowledge of psychology helps in reading other people's minds. Scope of psychology is very extensive. Behavior is associated with life and psychology with behavior. It studies all normal, abnormal, child, adult, man and animals and also compares them.

■ NEED OF PSYCHOLOGY IN NURSING

Nurses perform many important tasks in the care of patients. Interacting with patients from a diverse range of backgrounds allows nurses to provide better care. An educational background that includes psychology training can give you the tools that you need as a healthcare professional to provide the best care and accurately identify any mental health issues that a patient may have. Psychology in the nursing field is taught purposely. The contemporary scientific literature on counseling psychology and clinical psychology helps nurses perform their everyday tasks. They interact with patients on daily basis and it is easy for them to identify the signs of mental disturbances compared to other medical health aides. It ensures proper care to patients and professional services are given to them.

In hospitals and health centers, there are different kind of patients in intensive care unit (ICU), high dependency unit (HDU) and general ward. Nurses are assigned to work with patients, who are severely ill or have acute health issues. Every patient responds in a different manner, some might face illusions due to long-term use of ventilator, while others have unpredictable mood swings. Nurses are prepared to face such behaviors throughout their academic life. Along the process of treatment they create a strong relationship with the patients. As away from home they expect people to be friendly and compassionate to them. And nurses are taught to do so. Nurses should have some extraordinary traits such as patience, friendly nature, compassion, love for others and the ability to feel the pain of others.

PSYCHOLOGICAL ASPECTS OF NURSING

The nurse, because of the close personal relationship with the patient, must understand human emotional reactions as well as physical illness. Psychology is the key to this understanding. In this text, the authors deal with the subject in a clear, succinct, practical and scientific manner. From their wide experience in the clinical aspects of psychology and in the instruction of student and graduate nurses, they have recognized the needs of the nursing profession regarding the understanding of human behavior. This book was written specifically to meet these needs.

Following a concise treatise on the fundamental principles of psychology and their applications to the profession of nursing the authors proceed to give the student specific help in understanding various types of normal and abnormal patients. They stress all the important relationships between mind and body, 'psychosomatic unity' pointing out that the nurse must minister to the emotional as well as the physical needs of the patient. They emphasize the essential need for cooperation among the professions of nursing, m edicine, psychology, social work, occupational therapy, etc. in the effective treatment of the patient. Special interest in this connection will be the chapter orienting the nurse in regard to diagnostic procedures and therapeutic techniques.

Psychology seeks to understand why people behave, think and feel the way they do, individually and in groups, in all areas of life including change in behaviors to enhance well-being and quality of life. This can be seen to link very closely with what nurses do. Nurses and psychologists seek to understand the health needs of the people they work with, but also to change their behaviors, thoughts and feelings to enhance the well-being of the person, not only at this moment but also for the future. At times nurses need to provide very basic care for the people they work with, but they are always looking to develop the person's ability to be more independent in any area of their life.

NURSING APPLICATION TOWARD PSYCHOLOGICAL CONCEPTS/IMPORTANCE OF PSYCHOLOGY IN NURSING

The importance of psychology in nursing is to help the nurses deal with patients' emotional problems caused by their health problems. Most of the time poor health can lead to depression and nurses skilled in dealing with psychological problems are better equipped to handle that issue. Nursing application toward psychological concepts are:

1. The study of psychology will help the student nurse to appreciate the necessity for changing the environment or surroundings.
2. Psychology will help the nurse to understand the close relationship between body, mind and spirit.
3. Psychology will help to understand other people; one will learn why others

differ from his/her in their likes and dislikes, in their interests and abilities or in their reactions to others.

Nurses can use psychological research and theories to enhance their nursing practice, and most nursing practice has a foundation in psychology, sociology or biology. Nursing now has developed its own unique body of knowledge, but other sciences can still enhance nurses' understanding and practice.

When the nursing field incorporates psychology, it begins to resemble a field called biopsychology. The biopsychology attempts to understand behavior through biological theories. Nursing already has a biological base and when a nurse attempts to understand patients beyond a biological level, biopsychology begins to emerge. The expansion of fields such as biopsychology continues to be a key part in nursing and nurse training.

■ PSYCHOLOGICAL APPLICATION IN NURSING PRACTICE

Nurses have to take care of patients during severe health conditions and deal with their moods and behaviors. Patients begin to rely on nurses who try to lessen their mental stress. It has been seen in many cases that physical illness results in mental disturbance, at this stage nurses have to be compassionate and understanding. Nurses are trained in a manner that they support patients emotionally by addressing the mental changes.

Nurses perform many important tasks in the care of patients. Interacting with patients from a diverse range of backgrounds allows nurses to provide better care. An educational background that includes psychology training can give you the tools that you need as a healthcare professional to provide the best care and accurately identify any mental health issues that a patient may have.

Commonly referred to as bedside manner, the way that you communicate with and care for patients can have an impact on the patient's mental state and overall sense of well-being. Nurses, who can provide compassionate care to even the most challenging patients, have the ability to empathize with patients. This compassion can be discovered by studying psychology and how illness and disease changes the patient's mental states. Psychology course is a simple solution to learn how to promote positive thinking in patients, which can in turn decrease the amount of time spent in the hospital or other healthcare facility.

■ INTEGRATION OF PSYCHOLOGY IN NURSING

As the mind and body are intricately interwoven, it is nearly impossible to separate mental health from physical health. Given the profound influence elements of wellness have upon each other, it is important to understand the connection between psychology and nursing. The nurse, because of the close personal relationship with the patient, must understand human emotional reactions as well as physical illness. Psychology is the key to this understanding. In this text, the author deal with the subject in a clear, succinct, practical and scientific manner. From his wide experience in the clinical aspects of psychology and in giving the instructions to student and graduate nurses, he has recognized the needs of the nursing profession regarding the understanding of human behavior. This book was written specifically to meet these needs.

Nurses, who want to integrate more psychology into their practice, might choose to work as a psychiatric nurse, which may include taking care of suicidal patients, bipolar patients or patients with other forms of mental illness. In this field, an understanding of psychology is very important as well as a solid medical background, since amongst psychiatrists and psychologists, the psychiatric nurse may be the only one with a general medical background. Nurses who want to focus on using even more psychology into their practice would have to pursue a Master's Degree and become a mental health nurse practitioner, who would be able to diagnose illness and prescribe medication and other treatments.

The practical work or training of nurses is based on theoretical knowledge and the change of behavior they see in every patient. Biological psychology is used by the nurses to thoroughly analyze the association between human behavior and biological changes. Nurses are taught about the psychological illnesses and mood swings of patients caused by hormonal changes, neurological reactions and last, but not the least—genes. The study of psychodynamic psychology done by nurses is merely to spread the optimism among patients. It has been scientifically proven that positive thoughts affect the overall health of a person, which results in strong immune system.

■ RELATION BETWEEN PSYCHOLOGY AND NURSING PROCESS

Although a nurse's primary duties involve physical care such as administering medications, she also relies on psychology to help her evaluate patients' mental status and determine the most effective way to interact with them. Some nurses combine the two disciplines by working as psychiatric nurses, where they use their nursing and psychology training to help patients cope with mental health issues (Fig. 3.1).

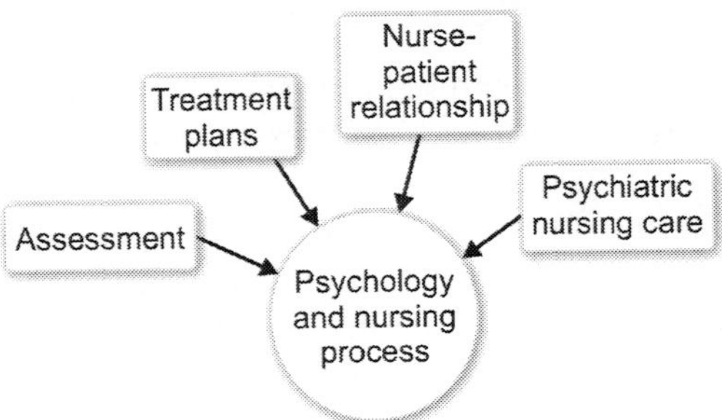

Figure 3.1: Relation between psychology and nursing process

Assessment

When evaluating a patient's condition, nurses not only consider the severity of the illness or the level of pain or discomfort, but they also examine the patient's response. Some patients, for example, remain optimistic no matter how sick they are or how bleak their prognosis. They may also cope well with pain or other symptoms accompanying their illnesses. Other patients, though, may respond by becoming angry or despondent, sometimes withdrawing or lashing out at hospital staff and even their families. They may also have more difficulty handling their symptoms and may report greater pain or discomfort than other patients. Nurses must recognize these mental and emotional issues and include them as part of the patient's evaluation.

Treatment Plans

Nurses must consider the entire patient, both physical and mental health, when creating treatment plans. A patient suffering anxiety over his/her illness, for example, may refuse to get out of bed, which could cause secondary complications such as respiratory infection or pneumonia. If a nurse suspects a patient will not participate in his/her recovery, she will need to provide emotional support and encouragement, while adapting his/her treatment plan to his/her psychological health. For example, he/she may set short-term goals that are easy for the patient to achieve, such as getting out of bed three times a day or sitting in a chair at least 15 minutes a day.

Nurse Patient Relationship

Psychology can help nurses adapt how they interact with patients based on factors such as age and personality. For example, when caring for pediatric patients, nurses must consider that younger patients may be more frightened than adults and may have more difficulty in understanding their situations. Nurses with knowledge of child development or psychology will better understand how to relate to patients in a way that eases their fears and alleviates their confusion. Psychology can improve their relationships with patients, making it more likely that patients will communicate openly with them about their symptoms. Nurses also rely on psychology to encourage patients to trust them by increasing the chances patients will follow the nurse's instructions and take more active roles in their own care.

Psychiatric Nursing Care

While some nurses use psychology as a secondary skill, others center their practice around it, helping patients to cope with everything from severe depression to substance abuse. Psychiatric nurses work with individuals and families in settings as diverse as hospitals, drug treatment facilities and home health agencies. They often work as case managers, creating and monitoring treatment plans, evaluating patient progress, providing counseling and crisis intervention, setting short-term goals and teaching long-term strategies for managing mental and emotional health issues.

■ CONCLUSION

Psychology seeks to understand why people behave, think and feel the way they do, individually and in groups, in all areas of life including change in behaviors to enhance well-being and quality of life.

■ REVIEW QUESTIONS

Long Essays

1. Explain the need of studying psychology in nursing.
2. Describe the importance of psychology in nursing.

Short Essays

3. Discuss the psychological aspects of nursing.
4. Psychological application in nursing practice.
5. Relationship between psychology and nursing process.
6. Integration of psychology in nursing.
7. Describe how psychology can be used in nursing.

Short Answers

8. Patient-nurse relationship.
9. Psychiatric nurses.
10. List the nurse's role in psychological treatments.
11. Importance of studying human behavior in nursing.
12. Relevance psychology in nursing.

CHAPTER 4

Methods of Psychology

■ INTRODUCTION

The scientific method is emphasized as the basis for investigation. The founding of Wundt's laboratory marked the beginning of the formal application of the scientific method to problems in psychology. This method is neither identified with any particular kind of equipment nor is it associated exclusively with specific research procedures.

■ DEFINITION

Method is defined as a systematic procedure involved in the investigation of facts and concepts. It also uses special techniques in psychology such as experimental method or the clinical method used to collect facts.

■ INTROSPECTION

The term introspection can be used to describe both an informal reflection process and a more formalized experimental approach. The first meaning is the one that most people are probably the most familiar with, which involves informally examining our own internal thoughts and feelings. When we reflect on our thoughts, emotions and memories, and examine what they mean, we are engaging in introspection. The definitions are as follows:

1. The process of 'looking inward' and examining one's self and one's own actions in order to gain insight. This was a central component to the early days of psychology during the structuralism period. Wundt and other psychologists had made people introspect and then report on their feelings, thoughts, etc.
2. The word introspection need hardly be defined—it means, of course, the looking into our own minds and reporting what we discover there.

Concept

1. Introspection is one of the oldest methods used for investigating consciousness. It is a process of analyzing a conscious experience by reporting the sensory qualities of the stimuli that are expressed.
2. The word introspection means 'to look within.' In introspection subjects were presented with a particular stimulus or task and asked to describe their mental state as thoroughly as possible.
3. This method is used to observe the individual, analyze and reports his/her own feelings, thought or all that passes in his/her mind during the course of a mental act or experience.

4. This method cannot be used by children or animals or of mental defectives because they cannot introspect. By the early 20th century psychologist recognizes the inadequacies of introspection.

Meaning

Introspection is self-observation, self-examination and self-reflection. It is the opposite of extrospection, which means looking outward. Introspection is studied and used in the profession of psychology, although not all psychologists agree as to its exact value therapeutically. The idea is thought to date back to the ancient Greek philosopher Socrates. He spent much of life being introspective as well as encouraging others to do so. Two of Socrates' most well-known quotes are 'know thyself' and 'the unexamined life is not worth living'.

Advantages

1. Introspection is the fundamental method of psychology. Observation and experiment are based upon introspection.
2. Introspection gives us direct, immediate and certain, and exact knowledge of our own mental processes.
3. It enables us to fully understand the behavior of an individual.
4. We cannot confine ourselves to mere objective and direct observation of a person we want to understand. We need to know what is going on in the mind of the person.
5. This method is inexpensive and does not require any apparatus or laboratory.

Disadvantages

1. This method cannot be used by children, animals, or mentally retards as they cannot introspect.
2. Something that is going on in another person's mind is not accessible to us because mental processes are vague and obscure, and cannot be observed. The introspective results cannot be, therefore, verified by other observers. Scientific results are always verifiable; hence introspection is an unscientific method.
3. Mental processes are fleeting and evanescent by their nature, they elude grasp of internal perception. Mild anger, fear and other emotions tend to disappear when they are attended to. Thoughts, feelings, emotions or desires change from moment to moment. If one does not want to change the mental process, one should study it after the process is finished, rather than during the process. This is called retrospection and requires clear memory.
4. Two psychologists cannot observe the same mental processes (e.g. fear). But they can observe the similar emotions of fear in their own minds and compare their experiences with one another. Introspection of a particular kind of mental process should be carried out by a number of experts in coordination; and they should compare the results of their introspection with one another.
5. Introspection implies a cleavage in the observing mind for the same mind in the observer and the observed. It requires the same mind be the observer and the observed. However, the same mind cannot divide itself into two parts, the knower and the known, the subject and the object. Therefore, introspection is difficult and sometimes almost impossible.
6. Introspection sometimes involves attention to a mental process (e.g. perception), which is produced by an external object. When we attend to the

mental process we withdraw attention from the object and as soon as we withdraw attention from the object the mental process vanishes, thus making introspection impossible.

■ OBSERVATIONAL METHOD

Observation is the objective method of studying the behavior of individuals. It consists of perception of an individual's behavior under natural conditions by the other individuals and the interpretation and analyses of this perceived behavior by them. It is essentially a way of perceiving the behavior like as it is. We can infer the mental processes of other persons through observation of their behavior.

Steps in Observation

- Observation of behavior
- Noting of behavior
- Interpretation and analysis of behavior
- Generalization.

Advantages

1. Observation is economical, natural, as well as flexible.
2. The data, which is studied through the observations, can be analyzed, measured, classified and interpreted.
3. The results can be verified and relied.
4. Observation method is quite suitable for observing the developmental characteristics such as children's habits and interests. For example, the effect of absence of a mother or father, or both on the child's development can be determined properly through observing the development of such deprived children. Similarly, a clinical psychologist may be able to collect the required data about abnormal behavior of an individual by observing him/her in day-to-day life under natural conditions.

Disadvantages

1. Through observation it is impossible to know what is happening in the minds of others; we can only observe this through external behavior. It is possible a person may be an expert in hiding his/her feelings and emotions from others.
2. Subjectivity factors on the part of the investigator as well as the process of observation, also affect the results of observation. For example, one may give overemphasis on a particular aspect of one's behavior and altogether neglect some other very important aspect.
3. Another serious limitation of the observation method lies in the fact that the behavior observed is dependent on the particular time and place, and on the particular individual or groups of individuals involved. It lacks repeatability as each natural situation can occur only once.
4. Another important limitation of the observation method is not being able to establish a proper cause and effect relationship. In case we observe two phenomena say poverty and delinquency behavior, invariably occurring together, we cannot infer from this that poverty is the sufficient and necessary cause of delinquent behavior or vice versa.

■ EXPERIMENTAL METHOD

Experimental method is considered as the most scientific and objective method of studying behavior. The word experiment comes from a Latin word meaning 'to try', or 'put to the test'. Therefore, in experimentation we try or put to test the material or phenomenon, the characteristics of consequences of which we wish to ascertain. The use of this method has raised psychology to the status of an experimental science such as physics, chemistry and physiology.

In psychology, experimental study is used to study the cause and effect relationship regarding the nature of human behavior, i.e. the effect of anxiety on the human behavior. To study the cause and effect relationship, the psychologists use objective observations under controlled conditions to observe actions or behaviors performed by individuals. From these observations certain conclusions are drawn and theories or principles established.

Essential Features

1. Requires two persons, the experimenter and the subject or the person whose behavior is observed.
2. Experimentation should be done on living organisms.
3. All experiments are conducted under controlled conditions.

Steps in Experimentation

Steps in experimentation are given in Figure 4.1:

1. **Stating problem:** The first step in an experiment is stating the problem. For example, stated as 'to study the effects of smoking on physical and mental health of students.'

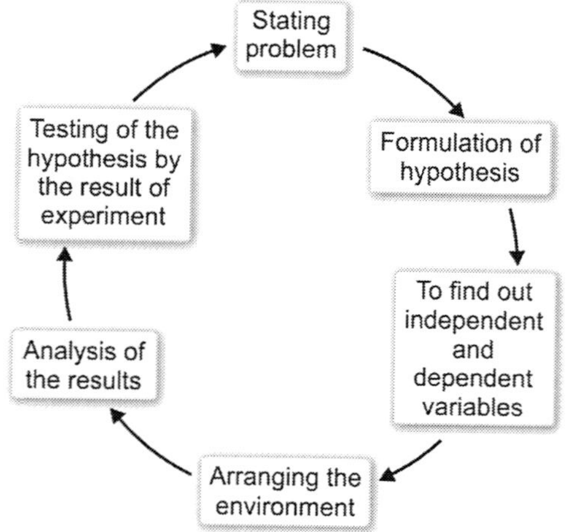

Figure 4.1: Steps in experimentation

2. **Formulation of hypothesis:** Hypothesis is a tentative answer to the problem. For the above example, the hypothesis can be—smoking is harmful for physical and mental health of students. This hypothesis will be tested.
3. **To find out independent and dependent variables:** The effect of which we want to study will be called the independent variable and the other the dependent variable. The independent variable stands for the cause and dependent variable is characterized as the effect of the cause. In the above example, physical and mental health will be dependent variables and smoking will be an independent variable.
4. **Arranging the environment:** Under controlled environment the variables are objectively observed. For example, physical and mental health of students (who are smoking) will be observed. In experimentation, it is important that only the specified independent variables be allowed to change. Factors other than the independent variable must be held constant.
5. **Analysis of the results:** Generally the subjects of the experiment are divided into two groups one controlled and other experimental. They can be compared statistically. For example, smokers' and nonsmokers,' mental and physical health can be compared.
6. **Testing of the hypothesis by the result of experiment:** The results may prove or disprove the hypothesis.

Advantages

- Scientific method
- Finds out cause and effect relationship
- Maximum control of phenomena
- Repetition is possible.

Disadvantages

1. Experimental method advocates the study of behavior under completely controlled rigid conditions. These conditions demand the creation of artificial situations or environment and the behavior studied under these conditions may be different from natural behavior. Thus, experimental method fails to study behavior in naturalistic conditions.
2. Difficulty in controlling or equalizing intervening variables.
3. All problems of psychology cannot be studied by this method, as we cannot perform experiments for all the problems.
4. The dynamic nature of human behavior does not always allow the independent variable leading to a change in the dependent variable.
5. Experimental method is a costly and time-consuming method. Moreover handling of this method demands specialized knowledge and skill. In the absence of such expertise this method is not functional.

In spite of various limitations, it is a fact that the results obtained by experimental method are reliable, verifiable, definite, precise and capable of quantitative treatment than those obtained by the use of other methods.

▪ CLINICAL/CASE STUDY METHOD

Clinical or case history method is used by clinical psychologists, psychiatrists, psychiatric social workers in child guidance clinics or mental hygiene clinics and the allied institutions. It aims at studying the cause and basis of people's anxieties, fears and personal maladjustments. A great deal of relevant data is collected by using case histories, interviews, home visits and psychological tests to draw valid inferences about the nature of the individual's difficulties and problems, the probable origin and course of development. This may suggest some course of action to be pursued in helping the individual.

In this technique, information is collected from the memory of the individual, his/her parents, members of family, friends, teachers and all other available records and reports. This enables us to understand the major forces and influences that have developed and shaped the individual's personality.

Case histories may also be based on a longitudinal study. This type of study follows an individual or group of individuals over an extended period of time, with measurements made at periodic intervals. The case history is constructed from actual observations made by the investigator according to a plan.

Advantages

1. Case histories will give the clinician an insight into the causes of the problem and suggest possible solutions.
2. Case studies can be productive sources of ideas for further investigation by other methods.

Disadvantage

The case history method depends largely on memory of incidents, which may have been observed inaccurately or over interpreted.

▪ SURVEY METHOD

All problems in psychology cannot be studied by experimental or other methods. Some problems such as study of opinions, attitudes, healthcare needs, etc. can be studied by means of survey method. This is commonly employed in social psychology.

Concepts

1. Surveys study large and small population of selected representative samples chosen from the population to discover the relative incidence, distribution and interrelation of psychological and sociological variables.
2. In survey research, the researcher simply collects data about psychological and sociological variables or characteristics of a sample that represents a known population in natural setting.
3. The survey research is concerned with conditions or relationships that exist, opinions that are held, processes that are going on, effects that are evident or trends that are developing.
4. That survey research, which involves samples, usually is called 'sample survey'.

The survey method involves collection or gathering of information from a large number of people by using questionnaires, inventories and interviews. An adequate survey requires a carefully pretested questionnaire, a group of interviewers trained in its use, a representative subject and appropriate methods of data analysis, so that the results are properly interpreted.

Merits and Demerits

Merits: A large amount of data can be collected in a shorter time.

Demerits: The behavior is not observed directly.

■ RATING SCALE AND CHECKLIST

1. Rating scale and checklist are commonly used devices of observing and evaluating personality or behavior traits. In rating scales, we rate on individual on the possession or absence of certain traits on a certain scale.
2. The measurement scale has five degree of the trait to be rated. This is a five-point scale. Some scales have three or seven degree.
3. In a checklist, examiners may be provided with a list of traits or qualities and may be asked to point out or checkup ones that apply to particular persons.

■ GENETIC OR DEVELOPMENTAL METHOD

1. Genetic or developmental method seeks to find out the causes of a complicated behavior in its simple beginning. It assumes that a full appreciation of each behavior patterns of an adult requires the study of simple behavior patterns.
2. These simple behavior pattern grow more complex gradually as the individual grows in age. For example, if we are interested in understanding the learning behavior of an adult, we should begin with the learning behavior in his/her preadolescence and in the light of these, arrive at some conclusions about the learning behaviors in adulthood.

Cross-sectional vs Longitudinal Research

Cross-sectional vs longitudinal research methods are employed to get information regarding the changes that take place in children's behavior over an extended period of time. Through the cross-sectional approach the children of different ages are observed and their behavior patterns noted. The changes, which occur from one age period to another give an idea of development of characteristics. For example, the emotional problems of children at various developmental periods may be solved by observing emotional behavior of the children during infancy, childhood, adolescence and adulthood.

In longitudinal approach, the same children are observed over an extended time span. The emotional development is studied by observing the same children from birth to their adulthood. This approach gives a good picture of the developmental process. Since, the subjects are the same, the influence of the environmental factors and other factors remain almost similar at all the stages of development.

Merits and Demerits

Cross-sectional research

Merits: As follows:

- Cost-effective
- Information can be collected easily.

Demerits: Influence of the environment over different children may be different, drawing conclusion is difficult.

Longitudinal study

Merits: Same subjects are followed over a period of time. The influence of environmental factors and other factors remains almost similar at all the stages of development.

Demerits: Longitudinal study is time consuming.

■ CONCLUSION

Psychology is a young science; a study of psychology can help to understand the self in better, understand other people, improve situations by helping others, solve problems and understand the close relationship between body, mind and spirit. Literary meaning of psychology is the science of mind. Some others have accepted it as the science of consciousness. Both of these meanings are not appropriate for psychology, as the modern psychology does not recognize mind and gives more importance to the mental processes or modes. According to modern concept, psychology is the study of human behavior. It includes stimulated behavior and internal mechanism. Psychology deals with the mind and its working, and that the knowledge of psychology helps in reading other people's minds. Scope of psychology is very extensive. Behavior is associated with life and psychology with behavior. It studies all normal/abnormal child, adult, man and animals and also compares them.

■ REVIEW QUESTIONS

Long Essays

1. Define methods of psychology. Discuss various methods in detail.
2. Discuss introspection method in detail with its advantages and disadvantages.

Short Essays

3. Observation method.
4. Discuss the steps of experimental method.
5. Clinical/Case study method.
6. Survey method.
7. Discuss about genetic/developmental method.
8. Rating scale and checklist method.

Short Answers

9. Scientific method.
10. Self-observation.
11. Retrospection.
12. Essential features of experimental method.
13. Cross-sectional research.

■ BIBLIOGRAPHY

1. Armstrong DM. A Materialist Theory of the Mind. 1968.
2. Burge T. Individualism and self-knowledge. Journal of Philosophy. 1988:85.

3. Chalmers D. The content and epistemology of phenomenal belief. In: Smith Q, Jokic A (Eds). Consciousness. New Philosophical Essays; 2002.
4. Dennett D. 'Who's on first? Heterophenomenology explained.' Journal of Consciousness Studies. 2003;10:9-10.
5. Gertler B. Introspecting Phenomenal States. Philosophy and Phenomenological Research. 2001. p. 63.
6. Rogers CR. The necessary and sufficient conditions of therapeutic personality change. J of Consult Psychol. 1957;21(2):95-103.
7. Rosenzweig MR, Breedlove SM, Watson NV. Biological Psychology: An Introduction to Behavioral and Cognitive Neuroscience, 4th edition. Sunderland: Sinauer Associates Inc; 2005. p. 137.
8. William James. Principles of Psychology. Cambridge: Harvard; 1890/1981. p. 85.

Section II

Biology of Behavior

CHAPTER 5

Mind-body Relationship

■ INTRODUCTION

Psychology studies the relationship between mind and body. Mind and body affect each other. The mind operates at the levels of thinking, emotion and action. The Western Greco-Roman approach to the mind-body connection differs from the Eastern meditation approach. In the West, natural philosophies always start with the physical. The ancient Greeks fully understood that the nearer one's physique approached the state of physical perfection, the nearer one's mind approached the state of mental perfection. They knew that the simultaneous and coequal development of one's ability voluntarily to control one's body and mind was a paramount law of nature.

■ BODY: THE INSTRUMENT OF THE MIND

The body is the most visible part. The body is the physical presentation, the material medium; it is merely the instrument of the mind. The thought or idea, i.e. consciously or unconsciously chosen and impressed upon the subconscious mind must move the body into action. The action determines the results. Within the conscious mind you have the ability to choose your thoughts and you can choose any thoughts you want.

The conscious mind has the power to either accept or reject any thought or idea that presents itself. So, if you have that choice, why not choose to build those big, beautiful, wonderful pictures of everything you want in your lives instead of choosing to build a picture of all things you do not want in your lives and all the reasons why something just is not going to work out. You can take the very worst of situations and choose to think something positive about it.

So if you have the ability to replace the thoughts of an empty bank account with one full of what you need, or you surrounded by loving and caring friends, or healthy and active, then this is what gets passed to your subconscious (remember it does not have a choice) and that leads to the results in your life.

Either way, the thoughts you choose to accept, whether they are positive or negative, are then impressed upon the subconscious mind and they dictate the way you feel. So, if you think positive thoughts such as "everything always works out for me," "life is great," "I am grateful," you are going to feel good and you will actually attract more of those thoughts and feelings into your life.

Effects of Mind Upon Body

Every action of the mind produces a certain effect in the body. When the mental action is weak or superficial, the physical effect may be too slight to be noticed, but when this action is both deep and strong, the results will be so clearly in evidence that any one can detect them. These effects, however, are neither simply functional, nor that the nervous system alone is acted upon. The power of the mind can (and does) affect everything in the body, frequently producing chemical changes that we have believed were possible only through the use of most powerful drugs. But the action of mind in the body always follows exact law; therefore when one knows the exact physical effect produced by each mental state, physical conditions can be largely determined by the intelligent use of the mind.

Every thought you entertain affects your body and your emotions. For example, thinking about your favorite food, especially if you feel hungry, will cause your mouth to water. Every physical action affects your mood and your thinking. Walk around, very slowly so that you are almost dragging your feet, with your spine slumped forwards and with your head hanging down and a notice how this affects your mood. It is pretty likely that it will drag you down emotionally.

You have no doubt recognized that when you feel physically tired or less than well this affects your mood. It is very difficult, e.g. to be cheerful and humorous when you are exhausted. Similarly your thinking affects your physical state. If you spend a while going around silently telling yourself that you cannot cope or that you are a failure or that 'it is all too much' then this will undoubtedly cause you to feel tense, demoralized and physically tired.

Theories of Mind-body Relationship

Mind-body is the relationship between a human body and its unique mind (Fig. 5.1). Theories of the mind-body relationship can be divided into two broad categories—monistic and dualistic theories.

Monistic Theories

Monistic theories suggest that mind and body are not separate substances. Thinkers such as Aristotle, Hobbs, Hegel and the behaviorists, collectively thought of as the materialists postulated that the mind was nothing more than a bodily function. A mind is generally thought to be of a substance other than a physical substance. Berkeley, Leibniz and Schopenhauer, collectively known as the idealists, were monists of a different sort; they theorized that the body was simply a mental representation. Spinoza proposed that mind and body were the manifestations of some third property—what he considered God! This is the theory of double aspectism, another monist view.

Dualistic Theories

According to the dualist view, mind is thought to be of a substance other than a

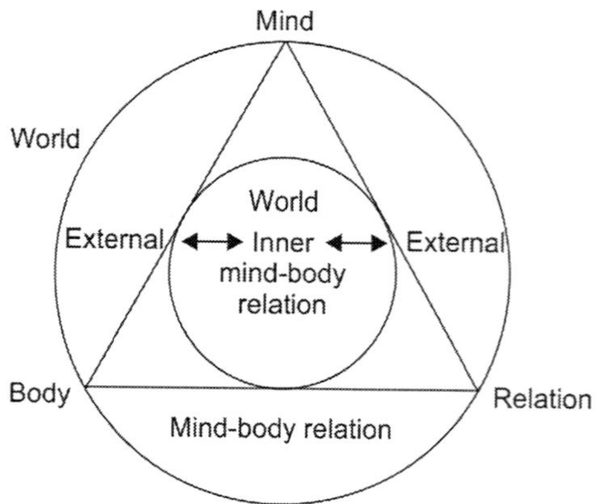

Figure 5.1: Mind-body relationship

physical substance. Popular dualists were Descartes, Locke and James, who collectively belong to the school of thought known as interactionism. Other dualistic views include parallelism, epiphenomenalism and occasionalism.

Different Positions of the Body and Mind

Various positions of body and mind according to the mind-body relationship theory in psychology are given in Table 5.1.

Double Aspectism

Mind and body are distinguishable, but inseparable. Cognitive and experiential aspects can be distinguished from physical aspects, so there is a separate mind and body sort of. The separate mind and body are two aspects of the state of being human. Spinoza explained it this way, 'thinking substance (the mind) and extended substance (the body) are one and the same thing'. For Spinoza, the single substance was God. This explanation of the mind-body connection may be the

Table 5.1: Varied positions of the mind-body relation in psychology

Position	Causal relation	Proponents
Interactive dualism	Both mind (soul) and body exist and causally interact—we are 'machines that think'	Descartes, La Mettrie
Epiphenomenalism	Mind real, but unimportant and not causal—study bodily mechanisms or behavioral 'operants'	Hobbes, Skinner
Reductive materialism	Mind does not exist—study bodily mechanisms, the nervous system, actions or behavior	Hobbes, French materialists (e.g. Pierre-Jean-Georges Cabanis), mid-19th century physiologists, Watson
Phenomenalism	Matter does not exist (theistic or logical immaterialism)—study sensations and habits	Berkeley, Hume and Condillac
Vitalism	No 'soul' but mind, body plus a 'life principle' —mind/consciousness relies on, but not reducible to a material nervous system	J Müller, early 19th century physiologists
Double aspect theory	Unity of body and mind, but not reducible—did not have or use evolutionary theory—study and measure the interaction of these aspects	Spinoza, Fechner, early Morgan CL, psychophysicists
Parallelism	Mind (consciousness) and body separate—who cares and why? Describe or measure each in their own way	British associationism, Wundt, structuralism, gestalt and humanistic psychology
Pre-established harmony	Both run in parallel according to God's (or nature's) initial winding of two clocks—study unconscious influences and character types	Leibniz, phrenologists, faculty psychologists
Occasionalism	Active God	Malebranche
Emergentism	Non-reductive functional relation between substantive body and mind as a transformative process—study the evolutionary development of the process	James, Dewey, later Morgan CL, functional psychologists, followers of dialectical materialism and activity theory

most difficult to understand, because it is perhaps the least clear.

Epiphenomenalism

The mind is really just a byproduct of the physical brain. Only physical events in the brain (e.g. neurons firing) have causal power. When we talk about the brain, we are speaking of a physical thing, so the brain is part of the body. This is very important to epiphenomenalism. If a human body were a TV set, the mind would simply be the picture you see when it is switched on. In this view the physical body affects (and even causes) the mind. However, because the mind is merely a byproduct, the mind does not affect the body. Huxley (1874) said that mental events are similar to a steam whistle that contributes nothing to the work of a locomotive. According to James (1879), mental events do not affect the brain activity that produces them as any more than a shadow reacts upon the steps of the traveler whom it accompanies.

Idealism

According to idealism, what one knows to be real is in some way confined to the contents of one's own mind. Anything we experience through our senses is colored by how our mind perceives it. We therefore cannot have access to external reality. Only thoughts and ideas that originate in the mind can be immediately experienced. Idealism stands in stark contrast to the theory of materialism, which endorses the physical, spatial, factual domain as the ultimate reality. Plato's theory of forms/ideas has been compared to idealism, although the forms were not confined to the mind, but existed independently of it. It has also been argued that Descartes contribution in which access to the mind is prioritized influenced idealism. Idealism has been pervasive since the 18th century, but has been less popular in recent times.

Interactionism

Sometimes the mind affects the body, and sometimes the body affects the mind. The body and the mind are separate, and they affect one another. Descartes laid the groundwork here. We are physical beings because we are extended in space. We are mental beings because we think. In Descartes' words, "I think, therefore I am" (Cogito Ergo Sum). Here is the problem we run into the mind is not physical in any way, and it exists separately from the body. So, how does the non-physical mind affect the physical body and vice versa? Descartes assumed that this interaction occurred in the pineal gland.

Materialism

Materialism is the view that only physical matter is real. The body is governed by strictly material, non-mental causes. Inasmuch as mental properties exist, they have no causal effect on the physical body. Strict materialists may hard-headedly deny that anything mental exists at all. Others may concede that the mind exists, but characterize it as being identical to the brain. The earliest exponents of something resembling materialism were the Greeks, Democritus and Aristotle. A specific type of materialism is epiphenomenalism, the view that the mind is a byproduct of physical processes. Another type of materialism is naturalism, the notion that nothing supernatural exists.

Occasionalism

Occasionalism seems that God is following us around all day, and when the mind gives the body some instruction, or vice versa, God makes it happen. Remember the problem we had with interactionism. We could not explain how the mind and body affected one another. Well, we have that all solved here. When your mind decides that it would like your body to be on the other side of the room it gets some Almighty intervention. Occasionalism was popularized by 17th century French philosopher, Nicolas Malebranche. The problem with occasionalism is that it not only supposes that there is a God but also that he has time to follow each and every one of us around.

Parallelism

Mind and body are separate, but they are perfectly synchronized. How do they affect one another? They do not, they only appear too. When your mind decides that it would like your body to be on the other side of the room it is just a coincidence that your body walks over there. Although the origin of this view can be traced back to GW Leibniz, he is also implicated in pre-established harmony, a view that implicates God in the correlation between mind and body.

Pre-established Harmony

Mind and body, at the time of their creation, were perfectly synchronized by God, as two clocks set for exactly the same time. Although they appear to correspond and interact, there is no causal relationship between mind and body. Pre-established harmony was a theory expounded by GW Leibniz, to oppose the theories of parallelism, occasionalism and interactionism. The problem with pre-established harmony is that it presupposes that there is a God.

Relationship Between Consciousness and Mind/Body

Thus the subconscious is that part of the body/mind that consciousness cannot access. As a person matures into adulthood, there is an intuitive sense that the subconscious grows. To state this differently, consciousness is gradually pushed out of more and more of the body/mind and into the head during maturation to adulthood. As this happens, it can be said that the subconscious mind grows as a person matures. It is not maturation itself that bring these changes about; rather it is the slow accumulation of difficult and unresolved experiences. It is this core shifting, changing relationship between consciousness and the body/mind that this work is about.

Mind-body Modalities

Most people acknowledge that there is a mind-body connection knowing how this communication occurs and assists in the understanding of the mind-body modalities (Fig. 5.2) of relaxation, meditation and imagery. Neuropeptides, the neurochemicals, are behaved to be the messenger molecules that connect body and mind. Neuropeptides have properties that allow them to affect neurological and physiologic tissue receptors.

Relaxation

Relaxation is the state of generalized decreased cognitive, physiological and/or behavioral arousal. The relaxation response is characterized by decreased heart and respiratory rates, blood pressure (BP), oxygen (O_2) consumption, and increased alpha brain activity and peripheral skin comparatives.

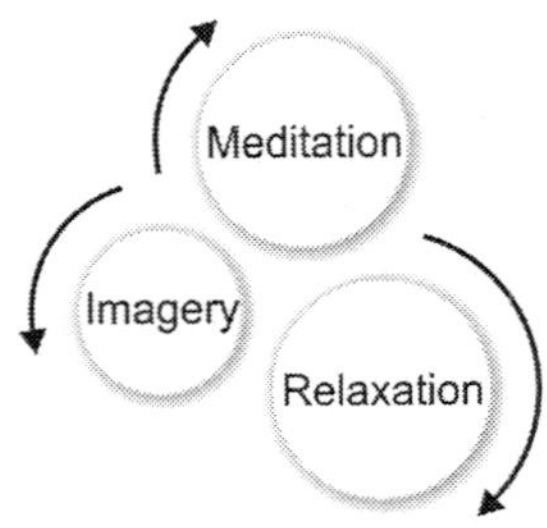

Figure 5.2: Mind-body modalities

The long-term goal of relaxation therapy is for the person to continually monitor himself or herself for indicatives of tension and to consciously let go and release the tension contained in various body parts.

Imagery

Visualization technique is the conscious mind to create mental images to evoke physical changes in the body, improve perceived well-being and/or enhance self-awareness. For example, the client may be directed to begin slow abdominal breathing, while focusing in the rhythm of breathing. The client then instructed to visualize occurrence of waves coming to slow with each inspiration and then speeding up with each expiration. Next the client is instructed to take notice of the smells and sounds that he is experiencing. As the imagery session progresses, the client may be instructed to visualize warmth entering the body during inspiration and tension leaving during expiration.

Meditation

Meditation seeks to change one's physiology to a more relaxed state and alter one's prescription to an increased acceptance of reality.

Nursing considerations

Patients seeking inpatient case might have a meditation practice that they want to continue. Nurses can provide the time necessary for this. Nursing is both an art and science that cares for the body, mind and spirit unity of persons in relation to their environment. Nursing is caring perspective views of human beings as persons in relation to every level of human existence and connection, individuals, families, groups and communities. The concept of human beings as persons-in-relation provides the framework from which nursing addresses the potential for promotion, maintenance and restoration of health. This framework underscores the importance of examining the political, economic and social forces that impact a person's agency and right to health. The infinite complexity of these forces creates a diversity of environments within which nursing seeks to maximize health at every level of human existence.

■ LEVELS OF CONSCIOUSNESS

The normal state of consciousness comprises either the state of wakefulness, awareness or alertness in which most human beings function, while not asleep or one of the recognized stages of normal sleep from which the person can be readily awakened. The abnormal state of consciousness is more difficult to define and characterize, as evidenced by the many terms applied to altered states of consciousness by various observers. Among such terms are clouding of consciousness, confusional state, delirium, lethargy, obtundation, stupor, dementia, hypersomnia, vegetative state, akinetic mutism, locked-in syndrome, coma and brain death. Many of these terms mean different things to different people, and may prove inaccurate when transmitting and recording information regarding the state of consciousness of a patient. Nevertheless, it is appropriate to define several of the terms as closely as possible.

Three Levels of Consciousness

The totality of our consciousness is comprised of three levels—the subconscious, the conscious and the superconscious (Fig. 5.3). These levels of consciousness represent different degrees of intensity of awareness. The first level, the subconscious is relatively dim in awareness; it is the stuff of which dreams are made. We may think of it as the repository of all remembered experiences, impressions left on the mind by those

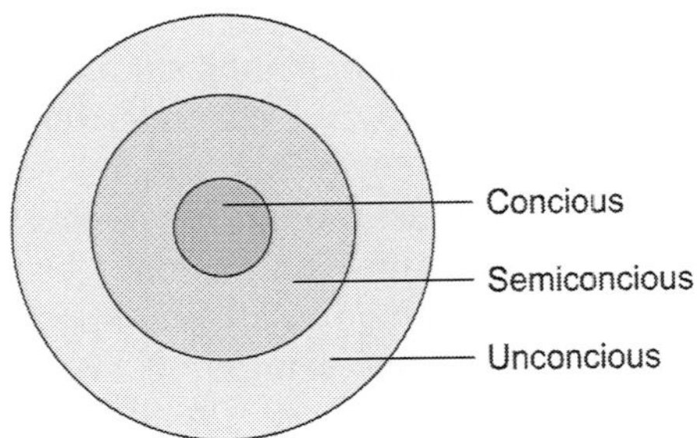

Figure 5.3: Three levels of consciousness

experiences and tendencies awakened or reinforced by those impressions. Every experience we have ever had, every thought, every impression of loss or gain, resides in the subconscious mind and determines our patterns of thought and behavior far more than we realize.

The subconscious, being unrestricted by the rigid demands of logic, permits a certain flow of ideas. This flow may border on intuition, but if the ideas are too circumscribed by subjectivity, they will not correspond with the external world around us. When we dream at night, we are mainly operating on the subconscious level.

The subconscious mind can all too easily intrude itself on our conscious awareness, tricking us into thinking. We are getting intuitive guidance, when actually we are merely being influenced by past impressions and unfulfilled desires. The subconscious mind is in some ways close to the superconscious, where real intuition resides. Both represent a flow of awareness without logical obstructions. The subconscious is therefore more open to the intuitions of the superconscious, and sometimes receives them, though usually mixed with confusing imagery. To be really clear in the guidance we receive is difficult, but very important. Calamitous decisions have been made in the belief that one was drawing on higher guidance, when in fact one was responding only to subconscious preconditioning.

The next level of consciousness from which we receive guidance is the conscious state, the rational awareness that usually guides our daily decisions. When we receive input from the senses, analyze the facts and makes decisions based on this information, we are using this conscious level of guidance. This process is also strongly affected by the opinions of others, which can cloud our ability to draw true guidance.

Dividing and separating the world into either/or categories, the conscious level of awareness is problem oriented. It is difficult to be completely certain of decisions drawn from this level, because the analytical mind can see all the possible solutions. But ultimately it does not have the ability to distinguish which one is best. If we rely exclusively on the conscious mind, we may find ourselves lacking in certainty and slipping into a state of perpetual indecision.

Intuition and heightened mental clarity flow from superconscious awareness. The conscious mind is limited by its analytical nature, and therefore sees all things as separate and distinct. We may be puzzled by a certain situation, but because it seems unrelated to other events, it is difficult to draw a clear course of action. By contrast, because the superconscious mind is unitive and sees all things as part of a whole, it can readily draw solutions. In superconsciousness the problem and the solution are seen as one, as though the solution was a natural outgrowth from the problem.

Altered Level of Consciousness

There is one more level of consciousness, altered level of consciousness. In this level, the person needs a stimulus to respond. Without any stimulus, the person is unable to respond. It can be further classified into state of confusion, stupor, delirium, coma and obtundation. This level can be a result of some brain injury or brain disorder such inadequate supply of O_2 in the brain or extreme pressure from the skull, etc.

We all are at different levels of consciousness at different time, so we possess different expressions and have a particular personality type. These levels sometimes become our identity, so we should always try to possess positive qualities as negative qualities not only impact us but also harm the sentiments of others. This is possible only when we always try to be in the state of consciousness. Altered level of consciousness include the following conditions (Fig. 5.4):

1. **Confusion:** A confused person cannot properly process all the information from their surroundings. Apathy and drowsiness are the most noticeable symptoms. The person may be disoriented, especially to time. A severely confused person is usually unable to carry out more than a few simple commands.
2. **Delirium:** This is a common and complicated problem, especially in the elderly. The signs of delirium include disorientation, which may be total. People with delirium may not remember who they are or may have delusions and hallucinations. People with delirium may also become drowsy or less alert at times.
3. **Obtundation:** A lower level of alertness typically characterizes this state. A person in this state often sleeps much more than usual, and when awakened, remains drowsy and confused. Wakefulness can only be maintained by continuously talking to the person or through constant painful stimulation.
4. **Stupor:** It is characterized by unresponsiveness from which a person can be aroused only by vigorous and repeated painful stimulation.
5. **Coma:** A person in a coma appears to be asleep, but cannot be awakened. Oftentimes reflexes are absent, and the legs and arms may be rigid. The respiration rate of someone in a coma is usually slowed.

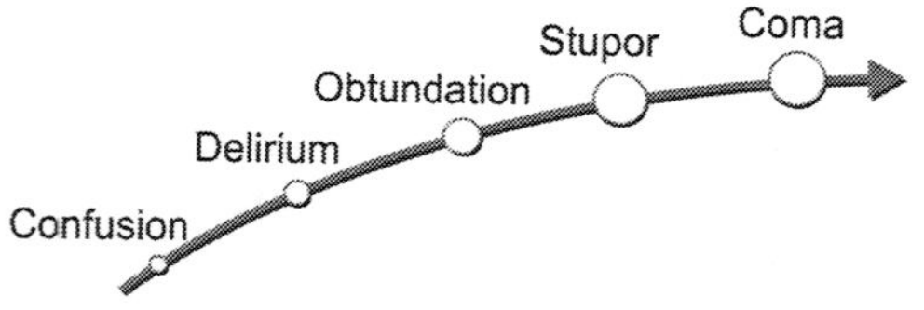

Figure 5.4: Altered level of consciousness

Causes

Mnemonic for causes of altered level of consciousness

A: Alcohol, acidosis, anoxia

E: Epilepsy, environment

I: Insulin (diabetes)

O: Overdose

U: Uremia (metabolic), underdose

T: Trauma, toxins, tumors

I: Infection (sepsis)

P: Psychiatric disorders

S: Stroke (CVA).

Trauma to the brain can cause impaired consciousness. Traumatic brain injury (TBI) is the leading cause of death and disability in young adults in the US. Several types of head trauma may cause TBI. For example, a closed head injury, the most common TBI can result if the head rapidly accelerates or decelerates, causing the brain to move through the fluid in the skull and strike the inside of the skull. Other causes include direct impact on the head or penetration by a foreign object such as a bullet. Infections are a common cause of impaired consciousness. The inflammation that accompanies infection is responsible for altered level of consciousness (ALC). Encephalitis and meningitis is two nervous system-specific infections that can cause ALC.

Defects in the metabolic system can lead to waste build-up that can cause ALC. As the body goes about the normal processes needed to keep us alive, chemicals and other by products are produced. In most cases, byproducts get into the bloodstream and are filtered by the liver, kidneys and other organs. If one of these systems fails, waste products can build-up and act as a poison that interferes with the brain's ability to function. The insulin/sugar imbalance of diabetes, for example, is a major metabolic problem that can cause impaired consciousness. Diabetics with low blood insulin levels produce ketones, a toxic by product of fat metabolism. Conversely, when there is too much insulin, cells begin to starve to death. Either case can result in ALC.

Drug exposure is a common cause for ALC. Drug-induced ALC can result from an overdose of either over-the-counter or illegal drugs. Alcohol intoxication is probably the most common cause of drug-induced ALC. Similarly, exposure to certain readily available home or industrial chemicals can lead to changes in consciousness or even to death.

Structural abnormalities of the brain can lead to ALC. Tumors (benign or cancerous) can form and crowd out the normal structures of the brain. As a result, weakness in the walls of the blood vessels in the brain (aneurysms) may begin to swell or may even break, causing blood to pool inside the head and push the brain against the bony wall of the skull. The resulting damage can then cause ALC.

Pathophysiology

Although the neural science behind alertness, wakefulness and arousal are not fully known, the reticular formation is known to play a role in these. The ascending reticular-activating system is a postulated group of neural connections that receives sensory input and projects to the cerebral cortex through the midbrain and thalamus from the reticular formation. Since this system is thought to modulate wakefulness and sleep, interference with it, such as injury, illness or metabolic disturbances could alter the level of consciousness.

Nurse's Roles and Responsibilities

Glasgow coma scale measurement

Over the years, many assessment tools have been developed to improve neurological assessment. The most popular and universally used tool is the Glasgow coma scale (GCS), developed in 1974 by Teasdale and Jennett.

The GCS is divided into three sections—eye opening, verbal responses and motor responses (Table 5.2). The patient is assessed and scored in each area and the scores are added together to give the patient's GCS score; the highest possible score is 15 and the lowest is 3. A patient, who is fully aware and orientated, will score 15; a lower score will reflect the patient's level of consciousness.

Pupil reaction is not included in the GCS, though it is often incorporated into locally adapted neurological observation charts.

Eye opening: This should be spontaneous when the patient is approached. If the patient's eyes do not open spontaneously, determine whether they open to speech or painful stimuli. If the eyes are open, do not assume that the patient is fully aware and orientated to their surroundings. Some patients with head injuries may have spontaneous blinking and eye movement; this does not indicate full consciousness (Muxlow, 2000).

Verbal response: This determines state of consciousness. Patients, who are fully orientated, will know their name, where they are, the date and year. A confused patient

Table 5.2: Glasgow coma scale

Features	Score
Eye opening	
Spontaneous	4
To sound	3
To pain	2
None	1
Best verbal response	
Oriented	5
Confused	4
Inappropriate words	3
Incomprehensible sounds	2
None	1
Best motor response	
Obeys command	6
Localizes stimulus	5
Withdrawal from stimulus	4
Abnormal flexion (decorticate)	3
Abnormal extension (decerebrate)	2
Flaccid	1
Total score possible	3 through 15

may be able to hold a conversation, but when asked questions may give replies, which are incorrect or inapt. They may use inappropriate words, which do not make sense to the assessor, or they may make incomprehensible sounds such as moans or groans. Some stimuli may be required to obtain a response from the patient; this type of patient is not aware of their surroundings.

Motor response: This is assessed by giving the patient some simple commands, such as 'squeeze my hand (both sides)', 'lift your legs up off the bed' and 'show your tongue'. The strength of the patient's limbs should be noted; it is essential to observe for weaknesses. When a patient does not respond to simple commands then response to painful stimuli is assessed. There are three recognized stimuli that can be used when assessing motor response.

The advantage of the GCS is that it is widely known and used, and provides a standardized assessment of neurological observations. It is simple to use and requires only a pen torch with a bright beam and a copy of the assessment tool. However, Ellis and Cavanagh (cited in Woodrow, 2000) have noted that there may be variations in the recording of pupil size and motor weakness.

Inaccurate and inconsistent recordings could have a detrimental effect on the patient's well-being and may affect their care plan. Nurses therefore need to be educated in the correct use of the tool, in order to address potential irregularities.

■ CONCLUSION

A behavior that is elicited by a stimulus is known as a response. Behavior has cognitive, affective and conative components. The process or result of the unification of these components into whole is called integrated response. The human being is capable of behavior and therefore is a living organism. The individual is in active relation with the environment and this environment influences and changes him/her.

■ REVIEW QUESTIONS

Long Essays

1. Describe in detail about body as a instrument of mind.
2. Explain the theories of mind and body relationship.

Short Essays

3. Describe the effects of mind upon body.
4. Relationship between consciousness and mind/body.
5. Mind and body modalities.
6. Levels of consciousness.
7. Altered levels of consciousness.
8. Glasgow coma scale measurement.

Short Answers

9. Epiphenomenalism.
10. Interactionism.
11. Materialism.
12. Imaginary.
13. Delirium.
14. Confusion.
15. Obtundation.

CHAPTER

6 Behavior and Neuroscience

■ INTRODUCTION

Behavior and neuroscience is the field of study that examines the biological roots of behavior. This interdisciplinary field includes the study of genetic factors, hormonal factors, neuroanatomy, drugs, development factors and environmental factors to team about brain-behavior relations. The human brain is the most complex of complicated structure in known universe. Scientists have estimated that the human brain is composed of 180 million nerve cells, 50 million of which are devoted to processing information.

■ MAJOR ACTIVITIES OF BRAIN

1. The brain monitors and controls our basic life support system, such as breathing and digesting.
2. It directs our movements and maintains our balance and posture.
3. It receives and interprets information from the world around us.
4. It records significant and sometimes insignificant event into our memory.
5. It allows us to solve problems, use language and think of new ideas.
6. It enables us to feel materials such as soft cotton and to experience emotions such as happiness and snows.
7. Working together with the glands of the endocrine system and the rest of the nervous system.

■ HISTORICAL REVIEW OF BIOLOGY AND BEHAVIOR

1. Early Greek and Roman physicians believed that behavioral problems were caused by imbalance of vital fluids that moved through the body and brain. Only after the renaissance did people accept the view that behaviors and thought were reduced by specific structures in the brain.
2. During the 19th century, neurologist performed autopsies on former patients and discovered the brain areas responsible for producing and comprehending speech. This work led to other discoveries, which specified that the psychological functions were associated with specific brain areas.
3. Early in the 20th century, research on the physiological basic of behavior showed that when an area of the brain is destroyed, sometimes remaining portions can take over its function. This view that different areas of the brain can be equivalent to one another is called equipotentiality theory.

4. According to integrationist theory, complex psychotically functions are based on number of basic abilities. These basic abilities may be involved in the same psychological function. Our thoughts and actions are a product of the functions of interrelated neural structures.
5. Today, neuropsychologists use a variety of procedures to learn about brain-behavior relation. Much of this work is based on studies of laboratory animals. They perform brain operations to see how the removal or destruction of brain tissue in a particular area affects. Now the medical imaging technique makes it possible to examine the living brain.

■ RELATIONSHIP BETWEEN MIND AND BODY

The nervous system is the primary seat of the vibrating mind in the human body. The nervous system is pervasive throughout the body. There are even nerves in the walls of arteries; thus there are few parts of the body that escape domination or at least contact by the mind. This means that the mind and body genuinely cannot be separated. Thus the relationship between them is that there is no relationship. They are the same thing at least for as long as the body is alive. Once a body dies, then the nervous system is left to physically decay with mind, long gone, or dissipated depending on beliefs.

■ NEURON

The nerve cells called 'neurons' are the basic units of operation in nervous system. By themselves, though they cannot explain the complexities of thought and emotion. It is only when the wires are arranged into complicated patterns thereby producing action and thought.

Basic Neural Processes (Fig. 6.1)

The nervous system is basically constellated from only two different types of cells.

Nerve cells: The neurons receive and transmit neural signals to other parts of the body.

Glial cells: The more numerous of the two, support and protect the neurons. Glial cells take their name from the French word glue. They form a connective network that holds together the brain's billions of neurons. The glial cells insulate the neuron from one another throughout the nervous system and clear away cellular debris when neurons degenerate and die. A continuous layer of glia surround the blood vessels in the brain to establish a blood-brain-barrier, a protective shield that prevents many harmful chemical substances passing from the blood to brain.

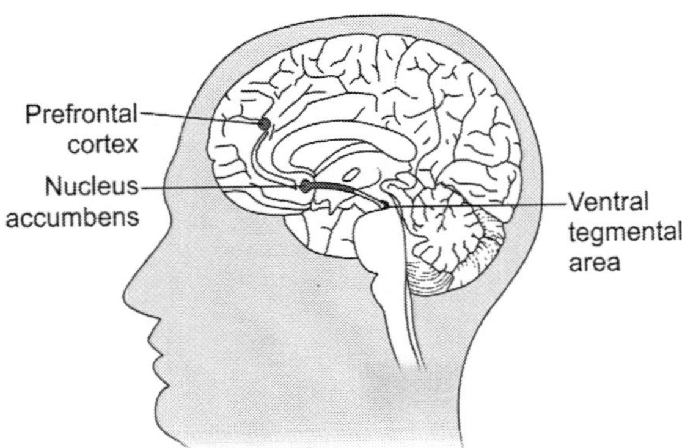

Figure 6.1: Basic neural process

Structure of Neuron (Fig. 6.2)

1. Neurons are of many different shapes and sizes, but they share certain anatomical features. Neurons have a cell body, dendrites and an axon.
2. The cell body consists of a membrane boundary that surrounds the nucleus and internal contents of the cell. The nucleus in the portion of cell contains deoxyribonucleic acid (DNA) strands for protein that holds the genetic blueprint for the cells makeup and function. Neuropsychological field of psychology that represents the convergence of this scientific discipline is called neuropsychology.
3. The cell also contains protoplasmic material that manufactures chemical substances used to communicate with other neurons.
4. Reaching out from the cell body, similar to the branches of the tree, dendrites receive information from other neurons. The longer and more complex a neuron's dendrites, the greater number of connections it can make with other cells.
5. Neural signals are transmitted to other cells by the axon, a single fiber that emerges from the cell body. Axons in the brain are usually less than 1 mm long. But axons from the spinal cord to the big toe can reach the length of 3 ft or more.
6. The chemical substances can travel in both directions along an axon and more than one type of chemical message can be passed to the receptors of an adjacent cell.
7. **Myelin sheath:** Axons are usually coated with an insulating material called myelin sheath that is produced by the glial cells. Myelin also helps prevent the scrambling of neural messages.
8. **Nodes of Ranvier:** Periodic breaks in the myelin sheath, which cause the axon to resemble a beaded necklace, are called nodes of Ranvier. These nodes allow axons with myelin insulation to

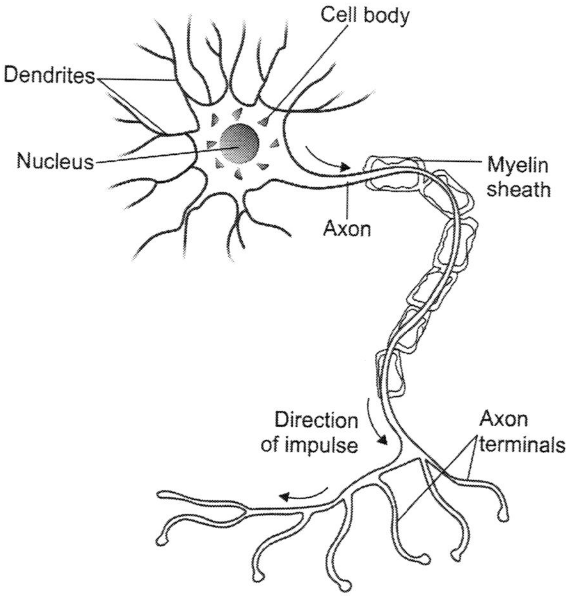

Figure 6.2: Structure of neuron

transmit neural signals faster than uninsulated axon because the signals can be transmitted along the axon by jumping from one note to the next.

Neural Impulses and Their Transmission

1. When a neuron is sufficiently stimulated by another neuron, there is an electrical reaction in the walls of the axon that travels over the entire length of the walls of axon till the terminals.
2. The electrical reaction is called neural impulse depending upon the diameter of the axon and thickness of the myelin sheath, a neural impulse travels at a rate of approximately 2–2,000 miles per hour.

Neural Firing

1. Neural impulses are generated by electrochemical processes involving the cell membrane.
2. When a nerve cell is strongly stimulated by another cell, there is a chemical change in the cell membrane, the membrane becomes permeable, causing positively charged ions from the outside to enter and negatively charged ions from the inside to exit.
3. This change quickly reverses the cell membrane's electrical change at the point of stimulation and causes the adjacent portion of the cell membrane to reverse its change as well.
4. For a neuron to generate an impulse, it must receive a certain level of stimulation. This is called threshold, which level the neuron fires in a uniform and unchanging way.
5. Neuron can fire even without outside stimulation. There is a baseline level of spontaneous activity in each neuron as it lies waiting for new stimulation. That stimulation may come in the form of excitatory influences that increases.
6. Drugs that have psychological effects often have an excitatory or inhibitory influence on neural firing. For example, the local anesthetic such as Novocain inhibits neural baring. Novocain blocks the conduction of the action potential along the axon.
7. Epilepsy itself provides a vivid example of the powerful influences that basic neural processes have on behavior. Dilantin is effective in berating firing of neurons.

Synoptic Transmission

1. Neurons not only fire, they communicate with other cells to generate or to create an informational network that links the various parts of our body.
2. The billions of neurons in the brain produce at least 10 billion synoptic connections. A typical neuron may have several thousands of these synapses, small gaps separating the nerve cells.
3. The electrical impulse, which has traveled down the axon of the transmitting cell, must be converted into a chemical messenger that stimulates another neuron across the synoptic junction.
4. In neurological terms, the transmitting cell is called the presynaptic neuron, the receiving cell is called the postsynaptic neuron and the chemical messenger is known as the neurotransmitter. Since neurotransmitter affects other cells chemically, this means that the most drug messengers are transmitted from one cell to another.

▪ NEUROTRANSMITTERS AND BEHAVIOR

Neurotransmitters are endogenous chemicals, which transmit signals from a neuron to a target cell across the synapse. Neurotransmitters are packaged into synaptic vesicles that cluster beneath the membrane on the presynaptic side of a synapse and are released into the synaptic cleft where they bind to receptors in the membrane on the postsynaptic side of the synapse.

Neurotransmitters are manufactured in the pragmatic neuron and stored in tiny sacs called vesicles located in the axon terminals of the pragmatic neuron. It forces the vesicles to break, similar to a cannon firing a burst of shells, and the vesicles shoot their chemical contents, the molecules of the neurotransmitter, into the synaptic junction.

A receptor site is simply a portion of an adjacent neuron that receives the molecules of a neurotransmitter. Since there are specific receptor sites different types of neurotransmitters will key into a given receptor site.

Criteria for a Neurotransmitter

- It should be produced and released from neuron
- It should be a precursor/synthesis enzyme in the presynaptic neuron
- It should be in the presynaptic neuron
- Sufficient amount should be available for the postsynaptic neuron
- It should bind to the postsynaptic receptors and show biological effect
- It must be inactivated.

Types of Neurotransmitters

1. **Excitatory:** It is responsible for the conduction of impulse from pre- to post-synaptic neurons resulting in the opening of sodium channels and the influx of sodium ions from extracellular fluid (ECF). This depolarization is called excitatory postsynaptic potential (EPSP).
2. **Inhibitory:** It inhibits the conduction of impulse from pre- to post-synaptic neurons causing opening of potassium channels and efflux of potassium ions. This hyperpolarized state is called inhibitory postsynaptic potential (IPSP).

Acetylcholine

1. **Location:** Brain, neuromuscular junction (Fig. 6.3) and in the peripheral nervous system; it may be critical for normal thinking.
2. **Effects:** Deficiency of acetylcholine (ACh) causes paralysis, Alzheimer's disease, etc. Excess may cause violent

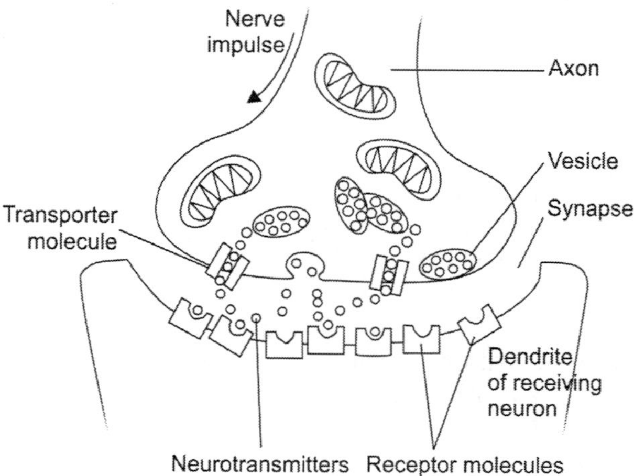

Figure 6.3: Neuromuscular junction

Enkephalins/GABA/Dopamine (Fig. 6.4)

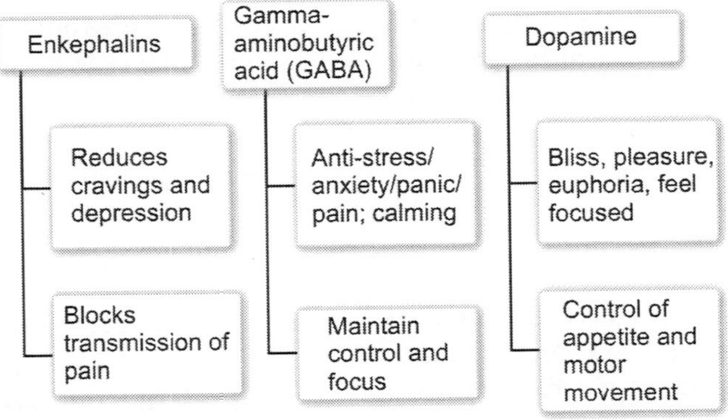

Figure 6.4: Functions of enkephalins, GABA and dopamine

muscle contractions. Drugs that increase ACh in cerebral cortex appear to help teaming and retention.

Amino Acids

1. **Location:** Brain; used by neurons for fast excitation and inhibition. Glutamic and aspartic acid for excitation. Gamma-aminobutyric acid areas and glycine are for inhibition.
2. **Effects:** These are linked to the control of anxiety. The deficiency causes mental deterioration (Huntington's chorea).

Neuropeptides

1. **Location:** Brain; released during painful or stressful situation, end options.
2. **Effects:** Neuropeptides causes pain reduction and may be involved in eating, memory, sexual behavior and mood.

Catecholamines (Fig. 6.5)

1. **Location:** Brain and peripheral nervous system; it includes acetylcholine, phenylethylamine and norepinephrine (NE).
2. **Effects:** Dopamine plays major role in the regulation of movement deficiencies

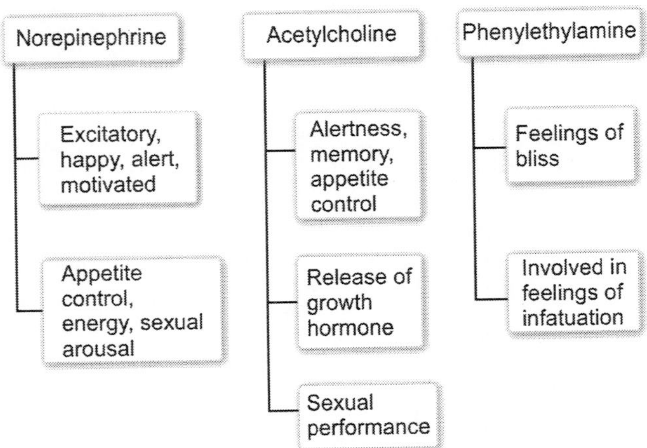

Figure 6.5: Action of norepinephrine, acetylcholine and phenylethylamine

causes Parkinson disease, excess may cause major disturbances of thought, perception and emotion behavior. Norepinephrine affects arousal and mood deficiency causes depression, agitation and manic condition.

Serotonin/Melatonin/ Oxytocin (Fig. 6.6)

1. **Location:** Central nervous system; influences sleep and body temperature.
2. **Effects:** Deficiency of serotonin causes depression.

Action of Neurotransmitters

1. The excitatory or inhibitory influence can change a neuron's threshold for firing. These excitatory or inhibitory influences are determined by the synaptic cells.
2. Synaptic sites at dendrites tend to be excitatory, while synaptic sites at the cell body tend to be inhibitory.
3. Consequently, a neurotransmitter at an inhibitory synapse will make it less likely to fire. At any given time, a cell receives neurotransmitters from various receptor sites.
4. The postsynaptic neuron analyzes the incoming excitatory and inhibitory signals and fires only if the net level of stimulation passes its firing threshold.
5. When this threshold is reached, the electrical to chemical and the chemical to electrical transmission process is almost complete.
6. All that remains are for the neurotransmitter to be deactivated to that the postsynaptic neuron can be stimulated again.

Deactivation or Reuptake

1. Deactivation can occur in one of the two ways, first an enzyme at the synapse can breakdown the neurotransmitters. The other one is to release the chemicals into synaptic cleft.
2. The neurotransmitter can return to the presynaptic neuron. This process is called reuptake and it is the most common form of deactivation.
3. Deactivation is crucial for without it the nervous system would become overstimulated, this would lead to tremors and eventually death.
4. Some insecticides and nerve gases produce their deadly effects by blocking the

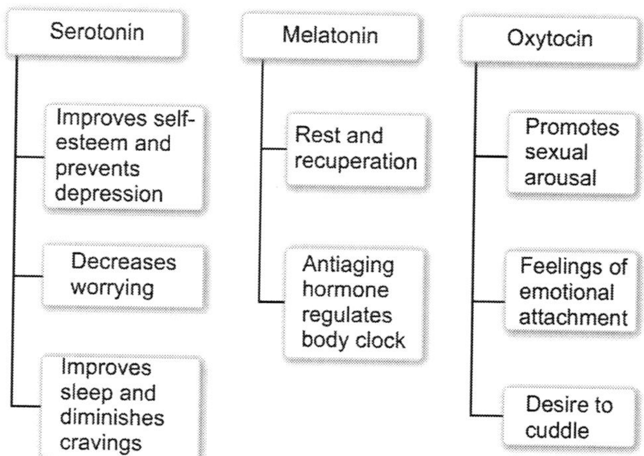

Figure 6.6: Functions of serotonin, melatonin and oxytocin

deactivation of neurotransmitters at the neuromuscular junctions, thus victims die of uncontrolled muscle spasms.

Neurotransmitters and Diseases

Depression

A group of drugs called tricyclics, among the most successful in relieving depression, are believed to increase the availability of both neurotransmitters in certain areas of the brain. The recent research that the antidepressant effects of these drugs may be related to increased sensitivity of the receptors for those two neurotransmitters (norepinephrine and serotonin) rather than a mere change in the actual levels of these brain chemicals.

Drug-related Behaviors

A wide variety of commonly used drugs have the effect of exchanging thought processes, emotional states or behaviors. Extensive research has linked the brain opiates to an array of behavioral and mental processes, including a sense of well-being and euphoria, counteracting the influence of stress, modulating food and liquid intake, facilitating learning and memory, and reducing anxiety.

■ ENDOCRINE SYSTEM AND BEHAVIOR (Fig. 6.7)

The endocrine system is a chemical communication network that sends messages throughout the nervous system and accretes hormone that affect body growth and functioning. Although the endocrine system is thought of a distinct from the brain, nervous system and sense organs, it has important functional relationships with these structures.

Concepts on Behaviors

The endocrine system includes all of the glands of the body and the hormones produced by those glands. The glands are controlled directly by stimulation from the nervous system as well as by chemical receptors in the blood and hormones produced by other glands. By regulating the functions of organs in the body, these glands help to maintain the body's homeostasis, cellular metabolism, reproduction, sexual development, sugar and mineral homeostasis, heart rate and digestion:

1. About 300 years ago, the French philosopher Rene Descartes proposed that the pineal gland is the point of interaction between the soul and the body.
2. The endocrine glands are distinguished from duct glands. Also they are said to be ductless because they secrete their products, chemical messengers called hormones, directly into the bloodstream.
3. The duct glands secrete their substances into body cavities or the surface of the body. Examples of duct glands are the salivary, digestive and tear glands.

Pituitary Gland

1. The pituitary gland is located at the base of the skull near the hypothalamus and is about the size of a pea. It is sometimes called master gland in view of the fact that its hormones often play the role of triggering the activity of other endocrine glands.
2. One of the key hormones released by the pituitary is the growth hormone, which controls a number of metabolic functions including the rate of growth of the bones and soft tissues.
3. The pituitary also produces a number of huge protein molecules called neuropeptides. These substances activities for

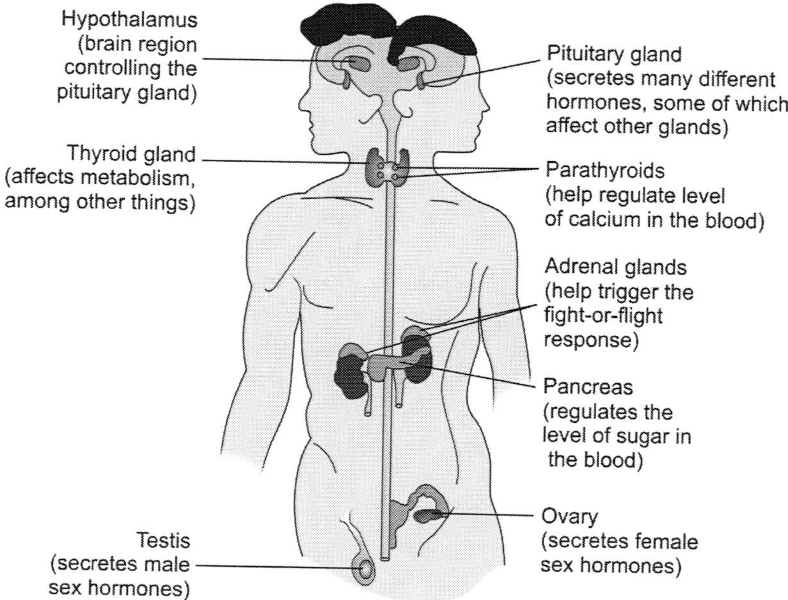

Figure 6.7: Functions of endocrine glands

eating and drinking, sexual behaviors, sleep, temperature regulation, pain reduction and responses to stimulus.

Thyroid Gland

The thyroid gland, located within the neck, response to pituitary stimulation by releasing the hormone thyroxine. The principal function associated with the thyroid gland is the control of body metabolism, the rate at which a person burns glucose circulating in the blood stream. The metabolism is in turn closely linked to motivational and mood states; the thyroid has important impact on behavior.

Parathyroid Glands

The four parathyroid glands are found behind the thyroid gland itself. They are small gland and they secrete a hormone that regulates a metabolism of calcium and phosphorus. Disorders of the parathyroid glands could bring about defective/hyper development during a child's early years of development.

Adrenal Gland

The adrenals are pair of glands, located just above each kidney that influences our emotional state, level of energy and ability to cope with stress. They consist of two parts, an inner core called adrenal medulla and outer layer called adrenal cortex. The medulla produces epinephrine and norepinephrine making the heart beat faster, diverting blood from the stomach and intestine to the voluntary muscles. At times of stress the hypothalamus causes the pituitary to release adrenocorticotropic hormone (ACTH), which in turn stimulates the adrenal cortex to increase its secretion of a number of hormones that influence metabolism.

Thymus Gland

1. The thymus gland is located below the thyroid gland and under the breast bone.
2. The thymus gland appears to play its major role in infancy and childhood.

Secretes a hormone associated with the body's capacity to resist infection. When a child has an infection, the thymus sends a message to the spleen and lymph node.

The message tells these structures that they should produce lymphocytes, the cleaning cells, which attack foreign organisms in the bloodstream. Once the body's immune system is developed, the thymus loses some of its functional role.

Pancreas Gland

The pancreas gland secretes two important hormones, insulin and glycogen. Insulin is the hormone that induces the oxidation or burning of blood sugar. If a person's pancreas is defective and it is unable to secrete adequate amount of insulin, the person will suffer from diabetes or chronic high blood sugar. Glycogen stores glucose in the liver.

Gonads

There are two types of gonads, i.e. the ovaries in female and testes in male. The ovaries are located in the vicinity of the uterus, one ovary on either side. In addition to producing egg cells, they also produce hormone. Estrogen is identified as playing a principal role in determining secondary female characteristics such as breast development and lack of facial hair.

Progesterone cooperates with estrogen in the regulation of ovulation and in the preparation of the uterus for pregnancy. Testosterone plays an important role in determining secondary male characteristics such as facial hair, voice depth and muscular development.

Body's Chemicals Help Control Behavior

The nervous system is designed to protect us from danger through its interpretation of and reactions to stimuli. But a primary function of the sympathetic and parasympathetic nervous systems is to interact with the endocrine system to elicit chemicals that provide another system for influencing the feelings and behaviors.

Gland

A group of cells in the endocrine system that functions to secrete hormones or chemicals that moves throughout the body to help regulate emotions and behaviors. When the hormones released by one gland arrive at receptor tissues or other glands, these receiving receptors may trigger the release of other hormones, resulting in a series of complex chemical chain reactions. The endocrine system works together with the nervous system to influence many aspects of human behavior including growth, reproduction and metabolism. And the endocrine system plays a vital role in emotions. Because the glands in men and women differ, hormones also help explain some of the observed behavioral differences between men and women.

Pituitary Gland

A small pea-sized gland located near the center of the brain that is responsible for controlling the body's growth, but it also has many other influences that make it of primary importance to regulating behavior. The pituitary secretes hormones that influence our responses to pain as well as hormones that signal the ovaries and testes to make sex hormones. The pituitary gland also controls ovulation and the menstrual cycle in women. Because the pituitary has such an important influence on other glands, it is sometimes known as 'master gland.'

Adrenal Glands

The body has two triangular adrenal glands, one atop each kidney. The adrenal glands produce hormones that regulate salt and water balance in the body, and are involved in metabolism, immune system and sexual development and function. The most important function of the adrenal glands is to secrete the hormones epinephrine (also known as adrenaline) and norepinephrine (also known as noradrenaline) when we are excited, threatened or stressed. Epinephrine and norepinephrine stimulate the sympathetic division of the autonomic nervous system (ANS) causing increased heart and lung activity, dilation of the pupils and increases blood sugar, which give the body a surge of energy to respond to a threat. The activity and role of the adrenal glands in response to stress provides an excellent example of the close relationship and interdependency of the nervous and endocrine systems. A quick-acting nervous system is essential for immediate activation of the adrenal glands, while the endocrine system mobilizes the body for action.

Male Sex Glands

The male sex glands are known as testes. The male sex glands secrete a number of hormones, the most important of which is testosterone. It regulates body changes associated with sexual development, including enlargement of the penis, deepening of the voice, growth of facial and pubic hair, and the increase in muscle growth and strength.

Female Sex Glands

The female sex glands known as ovaries are located in the pelvis. They produce eggs and secrete the female hormones estrogen and progesterone. Estrogen is involved in the development of female sexual features, including breast growth, the accumulation of body fat around the hips and thighs, and the growth spurt that occurs during puberty. Both estrogen and progesterone are also involved in pregnancy and the regulation of the menstrual cycle.

Other glands in the endocrine system include the pancreas, which secretes hormones designed to keep the body supplied with fuel to produce and maintain stores of energy; the pineal gland, located in the middle of the brain, which secretes melatonin, a hormone that helps regulate the wake-sleep cycle; and the thyroid and parathyroid glands, which are responsible for determining how quickly the body uses energy and hormones, and controlling the amount of calcium in the blood and bones.

▪ GENETICS AND BEHAVIOR

Genetics is the study of how traits are inherited or passed on from parent to child. The cells from which we started contain genes, which are the basic units of heredity. They determine the sequence of growth into a human baby. Genes determine the blood group, coloration and many other traits. In general, genes determine the resemblance between newborn and the parents.

General Concepts of Genetics

Behavior genetics, also called psychogenetics, is the study of the influence of an organism's genetic composition on its behavior and the interaction of heredity and environment insofar as they affect behavior. The question of the determinants of behavioral abilities and disabilities has commonly been referred to as the 'nature-nurture' controversy:

1. Genes are located in the nucleus of every cell in the body. They are composed of DNA, which contains blue prints for life. Living organisms are made of protein and DNA controls the way in which protein chains are built.
2. Material for constructing protein surrounds cells and DNA sends out messenger molecule ribonucleic acid (RNA) to control how the material is fashioned into specific kinds of protein chains.

3. Every living cell contains 20,000–25,000 genes grouped together in clusters of a thousand or more. They are arranged in thread-like chains called chromosomes.
4. The cells in human body have 46 chromosomes, arranged in 23 pairs. We inherit one member of each pair from our father and the other from our mother.
5. Genes are transmitted from generation to generation by means of sex cells. A female gamete is called ovum and a male gamete is called sperm.
6. Ovum and sperm combine their chromosomes when they unite to form one cell called zygote. Thus zygotes have 46 chromosomes, half from the father, which determine our genotype or genetic inheritance, for the rest of our lives.

Genetic Errors

1. Errors are made occasionally in transmitting genes from one generation to the next. As a result, children are sometimes born with abnormal chromosome structures, which are called mutations.
2. XXY/XYY mutations:
   a. Two Xs and one Y: People with an XXY mutation often have characteristics of both sexes. They might have developed breasts and small testicles.
   b. Two Ys and one X: Males with an extra Y chromosome (XYY) are often taller than other males. On the other hand XYY males in the general population are no more aggressive than normal males.
3. Another kind of genetic mutation is one in which a person has 47 chromosomes because of an extra one added to pair 21.
4. Children with chromosomal abnormalities suffer from Down syndrome, a disorder, which is characterized by the mental retardation and the unique physical appearances, including folds on the eyelid corners, a round face, a head with flattened back, a short neck and a small nose.

Causes of Mutation

1. Some people carry mutator genes that increase the rate of mutations in other genes.
2. High temperatures can increase mutation rate. Males generate sperm in their scrotum, a sac that is usually cooler than the rest of the body in mammals.
3. Radiation has been linked to mutation rate, X-rays are one source of radiation and pregnant mothers are advised to avoid them.
4. Radiation before pregnancy may also increase mutation rate. Recent evidence suggests that the exposure to radiation may explain the increased risk of having Down syndrome babies for older mothers.

Genetic and Behavioral Problems

Genetic Influences and Schizophrenia

While research and debate continue over the role of biological factors and life experience in schizophrenia, a consensus is in forming one major point that genetic factors play a role. One of studies that have convinced many people involves identical and fraternal twins. Identical twin pairs have identical heredity and fraternal twin pairs do not; so, schizophrenia is strongly influenced by genes.

Genetic Factors and Depression

The cognitive learning or life experience factors may be involved in depression; many investigations believe that biological factors also play a role. Some physiological deficit either inherited or acquired in other ways, is thought to make some people especially vulnerable to depressive episodes. It is known for sometime that hereditary factors play a role in some depression.

▪ CONCLUSION

The term behavior is usually extensive in psychology. Its scope is not limited to physical activities, but includes all sense organs (i.e. eyes, ear, tongue, skin, nose) and all activities of brain (i.e. concentration, imagination, thought, effort, memory intellect, etc.). Thus human behavior includes all activities and this indicates the concept of Woodworth that psychology is the science of activities. It is very important to study the health behavior of man from the point of community health because human behavior is a result of complex interaction between body and mind. The interrelation between physical and mental processes affects the total health of individual.

▪ REVIEW QUESTIONS

Long Essays

1. Explain the structure of neurons and neural impulse and its transmission.
2. Enumerate neurotransmitters with their functions in detail.

Short Essays

3. Nervous system and behavior.
4. Neurotransmitters and diseases.
5. Endocrine and behavior.
6. Role of genetics in behavior.
7. Functions of neuropeptides.
8. Synaptic transmission.

Short Answers

9. Causes of mutation.
10. Genetic error.
11. Genes.
12. Adrenal gland.
13. Catecholamines.

CHAPTER 7

Individual Differences

▪ INTRODUCTION

No two persons are born alike, but each differs from the other in natural endowments and individual differences; psychology focuses on this second level of study. It is also sometimes called differential psychology because researchers in this area study the ways in which individual people differ in their behavior. This is distinguished from other aspects of psychology in that although psychology is ostensibly a study of individuals, modern psychologists often study groups or biological underpinnings of cognition that people differ from each other is obvious. How and why they differ is less clear and is the subject of the study of individual differences (IDs)? Although to study individual differences seems to be to study variance, how are people different, it is also to study central tendency, how well can a person be described in terms of an overall within person average. Indeed, perhaps the most important question of individual differences is whether people are more similar to themselves overtime and across situations than they are to others, and whether the variation within a single person across time and situation is less than the variation between people. Individuals differ from each other. One individual is never similar to another in all respects. Each one has his/her own peculiarities, which presents him/her as a separate individual from the others. In psychological terminology, differences between individuals that distinguish or separate them from one another and make one distinct, unique and stand out from the rest are termed as individual differences.

▪ MEANING

Differences between the individual is normally attributed to both heredity and environment. A related question is that of similarity, for people differ in their similarities to each other. Questions of whether particular groups (e.g. groupings by sex, culture, age or ethnicity) are more similar within than between groups are also questions of individual differences. Research for individual differences typically includes personality, motivation, intelligence, ability, intelligence quotient (IQ), interests, values, self-concept, self-efficacy and self-esteem (to name just a few). There are few remaining 'differential psychology' programs in the United States, although research in this area is very active. Current researchers are found in a variety of applied and experimental programs, including educational psychology, individual psychology, industrial psychology, personality psychology, social psychology and developmental psychology programs, in the neo-Piagetian theories of cognitive development in particular. Earlier studies show us a higher risk with the factors of social and behavioral domains in young children with a single parent. However, the variety of single parent families regarding gender of the main parent has rarely been taken into reason when understanding the relation between family and child's negative outcomes. According to 'Dictionary of Education' by Carter B Good, 1959:

1. Individual differences stand for the variations or deviations among individuals in regard to a single characteristic or a number of characteristics.
2. Individual differences stand for those differences, which in their totality distinguish one individual from another.

Similarities among individuals:

1. Intellectual capacity: All individuals have sense organs, brain, muscles and glands. They have an intellectual capacity to gain through education and experiences.
2. All individuals have the emotions of love, fear and the feelings of pleasure and pain.
3. All individuals feel the need for independence, success, acceptance, etc.
4. All individuals are influenced by the traditions and customs of the society.
5. All individuals have some rights and the society imposes certain obligations upon them.

■ CAUSES

There are many factors that make a person unique from others (Fig. 7.1). These factors are related to family, trait, social life, situation, emotion, culture, etc. Person with different traits possess different personalities, this includes heredity, brain, physical trade (Table 7.1).

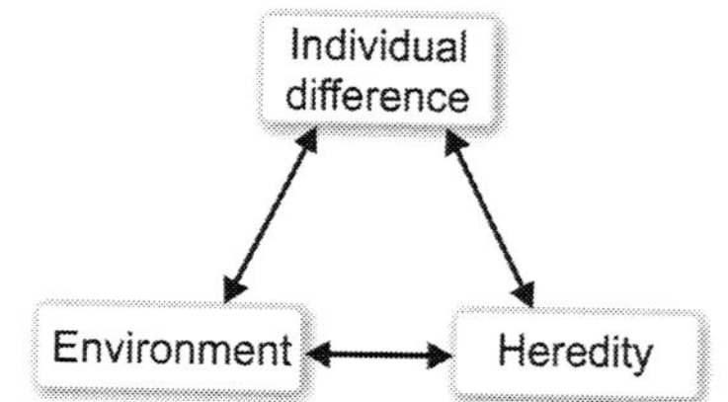

Figure 7.1: Causes of individual difference

Individual Differences

Individual differences are also caused by heredity and environmental factors. A child comes to this world with certain traits, which determine his/her individual capabilities and thus he/she differs from others on account of heredity.

Heredity

Heredity refers to the biological process of transmission of certain biological and psychological characteristics from parents to their children through genes. The hereditary decides the path of progress and development of an individual. Heredity provides the limits of one's growth and development in various dimensions, and aspects of one's personality and thus variations in hereditary characteristics causes differences between individuals.

Environment

The term 'environment' refers to such factors, in and around the individual, and brings about changes in the individual—physically and psychologically. The environment covers all the outside factors that act on the individual since, he/she begins life. The first environment for a child is the mother's womb. The fetus gets its nourishment from the bloodstream of its mothers. After birth, the child is expected to numerous environment factors such as food, water, climate, physical atmosphere at home, school, village, parents, members of the family, friends, neighbors, teachers, society, mass media, recreation, religious places, etc.

Table 7.2: Measurement of individual differences

Sl No.	Types	Description
1.	Intelligence	Stanford-Binet test Raven's progressive matrices Bhatia's battery of performance test of intelligence
2.	Aptitude test	Differential aptitude test (DAT): • Achievement tests • Term-end examinations
3.	Personality test	Self-reported or open reports Rating scales Questionnaires (Minnesota Multiphasic Personality Inventory, RB Cattell's 16 personal factors test and Eysenck's personality test) Projective tests (Rorschach inkblot test, thematic apperception test (TAT) Performance test Situational tests Interviews

■ TYPES (Table 7.2)

Table 7.2: Types of individual differences

Sl No.	Types	Description
1.	Physical/Physiological differences	Physical differences among individuals are related to the differences created on account of the differences in terms of physical make up of our bodies; individuals differ in height, weight, color of skin, color of eyes and hair, size of hands, arms, feet, mouth, nose, waistline, structure and functioning of internal organs, facial expression and mannerisms of speech, walk, hairstyle and other physical characteristics
2.	Psychological differences	Psychological make-up generates differences among us in terms of varying intellectual potentialities, interests, attitudes, emotions, social and moral development, etc.
3.	Gender	Men and women are different in every organ of the body even their skin; they are different at the cellular level and these differences may influence the variations in disease, treatment such as type and amount of medicine that are safe on the basis of gender
4.	Race	Racial differences can add up to significant group differences; many factors are involved such as socioeconomic factors, lifestyle, behaviors, social environment and access to preventive health services as well as treatment among other environmental differences
5.	Age	Age is an important factor, which decides the treatment and diagnosis of a disease in an individual; the mental, physical and intellectual abilities and the maturity level determine the individual variability according to the different age groups
6.	Intelligence	Individuals have difference in their general intelligence, e.g. it is not possible to send children with intelligence quotient of below 50 to school

Contd...

Contd...

Sl No.	Types	Description
7.	Nationality	Studies showed that individuals of different nations differ in respect to nature, physical and mental differences, interest and personality
8.	Personality	Personality is the total quality of an individual's behavior as is depicted in his/her habits of thinking, attitude, interest and his/her manner of acting, and his/her personal philosophy of life; personality is sum total of an individual's traits and characteristics, which is expressed through his/her behavior
9.	Abilities	Abilities will determine the individual for special professional and specialized fields of vocation
10.	Psychomotor activity	The individual's movements of the hand and feet, and other physical abilities are seen to be very individual and do not resemble to one another to a great extent
11.	Learning	Learning can be seen in children of different ages, but also among those in the same age group; it depends on their maturing and educational background
12.	Social background	Individual difference occurs based on types of family, culture, neighborhood and class, which manifests individual variations
13.	Economical status	Economic background creates differences in interest, tendencies, character, etc.
14.	Development	It is evident not only among those of different ages, but also in the individuals of same ages
15.	Mental differences	People differ in intellectual ability and capacities such as reasoning and thinking, power of imagination, creative expression, concentration, etc.
16.	Differences in attitudes	Individuals are found to possess varying attitudes toward different people, groups, objects and ideas; their attitudes may be positive, negative or somewhat different in nature
17.	Emotional differences	The individuals also differ in the manner they express their emotions; some are emotionally stable and mature, while others are emotionally unstable and immature

▪ HEREDITY

Heredity is considered as 'the sum total of inborn individual traits.' Biologically, it has been defined as 'the sum total of traits potentially present in the fertilized ovum.' According to Douglas and Holland, one's heredity consists of all the structures, physical characteristics, functions or capacities derived from parents, other ancestry or species. All organisms possess a life cycle, which includes growth, development, reproduction and decline. Though there is essential unity in life, the ways by which each organism exercises its capacities are different. These individual qualities of organisms and their basic properties are transmitted by means of heredity.

There is a popular notion that life begins at birth. But biologically life begins at the moment of fertilization (conception), i.e. when matured sperm of a man fuses with matured ovum of woman. It is most crucial events in the life of an individual because the biological substances present in the sperm and ovum determine the sex, biological, physiological and psychological characteristics of the emerging individual. Thus, biological heredity by interaction with the pre- and post-natal environment determines the potentialities of the individual. The knowledge of such hereditary factors and their functions help us to understand the growth, development, similarities and differences in physical, physiological and psychological makeup of an individual. Similarly the knowledge of the environment, which shapes the growth and development pattern of hereditary potentials, is necessary to understand the individual.

Hereditary Differences (Fig. 7.2)

Genetic Diversity

Genetic diversity is the amount of variation seen in a particular population. The differences occur in different communities, races or ethnic groups that lead to individual differences among population. The genes have an impact on the characteristics of human being, the Japanese and Chinese have significant appearance than Whites and Indians.

Genetic Variability

Genetic variability is a measure of the tendency of individual genotypes in a population to vary from one another. The genetic variability describes the susceptibility of organisms to disease and sensitivity to toxins or drugs.

Mechanism of Heredity

The life cycle of an individual begins with the fusion of a sperm and ovum. The origin of every human life can be traced to a single cell called zygote. When a sperm unites with an ovum, zygote is produced. The genes, which are

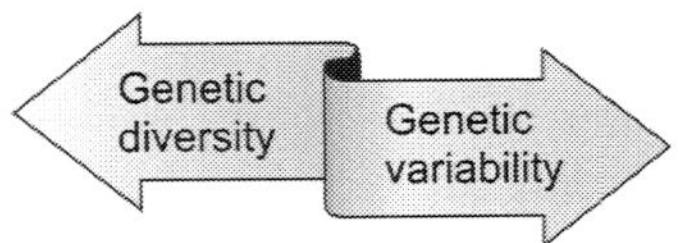

Figure 7.2: Hereditary differences

the carriers of distinctive traits are present both in the sperm and the ovum. In the fertilized ovum, there are 23 pairs of chromosomes, half of which are given by the father and the other half by the mother. While females have 23 pairs of XX chromosomes, males have 22 pairs of XX chromosomes plus two single chromosomes represented by X and Y. The X and Y are called sex chromosomes. Occasionally, through some unfortunate bodily error, aberrations in chromosomes appear. If an extra chromosome appears making the total 47 rather than the normal 46, mongolism (Down syndrome or trisomy 21 anomaly) results. A child with mongolism suffers from deceleration of growth during the prenatal period, which results in a highly complex, multidimensional disorder in which every organ is involved.

When chromosomes are studied under a microscope, bands of markings appear, representing an entity called genes, which appear to be the actual determiners of traits. Each chromosome is made up of many genes. Man has probably not less than 2,000 and not more than 50,000 genes in the chromosomes. Each gene is the determiner of a specific characteristic, such as straight nose or a deep lobed ear. At present, it appears that there is no simple one-to-one relationship between genes and traits that one gene may influence many characteristics or traits, or conversely many genes may combine to determine one characteristic.

Action of the genes on the cytoplasm changes the shape and other characteristics of the cells. The heredity basis of individual differences lies in the unlimited variety of possible gene combinations that can occur.

No two siblings get an identical heredity, as they do not get the same genes from the parents. Fraternal or dizygotic twins born to the same parents are different from each other because of different pairs of germ cells. However, identical or monozygotic twins develop from the same sperm and ovum, hence have exactly the same set of genes and therefore, resemble each other completely.

Determination of traits is not only due to combination of genes but also due to their dominant or recessive nature. In the color of the eye, e.g. brown is dominant over blue, if one parent carries only brown and the other only blue, their offspring will have brown eyes. Many people however, carry both and if two recessive blues happen to match up in the assorting process of meiosis and fertilization, the child would have blue eyes even though parents and all the immediate relatives have brown eyes.

Some characteristics are sex linked, i.e. one sex shows the characteristics, while the other sex not apparently affected is the carrier. One such trait is color blindness. For example, the sons of a color blind man and normal woman do not inherit the defect, but the daughters may be carriers of the disorder to another generation of males, their sons. Another example is hemophilia—a bleeding disorder, which rarely occurs in women, but is transmitted by them to their sons (Stern, 1960). Occasionally, in the reproductive cells of any living thing a change occurs, which causes the introduction of completely new traits in the next generation. Such changes are called mutations. Mutant plants and animals might have characteristics that breeders can use to improve existing varieties. In human beings, mutations are almost always undesirable. Their causes are not clear, but are known that they can be induced by atomic radiation.

Genetics and Behavior

Heredity is the basis for the development of human personality. It is similar to the raw material in the hands of the artist out of which the potter or tailor prepare the specific objects. Any amount of molding and treatment with special processes will still retain the basic properties of the raw material.

Many aspects of human behavior and development ranging from physical characteristics such as height, weight, eye and skin color, the complex patterns of social and intellectual behavior are influenced by person's genetic endowment. They also include physical deficiencies and the nature of glandular functioning. Heredity is a source of both similarities and differences among individuals.

Identity

'Like begets like'—the principle states that children have a tendency to be similar to their parents; the children of bright parents tend to be bright and those of dull, tend to be dull. But, this law is not universally true. It has exceptions. Sometimes we see white parents having black children. Such occurrences can be explained by the 'law of variation.'

Variation

The law of variation explains the causes of differences in the children of the same family. As the germ cells of the parents have genes, which unite in various ways, each combination produces a different quality of offspring, i.e. there will be as many variations as there are possible combination of genes. We sometimes find the same parents having children who are very different from one another. It is because of the different combinations of genes that different types of children are born, e.g. one combination would produce a white child, the other a dark one. We must remember that though the child of the same family is different in intellect, etc. yet they show a greater tendency to be similar to each other, than the children who are not related.

Sources of Variability in a Population (Table 7.3)

Table 7.3: Sources of variability in a population

Sl No.	Sources	Description
1.	Genetic recombination	During meiosis, two homologous chromosomes from male and female crossover one another and exchange gene sequences; the chromosomes than split apart and are ready to form an offspring; the crossover is random and is governed by its own set of genes that code from where crossovers can occur
2.	Immigration, emigration and translocation	Each of these is the movement of an individual into or out of a population; when an individual comes from a previous genetically isolated population into a new one, it will increase the genetic variability of the next generation if it reproduces
3.	Polyploidy	Having more than two homologous chromosomes allows for even more recombination during meiosis and allowing for even more genetic variability in one's offspring
4.	Diffuse centromeres	Being diffuse causes the chromatids to split apart in many different ways allowing for chromosome fragmentation and polyploidy hence creating more variability
5.	Genetic mutations	Contributed to the genetic variability within a population and can have positive, negative or neutral effects on the individual's fitness
6.	Correlated traits	Although some genes have only an effect on a single trait, many genes have an effect on various traits, so a change in a single gene will have an effect on all those traits
7.	Resemblance between relatives	A child has a father and mother, the child and father share 50% of their alleles, as do the child and the mother; however, the mother and father normally do not share genes as a result of shared ancestors; similarly two full siblings share on average 50% of alleles with each other, while half sibling only 25%

Regression

According to Sorenson, the tendency for the children of very bright parents to be less bright than parents and a comparable tendency for the children of very inferior parents to be less inferior is called regression.

Chromosomal Abnormalities

Cleft Palate

Cleft palate is an abnormal fissure in the palate of the mouth that is present at birth. It is caused by faulty development of the facial structure of the fetus. Very often a cleft palate is accompanied by a similar division in the upper lip called harelip. In the normal development separate tissues fuse together to form the palate, i.e. upper lip and upper jaw. Cleft palate occurs because the roof of the mouth does not develop completely and there will be a vertical gap (fissure) in the roof of the mouth.

Lobster Claw

Lobster hand is a rare congenital deformity of the hand. Here, the middle digit is missing. Lobster claw is an inherited condition. It often occurs both in males and females equally. The chance is 1 in 90,000 babies. It can be treated surgically to improve function and appearance, genetic counseling is given to parents who have genetic load. It is called by different names such as lobster claw hand, lobster hand, split hand deformity, cleft hand, etc.

Polydactyly or Syndactyly

Polydactyly or syndactyly is webbing between the fingers and toes. In most cases the condition is inherited. It usually affects both hands and feet. Syndactyly of the toes does not require treatment, but fingers can be corrected by surgery. Polydactylism is nothing, but having one or more extra fingers and/or toes. It is probably a most common abnormality of development found at birth. It occurs in about 2/1,000 children.

Hemophilia

Hemophilia is a congenital disorder, where the blood clotting is very slow. Due to this condition any wound or injury, even if it is a minor one, gives rise to prolonged bleeding. This individual will have a risk of anemia and dangerous loss in blood volume. Hemophilia is due to deficiency in one of the factors in blood plasma, which helps blood clotting normally. Hemophilia occurs almost exclusively in males (sex-linked trait); it is due to genetic defect, transmitted only by women.

Down Syndrome

Down syndrome is also known as mongolism or trisomy 21. It is called Down syndrome because this kind of mental retardation was first traced and studied by John Langdon-Downs. It is called mongolism because, these mentally retarded individuals will have the features of Mongolian race, i.e. short, broad face, round head, small lowest ears, flat nose, large tongue that protrudes from small mouth, a fold of skin at the inner corners of the eyes, short fingers, weak muscles. The child exhibits a marked degree of mental retardation with an IQ of 50 or below.

▪ ENVIRONMENT

Man cannot remain untouched by the environment in which he/she lives. If the environment is favorable, the impact is positive whereas in an unfavorable environment, man's development may be hindered or he/she may have to do more effort for adaptation. Environment is an extensive and broader concept, everything around us is environment. But, for physical scientists environment means only nature and physical conditions.

It may be any of every influence with which an individual comes into contact after the hereditary pattern has been received to the germ plasma. It includes the effects of training, trial and error learning influences of the home, school, neighborhood, hospital, church, playground, climate, geographical location and anything else that stimulates the senses in any way. Thus, the heredity plays its game only at the time of conception. What happens afterwards, i.e. after conception, is the game of environment. It affects the individual, his/her bodily structure and all of his/her personality make up and behavior.

Definition

1. Total environment includes physical and social aspects—Maclver and Page.
2. The environment can be explained as natural environment and sociocultural environment.

Types

According to Landis, environment can be divided into three parts such as natural, social and cultural (Fig. 7.3).

Natural environment: Physical environment, all natural life conditions, forces and objects, which influences life are included.

Social environment: It consists of three environments such as social organization, institutions and social relationship.

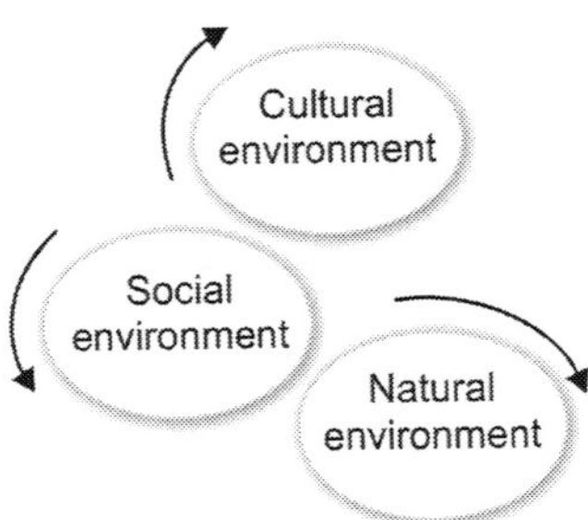

Figure 7.3: Types of environment

Cultural environment: It includes customs, tradition, usages, pattern and values.

Environmental Forces Categorization

Environmental forces can be categorized into two, internal and external environment.

Internal Environment

The internal environment refers to the prenatal environment. The nucleus with its chromosomes and their genes is surrounded by a jelly-like substance known as cytoplasm. Cytoplasm is considered as an intercellular environment. This environment influences the genes and thereby the traits they carry. In fact, what the organism becomes is determined by its cytoplasm and its heredity. Further the cells press upon one another and influence their neighboring cells chemically and electrically. This intracellular environment has an effect on the developing embryo. The cells in each area will develop into the respective organ.

The environment received by the individual from his/her conception in the womb of the mother till his/her birth, i.e. a period of about 10 months is called internal environment.

In this environment, the embryo receives the nutrition through the bloodstream of his/her mother. The physical and mental health of the mother including her habits, attitudes and interests, etc. all constitutes the inner surrounding or internal environment that affects the growth and development of the fetus along with the emerging behavior in future.

The role of heredity and environment in the development of personality and behavior has been extensively searched in the form of twins and family studies, and on experimenting selective breeding. The results have failed to establish a clear cut role of either presence of particular behavior or trait in an individual. What behaviors are learned or what are inherited is a controversial question that can only be answered through a reasonable understanding that once his/her behavior or development of a specific personality trait is always a result of the interaction of the environmental process on the genetically inherited characteristics.

External Environment

After the birth what the child gets in terms of environmental influences is purely external in nature. These can be physical and social or cultural influences. The physical environment are earth, river, mountains, weather and climatic conditions, food, water, etc. The parents, family members, friends, classmates, teachers, members of community and society, the means of mass communication and recreation, religious places, etc. include with social and cultural environment helping to shape the personality and behavior.

The environment after birth is more complex and powerful. It involves immense variety of physical and social contacts. This is what we customarily call 'environment'. The social environment includes language, customs, tradition and many cultural aspects such as values, moral, religion, etc. further schools, community, family, peer group, neighborhood also influence the individual. The physical environment involves stimuli such as the food we eat, the drinks we take, the cloths we wear, the shelter we live in, light, sound, smell, taste, etc. will have their own impact on the individual.

▪ RELATIVE IMPORTANCE OF HEREDITY AND ENVIRONMENT

The relative importance of heredity and environment is rather disputable because both heredity and environment factors are equally important in the individual. They interact in such a way that influence of each factor is dependent on the contribution of the others. Any single hereditary factor operates differently under different environmental conditions. In the same way the environmental conditions differ in their relative influences depending upon the hereditary factors involved. However, heredity and certain abnormalities prove the importance of hereditary; monsters prove the importance of environment. Hybrid is a product of two different species, which are similar to each other.

▪ INTERACTION BETWEEN HEREDITY AND ENVIRONMENT

Each individual enters the world with certain hereditary characteristics transmitted to him/her through parents. He grows up in a certain environment with its human, social and material surroundings. Everything he/she does as a child or adult results from the complex interactions between heredity and environment:

1. The relative influence of heredity and environment differs from one individual to another and from one human trait or condition to another.
2. Heredity and environment are interdependent forces. Inheritance is an important factor in the development of the artistic abilities, i.e. music. Heredity supplies the potential talent, while favorable environment brings it out.
3. Heredity and environment are equally important in shaping the temperament of the child. Heredity lays down the essential foundations, while environment can change these foundations for better or worse.
4. Heredity provides the raw material from which a person is made. How the material is molded, and what he/she becomes, depend chiefly on the environment. Good materials placed in good hands result in a fine finished product. Poor material, no matter how carefully fashioned can never become a first-rate product.
5. Our inheritance prescribes the limits beyond which it may not be possible for any individual to develop, however wholesome and stimulating the environment may be.

Today no one believes that nurture alone completely determine the course of our development. Psychologists agree development is shaped by the interaction of heredity and the environment. Within this interaction, our genetic endowment for many characteristics provides us with a reaction range of possible levels that we may ultimately reach depending on the quality of our experience in the environment. Heredity and environment are interdependent forces. The influence of heredity and environment are so interrelated that they are practically inseparable.

The knowledge of the mechanism of heredity and the influence of environment on the personality development is important for a nurse to understand the behavior of a patient.

▪ INDIVIDUAL DIFFERENCES IN HEALTH AND ILLNESS

Understand the Child's Abilities

Individual differs in intelligence. It is not possible to send children with an IQ of below 50 to schools. Children with a higher IQ go to school. Children with IQ's between 50 and 70 can learn only the simplest tasks (Fig. 7.4).

Even the small schools trouble children whose IQ varies between 70 and 80. Children with IQ varying between 115 and 120 are considered brilliant or intelligent. Very low and

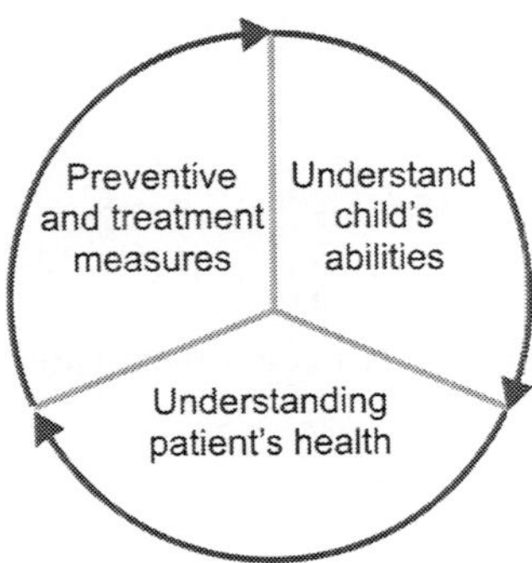

Figure 7.4: Individual difference in health and illness

high IQ children have difficulty in learning with those having average IQ. Generally, 40–60% of the children in school have IQs varying between 95 and 105, being the children with average intelligence who form the basis for the formulation of the syllabus and curriculum as well as the method of teaching:

1. Individuals with special abilities are helpful to judge special professions and specialized fields of vocation.
2. Mental ages and education are intimately related. The child's level of education is determined according to his/her mental age.
3. Children's interests, tendencies and character can also be seen influenced by economic situation, which would affect the learning and special abilities.

Understanding the Patient's Health

1. Individual differences are useful for explaining and predicting behavior and performance.
2. People vary on a range of psychological attributes. Thus, it is possible to measure and study these individual differences.
3. It helps to understand the behavior, feeling, thinking and attitude of patients during sickness.
4. Gene-environment interaction means some people carry genetic factors that cause susceptibility or resistance to a certain disorder in a particular environment. It may be significant public health benefits in using genetic information to decide environmental interventions that prevent disease.

Preventive and Treatment Measures

1. It can assess the health promoting or treatment behaviors such as medication taking, proper diet and engaging in physical activity through patient perceptions of health and threat of disease and barriers in a patient's social or cultural environment.
2. It helps in evaluating the effectiveness of a new therapy on the group.
3. Treatment with drugs can be made safer and more effective when the patient's genotype is known. Pharmacokinetics studies the genetic variation that causes people to respond differently to drugs.

■ CONCLUSION

Thus, the individual from the time of conception to death is subjected to environmental influences. So, we find that the continuous interplay of the heredity endowments and the environment factors are in determining the physical, physiological, social and psychological growth, and development of the individual. So, man is a product of the interplay of heredity and environment.

■ REVIEW QUESTIONS

Long Essays

1. Define individual difference. Explain meaning and types of individual differences.

2. Explain heredity and environment, and discuss their role in causing individual differences.

Short Essays

3. Measurement of individual difference.
4. Mechanism of heredity.
5. Chromosomal abnormalities.
6. Sources of variability in population.
7. Explain the role of environment in causing individual difference.
8. Individual difference in health and illness.

Short Notes

9. Psychological difference.
10. List down the factors causing individual difference.
11. Genetic diversity.
12. Hemophilia.
13. Types of environment.

CHAPTER

8 Sensation

■ INTRODUCTION

A term sensation commonly used to refer to the subjective experience resulting from stimulation of a sense organ (Fig. 8.1), for instance, a sensation of warm, sour or green. As a general scientific category, the study of sensation is the study of the operation of the senses. Sense receptors are the means by which information presented as one form of energy. For example, light is converted to information in the form used by the nervous system, i.e. impulses traveling along nerve fibers. Each sense has mechanisms and characteristics peculiar to itself, but all display the phenomena of absolute threshold, differential threshold and adaptation. Not until sufficient stimulation impinges on a receptor can the presence of a stimulus be detected. The quantity of stimulation required is known as the absolute threshold. Not until a sufficient change occurs in some aspect of a stimulus can the change be detected. The magnitude of the change required is called differential threshold. Under steady stimulation, there is a decrease in sensitivity of the corresponding sense, as indicated by a shift in the absolute threshold and in the magnitude of sensation. After the stimulation ceases, sensitivity increases. An obvious example of visual adaptation occurs when one goes from bright to dim surroundings or vice versa.

■ DEFINITIONS

1. Sensations can be defined as the passive process of bringing information from the outside world into the body and to the brain. The process is passive in the sense that we do not have to be consciously engaging in a sensing process.
2. Sensation is defined as the process by which our sensory receptors and nervous system receive and represent stimulus energies from our environment.

■ MEANING AND CONCEPTS OF SENSATION

In psychology, sensation is the first stage in the biochemical and neurological events that begins with the impinging of a stimulus upon the receptor cells of a sensory organ, which then leads to perception, the mental state that is reflected in statements "I see a uniformly blue wall."

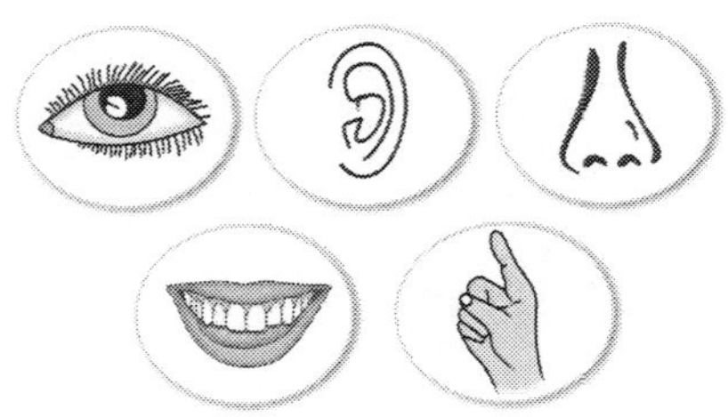

Figure 8.1: Sense organs

A sensation that might lead to that statement could include the excitation of cone cells in the retina, spatially varying in the proportion of blue and green cone excitation due to portions of the wall receiving different proportions of yellowish artificial and bluish skylight; it is common for these variations to be compensated for, within the brain, so that the non-uniform sensation yields a perception of uniform color.

Sensation is the process by which our senses gather information and send it to the brain. A large amount of information is being sensed at any one time such as room temperature, brightness of the lights, someone talking, a distant train or the smell of perfume. With all this information coming into our senses, the majority of our world never gets recognized. We do not notice radio waves, X-rays or the microscopic parasites crawling on our skin. We do not sense all the odors around us or taste every individual spice in our gourmet dinner. We only sense those things we are able to, since we do not have the sense of smell as has a bloodhound or the sense of sight as that of hawk; our thresholds are different from these animals and often even from each other.

■ STEPS INVOLVED IN SENSATION (Fig. 8.2)

There are four essential steps involved if stimulation is to lead to sensation (Floyd L Ruch, 1970); if any one of these four steps is missing there will be no sensation at all:

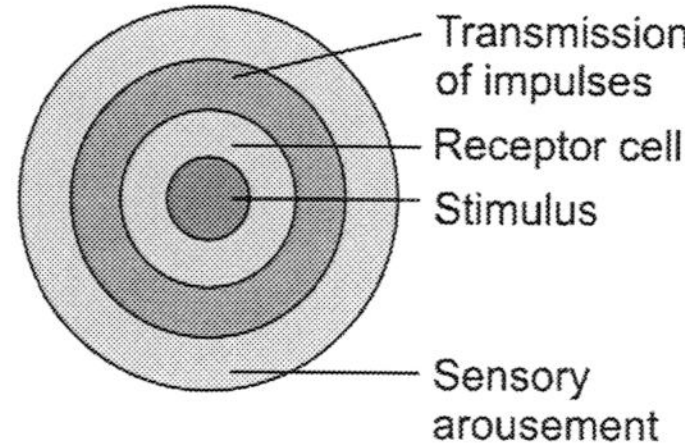

Figure 8.2: Steps involved in sensation

1. **Stimulus:** It must be applied internally or externally. A stimulus is some kind of radiant, mechanical or other energy, which activates the receptors of the concerned sense organ.
2. **Receptor cell:** The stimulus must stir certain receptors cells or nerve endings into activity. Usually, a receptors cell is activated only by a particular form of energy. For example, visual receptors are stimulated by light waves; auditory receptors are stimulated by sound waves and so on.
3. **Transmission of impulses:** The neural impulses released must travel from the receptor cells to brain through nerves.
4. **Sensory arousement:** Activity must be aroused in the sensory arose of the brain proceeding conscious sensations and has its own special conscious sensations. Each sensory activity has its own special areas in the cerebrum or brain.

■ CLASSIFICATIONS OF SENSATIONS

One convenient method of classifying sensations is to categorize them according to the location of the receptor. On this basis, receptors may be classified as exteroceptors, visceroceptors and proprioceptors (Fig. 8.3):

1. **Exteroceptors:** These are located near the surface of the body, provide information about the external environment. They receive stimuli from outside the body and transmit sensations of hearing, sight, touch, pressure, temperature and pain on the skin.
2. **Visceroceptors:** These are located in blood vessels and viscera, provide information about the internal environment. This information arises from within the body and may be felt as pain, taste, fatigue, hunger, thirst and nausea.

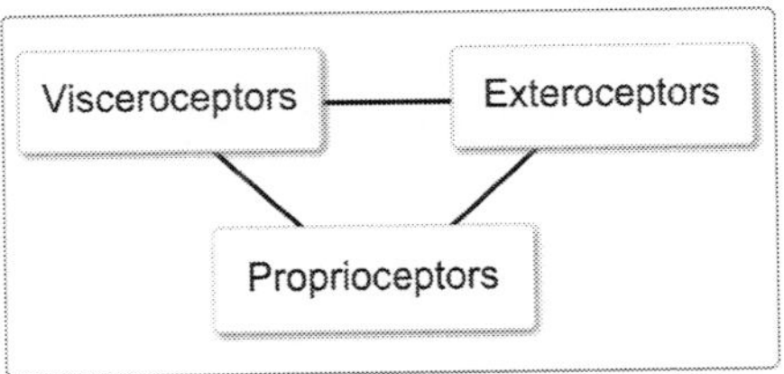

Figure 8.3: Classifications of sensation

3. **Proprioceptors:** These are located in muscles, tendons and joints; allow us to feel sensations of position, movement, equilibrium and tension of muscles and joints through the stretching or movement of parts where these receptors are located.

■ GENERAL CHARACTERISTICS OF SENSATION

The sensation whether it is visual, auditory or gustatory, or any other form has certain fundamental characteristics common to all, some of them are detailed in Table 8.1.

■ SENSE ORGANS AND THEIR FUNCTIONS

Visual Sense

The eye is the organ of vision. It has a complex structure consisting of a transparent lens that focuses light on the retina. The retina is covered with two basic types of light-sensitive cells such as rods and cones. The cone cells are sensitive to color and are located in the part of the retina called fovea, where the light is focused by the lens. The rod cells are not sensitive to color, but have greater sensitivity to light than the cone cells. These cells are located around the fovea and are responsible for peripheral vision and night vision. The eye is connected to the brain through the optic nerve. The point of this connection is called blind spot, because it is insensitive to light. Experiments have shown that the back of the brain maps the visual input from the eyes.

The brain combines the input of our two eyes into a single three-dimensional image. In addition, even though the image on the retina is upside down. Because of the focusing action of the lens, the brain compensates and provides the right-side-up perception. Experiments have been done with subjects fitted with prisms that invert the images. The subjects go through an initial period of great confusion, but subsequently they perceive the images as right-side-up.

The range of perception of the eye is phenomenal. In the dark, a substance produced by the rod cells increases the sensitivity of the eye so that it is possible to detect very dim light. In strong light, the iris contracts reducing the size of the aperture that admits light into the eye and a protective obscure substance reduces the exposure of the light-sensitive cells. The spectrum of light to which the eye is sensitive varies from the red to the violet. Lower electromagnetic frequencies in the infrared are sensed as heat, but cannot be seen. Higher frequencies in the ultraviolet (UV) and beyond cannot be seen either, but can be sensed as tingling of the skin or eyes depending on the frequency. The human eye is not sensitive to the polarization of light, i.e. light that oscillates on a specific plane. Bees, on the other hand, are sensitive to polarized light and have a visual range that extends into the UV. Some kinds of snakes have special infrared sensors that enable them to hunt in absolute darkness using only the heat emitted by their prey. Birds have a higher density of light-sensing cells than humans do in their retinas and therefore higher visual acuity (Fig. 8.4).

Hearing Sense

The ear is the organ of hearing. The outer ear protrudes away from the head and is shaped as a cup to direct sounds toward

Table 8.1: General characteristics of sensations

Sl No.	Characteristics	Description
1.	Stimulation	Sensation is a change brought about in us by a stimulus; we may call it as stimulation It makes us aware of certain facts either in the world outside or within us; they come in the form of air waves, light waves or heat waves, etc.
2.	Intensity	Within each modality sensations vary in intensity from low to high, thus, we experience mid pain or severe pain For sensation to be effective, it must possess some amount of intensity It should not be very faint or very intense, e.g. a very faint sound may not be heard or very faint light may not be seen On the other hand, if it is very intense beyond certain limits, it gives raise to some other experience than what it has to, e.g. sound of very-high intensity causes pain in the ear instead of causing the experience of sound
3.	Limen	The point below which a sensation has no effect is known as limen or lower limit The point above which it because painful is known as upper limit In between these two limits there is much sensory intensity
4.	Threshold	The upper and lower limits are known as also known as the threshold The stimulus, which is below the threshold causes no response It is known as subliminal stimulus Two or more subliminal stimuli, combining together, may produce a single strong reaction This phenomenon is known as the summation of stimuli
5.	Latency period	It is the time that lapses between the stimuli presented and the responses shown The stimulus takes a certain length of time, i.e. roughly 0.005–0.1 second to arouse a sense organ Then, it takes time to arouse nerve fibers that lead to the brain Further, the brain connections, the motor nerves and the muscles also take time to respond Thus, there is bound to be lapse of time between the awareness of the sensation and consequent imitation of action Usually, the response and the stimulus appear to take place simultaneously, but there is always some lapse of time, which is known as latency period, this can be measured by reaction time apparatus
6.	Duration	If a stimulus is to be effective, it must be presented for a certain length of time It should be neither too short nor too long, if it is too short, it does not act upon the sense organs effectively and produce the desired sensation If it is too long, the concentration of sense organs either gets fatigue or their will be adopted in the sense organ and hence there will be no sensation and no response For example, continuous presentation of an odor or sound for a long period causes negative adaptation and will not provoke the expected response

Contd...

Contd...

Sl No.	Characteristics	Description
7.	Extensity	It refers to the amount of space that the stimulus occupies In fact, many sensations will have extensity Bigger stimulus occupies larger space and smaller stimulus occupies larger space smaller areas For example, hot water bath occupies larger space in the skin and a pin prick occupies smaller larger spaces in the skin High intensity of sound occupies areas of the basilar membrane and low intensity occupies smaller area of the basilar membranes
8.	Quality	Every sensation has quality in addition to quality, the quality tells us the kind of sensation and the quality refers to the amount of sensation For example, two colors of same saturation and brightness values may still differ in color Similarly, tones of different instruments, though they are equal in intensity and frequency of sound waves differ in their tonal quality, which is distinguishable
9.	Absolute threshold	For any sensation to be aroused, the stimulus (light, sound, touch, etc.) must have a minimum intensity called absolute threshold The absolute threshold is different for each individuals; it also changes from time to time for the same person Absolute threshold for the sense can be lower or higher in times of illness and fatigue When we are much tried our senses need fewer or greater stimuli to arouse them A moderate sound may seem very loud, a weak light or small wrinkle in the sheet may irritate an ill person Absolute threshold varies depending upon the individuals physical conditions under which the observations are made
10.	Difference threshold	Just as there must be a certain minimum amount of stimulation to evoke a sensory experience, so there must also be certain magnitude of difference between two stimuli before one can be distinguished from the other The minimum amount of stimulation necessary to tell two stimuli apart is known as the difference threshold

the tympanic membrane, which transmits vibrations to the inner ear through a series of small bones in the middle ear called malleus, incus and stapes. The inner ear or cochlea, is a spiral-shaped chamber covered internally by nerve fibers that react to the vibrations and transmit impulses to the brain via the auditory nerve. The brain combines the input of our two ears to determine the direction and distance of sounds.

The inner ear has a vestibular system formed by three semicircular canals that are approximately at right angles to each other, which are responsible for the sense of balance and spatial orientation. The inner ear has chambers filled with a viscous fluid and small particles (otoliths) containing calcium carbonate. The movement of these particles over small hair cells in the inner ear sends signals to the brain that are interpreted as motion and acceleration (Fig. 8.5).

The human ear can perceive frequencies from 16 cycles per second, which is a very deep bass to 28,000 cycles per second,

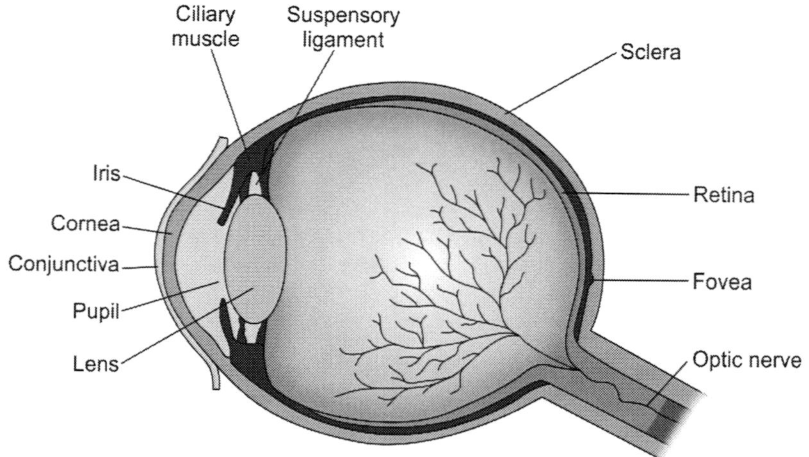

Figure 8.4: Anatomy of eye

which is a very high pitch. Bats and dolphins can detect frequencies higher than 100,000 cycles per second. The human ear can detect pitch changes as small as hundredths of 1% of the original frequency in some frequency ranges. Some people have perfect pitch, which is the ability to map a tone precisely on the musical scale without reference to an external standard. It is estimated that less than 1 in 10,000 people have perfect pitch, but speakers of tonal languages such as Vietnamese and Mandarin show remarkably precise absolute pitch in reading out lists of words because pitch is an essential feature in conveying the meaning of words in tone languages. The Eguchi Method teaches perfect pitch to children starting before they are 4 years old. After age 7, the ability to recognize notes does not improve much.

Gustatory

Taste or gustation is the ability to detect sensory changes in the tongue, through the use

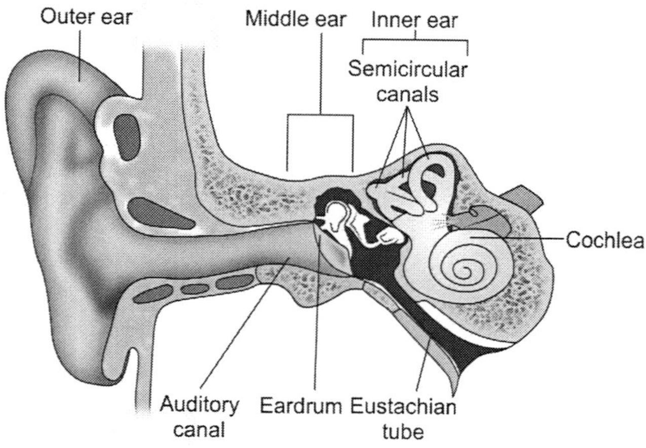

Figure 8.5: Anatomy of ear

of taste buds, situated deep into the papillae. Intriguingly, the sense called gustation is a fact comprised of varying ratios of multiple sensory systems, shifting in importance and attention as food is chewed, tasted and swallowed.

These include the taste buds, the sense of touch in the structures of the mouth and digestive system, chemical sensation of irritation in the trigeminal nerve system and unique receptors for sensing the properties of water located at the rear of the oral cavity. The receptors for taste called taste buds are situated chiefly in the tongue, but they are also located in the roof of the mouth and near the pharynx. They are able to detect four basic tastes, i.e. salty, sweet, bitter and sour.

The tongue also can detect a sensation called umami from taste receptors sensitive to amino acids. Generally, the taste buds close to the tip of the tongue are sensitive to sweet tastes, whereas those in the back of the tongue are sensitive to bitter tastes. The taste buds on top and on the side of the tongue are sensitive to salty and sour tastes. At the base of each taste bud there is a nerve that sends the sensations to the brain. The sense of taste functions in coordination with the sense of smell. The number of taste buds varies substantially from individual to individual, but greater numbers increase sensitivity. Women, in general, have a greater number of taste buds than men. As in the case of color blindness, some people are insensitive to some tastes (Fig. 8.6).

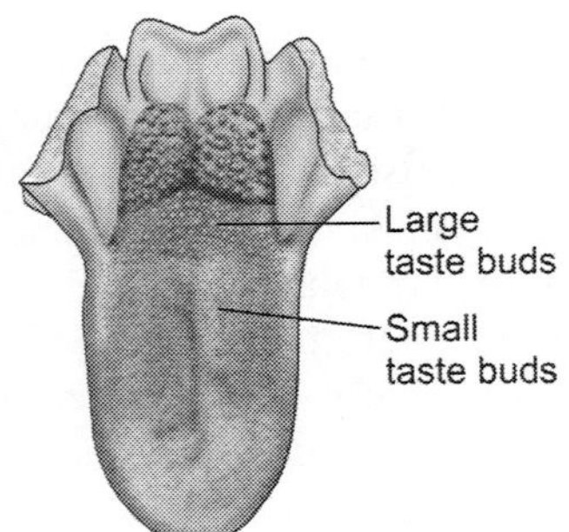

Figure 8.6: Anatomy of tongue

Olfactory Sense

Smell or olfaction is received by the olfactory bulb and are connected to the brain by the olfactory nerve, the I cranial nerve of the brain, just after the nasal turbinates of the nose warm, strain and filter the air (Fig. 8.7).

The nose is the organ responsible for the sense of smell. The cavity of the nose is lined with mucous membranes that have smell receptors connected to the olfactory nerve. The smells themselves consist of vapors of

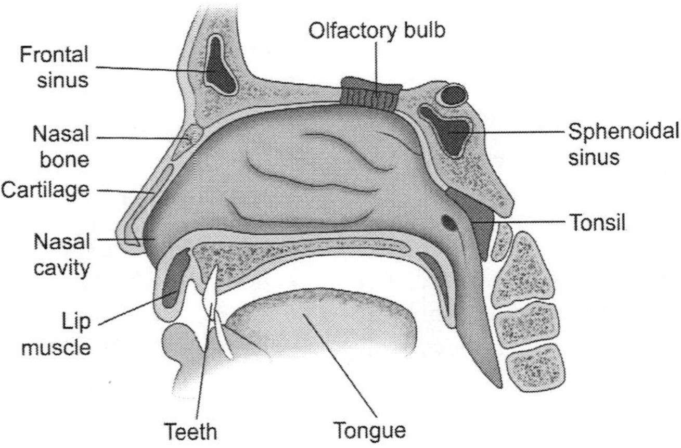

Figure 8.7: Anatomy of nose

various substances. The smell receptors interact with the molecules of these vapors and transmit the sensations to the brain.

The nose also has a structure called vomeronasal organ whose function has not been determined, but which is suspected of being sensitive to pheromones that influence the reproductive cycle. The smell receptors are sensitive to seven types of sensations that can be characterized as camphor, musk, flower, mint, ether, acrid and putrid. The sense of smell is sometimes temporarily lost when a person has a cold. Dogs have a sense of smell that is many times more sensitive than human being.

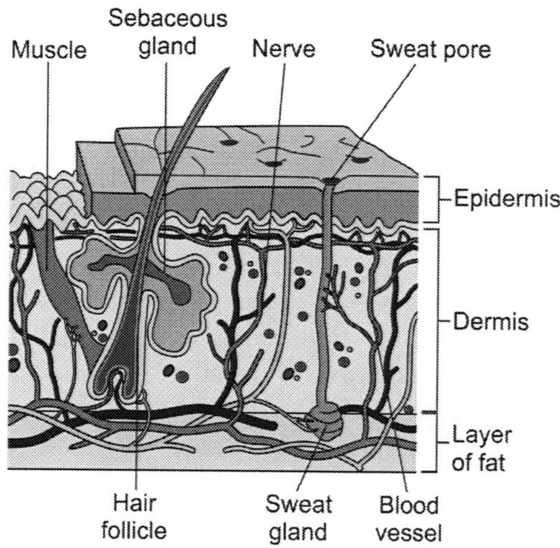

Figure 8.8: Anatomy of skin

Skin (Touch)

The sense of touch is distributed throughout the body. Nerve endings in the skin and other parts of the body transmit sensations to the brain. Some parts of the body have a larger number of nerve endings and therefore are more sensitive.

Four kinds of touch sensations can be identified are cold, heat, contact and pain. Hairs on the skin magnify the sensitivity and act as an early warning system for the body. The fingertips and the sexual organs have the greatest concentration of nerve endings. The sexual organs have erogenous zones that when stimulated start a series of endocrine reactions and motor responses resulting in orgasm (Fig. 8.8).

Beyond the Five Sense Organs

In addition to sight, smell, taste, touch and hearing, the humans also have awareness of balance (equilibrioception), pressure, temperature (thermoception), pain (nociception) and motion to all of which may involve the coordinated use of multiple sensory organs. The sense of balance is maintained by a complex interaction of visual inputs, the proprioceptive sensors (which are affected by gravity and stretch sensors found in muscles, skin and joints), the inner ear vestibular system and the central nervous system. Disturbances occurring in any part of the balance system or even within the brain's integration of inputs can cause the feeling of dizziness or unsteadiness.

Kinesthesia

Kinesthesia is the precise awareness of muscle and joint movement that allows us to coordinate our muscles when we walk, talk and use our hands. It is the sense of kinesthesia that enables us to touch the tip of our nose with our eyes closed or to know, which part of the body we should scratch when we itch.

Synesthesia

Some people experience a phenomenon called synesthesia in which one type of stimulation evokes the sensation of another. For example, the hearing of a sound may result in the sensation of the visualization of a color or a shape may be sensed as a smell. Synesthesia is hereditary and it is estimated that it occurs in 1 out of 1,000 individuals with variations of type and intensity. The most common forms of synesthesia link numbers or letters with colors.

■ LOSS OF SENSATION

Many types of sense loss occur due to a dysfunctional sensation process, whether it is ineffective receptors, nerve damage or cerebral impairment (Fig. 8.9). Unlike agnosia, these impairments are due to damages prior to the perception process.

Vision Loss

Degrees of vision loss vary dramatically, although the International Classification of Diseases-9 (ICD-9) released in 1979 categorized them into three tiers normal vision, low vision and blindness. Two significant causes of vision loss due to sensory failures include media opacity and optic nerve diseases, although hypoxia and retinal disease can also lead to blindness. Most causes of vision loss can cause varying degrees of damage from total blindness to a negligible effect. Media opacity occurs in the presence of opacities in the eye media, distorting and/or blocking the image prior to contact with the photoreceptor cells. Vision loss due to media opacity often results despite correctly functioning retinal receptors. Optic nerve diseases such as optic neuritis or retrobulbar neuritis lead to dysfunction in the afferent nerve pathway once the signal has been correctly transmitted from retinal photoreceptors.

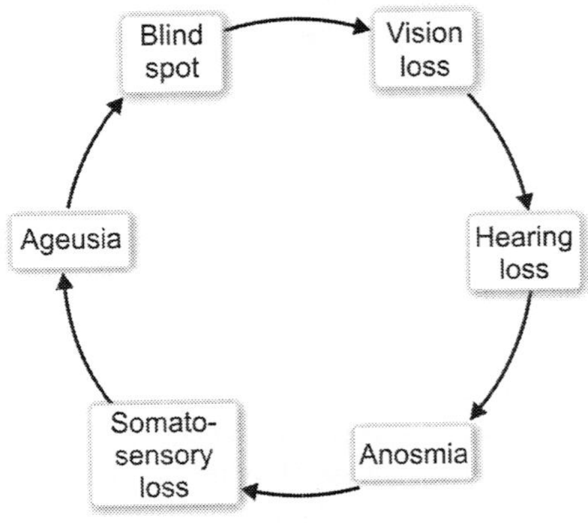

Figure 8.9: Problems of sensation

Hearing Loss

Similarly to vision loss, hearing loss can vary from full or partial inability to detect some or all frequencies of sound, which can typically be heard by members of their species. For humans, this range is approximately 20 Hz to 20 kHz at ~6.5 dB, although a 10 dB correction is often allowed for the elderly. Primary causes of hearing loss due to an impaired sensory system include long-term exposure to environmental noise, which can damage the mechanoreceptors responsible for receiving sound vibrations, as well as multiple diseases such as human immunodeficiency virus (HIV) or meningitis, which damage the cochlea and auditory nerve, respectively.

Anosmia

Primary causes of anosmia, a loss of smell, due to sensory damage involve the death of olfactory receptor neurons, often from nasal polyps or upper respiratory tract infections, as well as damage to the olfactory nerve, often from hypothyroidism or physical trauma. Unfortunately, anosmia is strongly correlated with a loss of taste.

Somatosensory Loss

Insensitivity to somatosensory stimuli such as heat, cold, touch and pain are most commonly a result of a more general physical impairment associated with paralysis. Damage to the spinal cord or other major nerve fiber may lead to a termination of both afferent and efferent signals to varying areas of the body causing both a loss of touch and a loss of motor coordination. Other types of somatosensory loss include hereditary sensory and automatic neuropathy, which consists of ineffective afferent neurons with fully functioning efferent neurons; essentially, motor movement without somatosensation.

Ageusia

Taste loss can vary from true ageusia, a complete loss of taste, to hypogeusia, a partial loss of taste, to dysgeusia, a distortion or alteration of taste. The primary cause of ageusia involves damage to the lingual nerve, which receives the stimuli from taste buds for the front two thirds of the tongue or the glossopharyngeal nerve, which acts similarly for the back third. Damage may be due to neurological disorders such as Bell's palsy or multiple sclerosis, as well as infectious diseases such as meningoencephalitis. Other causes include a vitamin B deficiency, as well as taste bud death due to acidic/spicy foods, radiation and/or tobacco use.

Blind Spot

Blind spot is a small area in each eye, which is completely blind. The area is completely free of rods and cones, and hence it is not sensitive to visualize stimulation. It is located in the place where the optic nerves leave the retina to the visual cortex.

■ REVIEW QUESTIONS

Long Essays

1. Define sensation. Explain meaning and concepts of sensation. Describe the classifications of sensation.
2. Describe sensory disorders. Explain nursing implications for sensory abnormalities.

Short Essays

3. Enumerate steps involved in sensation.
4. Describe functions of sense organs.
5. General characteristics of sensation.

Short Answers

6. Threshold.
7. Gustatory.
8. Blind spot.
9. Ageusia.
10. Anosmia.
11. Synesthesia.
12. Kinesthesia.

■ BIBLIOGRAPHY

1. Adles C, Adles S. Biofeedback and Psychosomatic Disorders, 2nd edition. Baltimore: Lippincott Williams & Wilkins; 1989. pp. 10-89.
2. Arnold MB, Gasson JA. Feelings and emotions as dynamic factors in personality integration. In: Arnold MB (Ed). The Nature of Emotion. London-Baltimore: Penguin; 1968.
3. Bandura A. Principles of Behavior Modifications. New York: Holt Rinehart & Winston; 1969.
4. Brody N, Ehrlichman H. A Thoughtful Introduction to the Broad Field of Personality. Personality Psychology: Science of Individuality: Prentice Hall Press; 1997.
5. Carlson NR. Psychology of Behavior. Boston: Allyn & Bacon; 1977.
6. Carol Taylor, Carol Lillis, LeMone P. Fundamentals of Nursing: The Art and Science of Nursing Care, 5th edition. Philadelphia: Lippircott Williams & Wilkins; 2004. pp. 685-705.
7. Cooper C. A broad overview of the field that includes a review of measurement methodologies. Individual Differences. London: Arnold; 1997.
8. Descartes René. Philosophical Essays and Correspondence. Indianapolis: Hackett; 1649.
9. Dossey MB, Keegan L, Shields D, et al. Holistic Nursing; A Handbook for Practice, 4th edition. Massachusetts: Jones & Bartlett Publishers; 2004. pp. 5-898.
10. Edelman, Gerald M. Wider Than the Sky: The Phenomenal Gift of Consciousness. New Haven: Yale University Press; 2004.

11. Eysenck HM, Eysenck MW. Personality and Individual Differences: A Natural Science Approach. New York: Plenum; 1985.
12. Eysenck HJ. Personality: Biological foundations. In: Vernon PA (Ed). The Neuropsychology of Individual Differences. London: Academic Press; 1994.
13. Ferguson ED. Motivation: An Experimental Approach. New York: Holt Rinehart and Winston; 1976.
14. Gale A, Eysenck MW. Handbook of Individual Differences: Biological Perspectives. Chichester: Wiley; 1991.
15. Galton F. Measurement of Character; 1884. pp. 179-85.
16. Goddard FA. The Human Senses, 2nd edition. New York: Wiley; 1972.
17. Goldberg LR. The Structure of Phenotypic Personality Traits. American Psychologist, 48; 1993. pp. 26-34.
18. Hochberg JE. Perception, 2nd edition. Englewood Cliffs, New Jersey: Prentice Hall; 1978.
19. Hogan R, Johnson J, Briggs S. The Definitive Handbook of the Field Includes Chapters on Evolutionary, Biological, and Social Bases of Individual Differences. Handbook of Personality Psychology. San Diego: Academic Press; 1997.
20. Jaegwon Kim, Ted Honderich. Problems in the Philosophy of Mind, in Oxford Companion to Philosophy Oxford: Oxford University Press.
21. Jensen AR. The G Factor: The Science of Mental Ability. Westport: Praeger; 1998.
22. Kim J. Problems in the Philosophy of Mind. Oxford Companion to Philosophy. Oxford: Oxford University Press; 1995.
23. Kim J. Physicalism or Something Near Enough. Princeton, New Jersey: Princeton University Press; 2005.
24. Korman AK. The Psychology of Motivation. Englewood Cliffs, New Jersey: Prentice Hall; 1974.
25. Lewith G, Kenyon J, Lewis P. Complementary Medicine: An Integrated Approach. Oxford: Oxford University Press; 1998. pp. 36-8.
26. Lindsay PH, Norman DA. Human Information Processing, 2nd edition. New York: Academic Press; 1977.
27. Loehlin JC. Genes and Environment in Personality Development. A Concise Tutorial on Genetic Modeling and Personality Taxonomies. Newbury Park: Sage; 1992.
28. Maltby J, Day L, Macaskill A. Personality, Individual Differences and Intelligence. London: Pearson Education; 2007.
29. Morgan CT. A Brief Introduction to Psychology. New Delhi: McGraw-Hill; 1975.
30. Morgan CT, King RA, Weizz JR, et al. Introduction to Psychology, 6th edition. New Delhi: McGraw-Hill; 1982.
31. Mueller CG. Sensory Psychology. Englewood Cliffs, New Jersey: Prentice Hall; 1965.
32. Munn, Norman L. Introduction to Psychology. New Delhi: Oxford & IBH; 1973.
33. Potter PA, Perry AG. Fundamentals of Nursing, 6th edition. Missouri: Elsevier-Health Sciences; 2005. pp. 968-87.
34. Robinson DN. An Intellectual History of Psychology. New York: Macmillan; 1976.
35. Saklofske DH, Zeidner M. International Handbook of Personality and Intelligence. New York: Plenum; 1995.
36. Seager W. Theories of Consciousness: An Introduction and Assessment. London: Routledge; 1999.
37. Strongman KT. The Psychology of Emotion: from Everyday Life of Theory. New York: Wiley; 1973.
38. Thompson RF. Introduction to Psychological Psychology. New York: Harper & Row; 1975.
39. Tyler LE. The Psychology of Human Differences. New York: Appleton-Century-Crofts; 1965.
40. Velmans, Max, Susan Schneider. Blackwell Companion to Consciousness. Malden, MA: Blackwell; 2007.
41. Watson J. Applying the Art and Science of Human Caring. New York: National League for Nursing; 1994.
42. White L. Basic Nursing: Foundations of Skills and Concept. Albany: Delmas Ine; 2002. pp. 345-69.
43. Zelazo, Philip David, Morris Moscovitch, Evan Thompson. Handbook of Consciousness. Cambridge: Cambridge University Press; 2007.

Section III

Cognitive Process

CHAPTER 9

Attention

■ INTRODUCTION

We are constantly being exposed to an extensive environment. Stimuli impinging upon us at a given moment are beyond exhaustive enlistment. It is a practical impossibility for a man to take note of all these stimuli collectively. Hence, he/she selects single stimuli or a few stimuli for observation. This purposive selection of stimuli for observation is called attention. During attention there is a mobilization of various parts of the body muscles and sense organs toward the object of attention. That is why attention is often described as a process of adjustment of the entire body.

■ MEANING

1. Attention is the focusing of consciousness on a particular object or idea at a particular time, to the exclusion of all other objects or ideas.
2. Attention is a selective mental activity; it constantly shifts from one object to another or from one aspect of the situation to another. The process of attention involves motor adjustments on the part of the person who is attending.
3. Our attention is controlled and directed by the intensity of the stimulus as well as a variation in intensity.
4. Attention is the chief characteristic of the conscious mind and is essential to acquiring knowledge.
5. The specific portion, which is selected for clear perception is called the focus of attention. Remaining part of the field is called the margin of attention.
6. Attention is not only merely a cognitive function but also essentially determined by emotional and conational factors of interest attitude and striving.

■ DEFINITION

1. Attention is process of getting an object or thought clearly before the mind.

   —*Ross*
2. Attention is the concentration of consciousness upon one object rather than upon another. —*Dumville*
3. Attention is being keenly alive to some specific factor in our environment. It is a preparatory adjustment for response.

   —*Morgan and Gilliland*

■ IMPORTANCE

Attention is the focus of consciousness, which is compared with a stream that flows constantly. All our thoughts, sensation, ideas and experience constitute this stream of consciousness. Attention enables the individual to gain these experiences. It also involves specific physical adjustments. When we see an attentive class with pin-drop silence, we can have picture of such adjustments, which help attention. These physical adjustments are necessary for bringing out the importance of attention:

1. Firstly, attention increases efficiency. Woodworth shows that familiar instances of readiness or preparedness for action in the military command of 'attention' and the athletic call of 'ready.' These signals bring about an increased state of motor readiness for responding very quickly to the instruction, 'go.'
2. Secondly, attention improves sensory discrimination. Like a bright searchlight, it shows the details of the landscape. All objects given attention are shown prominent or standout more prominently. They enter into the focus of consciousness and thus sensory discrimination is improved by attention.
3. Thirdly, attention is useful for acquisition of skill. The typist or the cyclist, or the cricket player pays attention to the hands and movements, to coordination and control. When the skill is adequately developed such attention is no longer required.
4. Lastly, attention is helpful for remembering. When attention is paid to certain specific areas or objects, concentration helps to know the details and retain them accurately. Other things, which are not properly attended to be not remembered well and as such are forgotten as soon as possible. Some common functions are:
   a. Attention helps in bringing mental alertness and preparedness.
   b. Attention helps in our awareness or consciousness of our environment.
   c. It makes us better equipped for distinguishing or discriminating the object of attention from others.
   d. Attention acts as a reinforcement of sensory process and help in the better organization of the perceptual field for the maximum clarity and understanding of the object or phenomenon.
   e. Attention helps in providing proper deep concentration by focusing one's consciousness up on one object at a time rather than two.

■ TYPES

Types of attention are as follows (Fig. 9.1):

- Non-volitional or involuntary attention
- Volitional or voluntary attention
- Habitual attention.

Non-volitional or Involuntary Attention

1. Non-volitional type of attention is aroused without the play or will.
2. Non-volitional attention can be aroused by our instincts as also by our sentiments.
3. Here, we attend to an object or an idea without making any conscious efforts on our parts.
4. For example, involuntary attention is mother's attention toward her crying child, attention toward the members of the opposite sex, sudden loud noise, bright colors, etc.
5. Involuntary attention does not require any conscious effort on our part; we cannot ignore the stimulus because of its intensity.

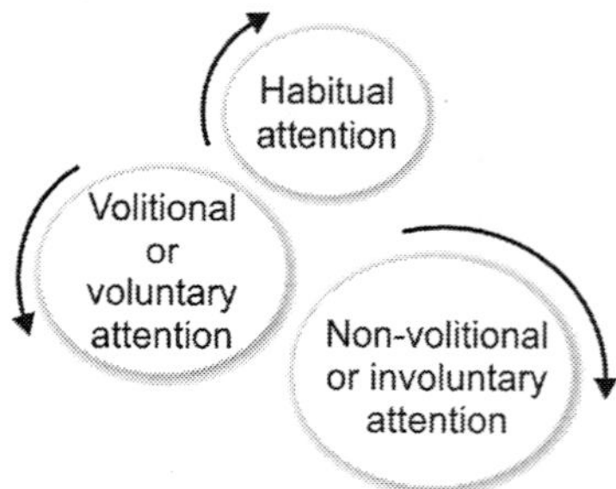

Figure 9.1: Types of attention

Volitional or Voluntary Attention

1. Voluntary attention demands the conscious efforts on our part. A habit is a learned mode of behaving that is relatively fixed and reliably occurs in certain situations. Frequent repetition or physiological exposure that shows itself in regularity of response acquires a behavior pattern.
2. Volitional attention is further subdivided in to two categories such as implicit volitional attention and explicit volitional attention.
3. Implicit volitional attention is single actor volition is sufficient to bring about attention.
4. Explicit volitional attention is obtained by repeated acts of will. One as to struggle hard for keeping one's self-attentive. It requires strong will power, keen attention and strong motives for the accomplishment of the task.
5. Voluntary attention is not given wholeheartedly or spontaneously. It has been given to interesting objects uninteresting locators, difficult assignments, which have to be done at time when you would like to be doing something else.

Habitual Attention

1. Habitual attention occurs by nature, inclined to take special note of certain things since we have natural interest them.
2. Our physiological make up is such that, we are dragged toward them. Thus food, drinks, etc. are things in which we have natural interest.
3. Factors determining attention is a selective mental process by which we attend to a particular stimulus is determined by a number of factors. We select one and give up others. It means there is something in these stimuli that makes us attend to them.

■ FACTORS INFLUENCE ATTENTION (Fig. 9.2)

Objective Factors

Intensity: It is a fact of our everyday experience that a louder sound attracts our attention easily. Similarly a dark color is more effective than a lighter shade.

Size: Sometimes size also determines the selection of a stimulus. Bigger patch of color would certainly draw our attention more easily than a smaller patch of the same color even of brighter shade.

Repetition: Certain stimuli are seen to attract our attention only on the strength of their repetition. They may be neither intense nor large size. When we knock at the door, it is habitual to repeat the knocking. For example, we take very little notice of the continuous ticking of the clock in our roomer of the dripping of the tap in our bathroom.

Change: Although we pay very little attention to the ticking of the clock, we may all of a sudden become aware of it, if it stops. Here, the factor that operates is change. Many fissions attract attention because of the change involved them.

Movement: Anything that moves has an attention value. Electronic signs are always made to move for attraction better attention. We often see infants attending not only to big and bright object but also to tiny insects that move.

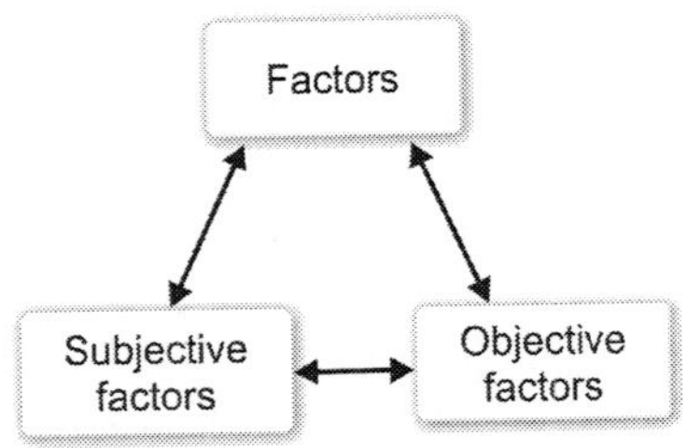

Figure 9.2: Factors affecting attention

Novelty: Attention is always aroused by something new. Some unfamiliar or strange object or a familiar one in some new setting catches attention.

Systematic forms: Among different things that arouse sensation, we may probably attend to those, which have definite systematic pattern or rhythm. A soft melodious tune may be easily heard in the midst of loud noises.

Subjective Factors

Interest: A person who is interested in a particular field, attend to object related to that field. For example, one who is interested in gardening is attracted by a new kind of plant or a girl who is interested in dresses will promptly observe a novel pattern of dress.

Motive: Our inner motive and desires also determine to a great extent what things we attend to. A sleeping mother may not be disturbed by the loud noises of traffic outside, but she may be easily aroused by even a faint cry of her baby. Appeal to certain important motives such as self-assertion, security or sex are also observed to arouse quick attention.

Organic state: A person's organic state to determine his/her attention. Thus, a hungry person is easily attracted by the flavor or sight of eatables.

Moods and attitudes: If one is in an angry mood, he/she is proving to notice even the minor mistake of others, but if he/she is in happy mood he/she usually overlooks them. Similarly attitudes toward people and object also determine attention.

Habits: These are enduring types of behavior, which becomes a part of a person. Habits are acquired over period of time in the object at a glance. For example, a person who has developed the habit of reading sports forest in a paper would look for the sports column in the newspaper.

■ SPAN

The maximum number of letters of numbers of figures that an individual can notice or apprehends at a glance is known as span of attention. According to this definition of attention, one can attend to only one stimulus or only one object at a glance. So, what we call as span of attention is only a span of apprehension and what we measure in the laboratory is not even span of apprehension, but its reproduction:

1. One more interesting problem of attention is the span of attention, which is also called the span of apprehension. While defining attention we have emphasized that in strict physiological sense only one object, idea or fact can be the center of consciousness at one particular movement and consequently we can attend to only one thing at time.
2. One of the oldest experiments in the physiological laboratory is concerned with determining how many separate items can thus be apprehended in a single glance. Sir William Hamilton, who in the year 1859, first of all tried to perform experiments on the span of attention.
3. Experiments to study the span of visual attention are carried out with the help of an instrument known as tachistoscope. The apparatus tachistoscope gives a quick exposure of cards containing number of dots or other figures only for a fraction of second. The maximum number of dots or figures that an individual can discarnate correctly gives his/her span of attention. There are individual differences, but usually four to five letters or numbers can be apprehended by an average individual.
4. The term span of attention may be defined in terms of the quality, size are extent to which the perceptual field of an individual can be effectively organized

in order to enable him/her to attend a number of things in a given spell of short duration.

Objectives and Subjective Factors

The span of an individual is determined by many objectives and subjective factors:

1. Grouping and organization of the materials facilitate span of apprehension than scattering and disorganization.
2. Pre- and post-exposure field, if free from glare and other distractions, they facilitate span.
3. If the duration of exposure period is a little more than the optimum time, the span will be more and if it is less than the optimum time the span will be less.
4. Optimum and constant interval between the ready signal and exposure of the material facilitate span.
5. Size of the stimulus, practice and meaning in the materials exposed add to the span.
6. Age, mental condition, memory images of materials observed, fatigue, familiarity and past experience also affect the span of apprehension.

■ SHIFTING OR FLUCTUATION

1. It is a fact of our experiences that we cannot attend to a certain stimulus for a longer time. Our attention oscillates among the stimuli around. Sometimes the center of our consciousness keeps on fluctuating from one stimulus to another or on the different parts of a stimulus; this is known as fluctuation of attention.
2. Fluctuation of attention also involves rapid change in the intensity of the attention. The intensity increases or decreases ranging between the paying of attention and no attention or at least of less attention.
3. While paying attention toward an object, event or phenomenon, it is not possible for us to hold it continuously with the same intensity for a longer duration. In course of time in the center of our consciousness either shifts from one stimulus to another or from one part of the same stimulus to another part, this is called shifting of our attention.
4. The phenomenon of fluctuation of attention was experimentally recorded for the first time by a psychologist named Urbantschitsch (1875). While testing the auditory sensation, he/she observed that the subject was not able to hear the tick continuously of an alarm clock kept at a distance.

■ DIVISION

Division of attention means attending two tasks simultaneously, with equal attention and efficiency (Fig. 9.3). We hear people telling that they can attend two tasks simultaneously with equal efficiency. They say that they read a novel and knit a sweater or listen to a radio program and knitting. As against this, studies have proved beyond doubt that one can attend only one task at a time. If anybody tries to attend two tasks at a time the work suffers either in quality or in quantity or both:

1. The attention is divided between two tasks, if more than two tasks are attended and performed simultaneously then the attention will have to be divided among those tasks.
2. Many researchers have tried to study the effect of the division of attention on the work product. It has been found that the work products suffer less, if both the

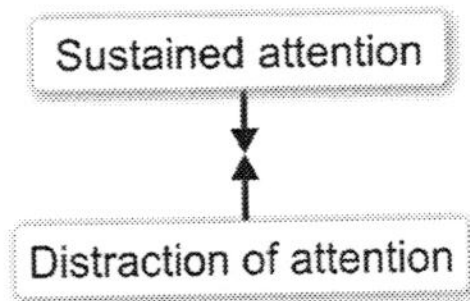

Figure 9.3: Division of attention

tasks are simpler, but in the case of difficult and similar tasks, the division of attempts proves disadvantages.

Sustained Attention

1. Sustained attention occurs, if one desires to be successful in the operation of a task, he/she has to begin with paying attention or concentrating his/her energies on the operation of that task, but the beginning of a process and not the end.
2. After paying initial attention, care is to be taken to hold it for a long enough duration. The individual should be absolutely absorbed in handling the task, unmindful of anything else going on, without getting disturbed in the least.
3. One has to make serious and deliberate efforts for sustaining ones attention by taking care of all the factors responsible for maintaining attention and eliminating or reducing the forces of distraction.

Distraction of Attention

1. Distraction may be defined as any stimulus whose presence interference with the process of attention or draws away attention from the object, which we wish to attend.
2. Distraction represents a sort of interference with our attention. The source of distraction may be external (e.g. noise, improper lighting, uncomfortable seats, etc.) and internal (e.g. lack of motivation, emotional disturbances, ill-health, boredom of fatigue, etc.).

■ CONCLUSION

Attention is the concentration of mental effort on sensory or mental events involving possession by the mind, in clear and vivid form, of one out of what seems to be several simultaneously possible objects or train of thoughts. It constantly shifts from one object to another or from one aspect of the situation to another. The process of attention involves motor adjustments on the part of person who is attending. Many researchers have tried to study the effect of the division of attention on the work product. It has been found that the work products suffer less, if both the tasks are simpler; but in the case of difficult and similar tasks, the division of attempts proves disadvantageous.

■ REVIEW QUESTIONS

Long Essays

1. Define attention. Explain the meaning and importance of attention.
2. Describe the factors influencing attention in detail.

Short Essays

3. Describe the types of attention.
4. Shifting and influctuations in attention.
5. Division of attention.
6. Distraction of attention.

Short Answers

7. Involuntary attention.
8. Habitual attention.
9. Span of attention.
10. Sustained attention.

CHAPTER

10 Perception

■ INTRODUCTION

Perception is the selection, organization and interpretation of sensory input. It involves giving meaning to sensations. Sensation refers to the immediate experiences that are generated by simple and isolated stimuli. Perception involves the organization and interpretation of these stimuli to give them meaning. For instance, in listening to a person who sings, we experience the qualities of loudness and pitch as sensations, while our ability to hear the sequence of sounds as a song is an act of perception. At the next level, if we understand and recognize the words of the song, our perception blends into 'cognition,' a more complex interpretive process that involves memory and thought.

■ MEANING

1. Perception is the selection, organization and interpretation of sensory input. It involves giving meaning to sensations. In other words, it is the activity of selecting, organizing and interpreting sensations with one's past experiences.
2. Perception is very essential to deal with the world around us, as it influences the memory, thinking, reasoning emotions, etc. The behavior is very much a reflection of how we react to an interpreted stimuli from the world around us. The process of perception helps in becoming aware of object's quality or relations by way of sense organs.
3. Perception is an intellectual and psychological process because it is a subjective process based on different people; here they assume according to their environment and interpret accordingly to their own views.
4. Perception is the intellectual process through which a person selects the date from the environment, organizes it and obtains meaning from it. Sensations are the first stage of receiving stimuli; it is the experience we get, when the receptors of the sense organs send impulses to specific areas of the brain. The activity of the organism is converting a sense impression into the awareness of some meaningful situation is called perception.
5. Perception is a highly individualized process that helps an organism, in organizing and interpreting one complex pattern of sensory stimulation for giving them, the necessary pattern meaning to initiate his behavioral responses.
6. It is a complex process, determined by both physiological and psychological characteristics of the organism.

■ DEFINITION

1. Perception is a process by which individual organize and interpret their sensory impressions in order to give meaning to their environment.
2. It is the appearance of things that is the focus of attention rather than objective reality.
3. It is the experience of objects, events or relationships obtained by extracting information from and interpreting sensations.
4. It is the organizing process by which interprets our sensory input.
5. Perception defined as all the processes involved in creating meaningful patterns out a jumble of sensory impressions, which fall under the general category of perception.
6. It is an individual's awareness aspects of behavior, for it is the way each person processes the raw data, he/she receives from the environment, into meaningful patterns.
7. It is the intellectual process by which an individual screens, selects, organizes and interprets the stimuli in order to give meaning to their environment.
8. Perception can be defined as the active process of selecting, organizing and interpreting the information brought to the brain by the senses.

■ NATURE OF PERCEPTION

1. Perception is a process: It is essentially a process rather than being a product or outcome of some psychological phenomenon.
2. Perception is the information extractor: Out sensory receptors are bombarded continuously by various stimuli present in the environment. Perception performs this duty by extracting relevant information out of a jumble of sensory impressions and converting them into some meaningful pattern.
3. Perception is the first event in the chain, which leads from the stimulus to action.
4. Perception is the act of interpreting a stimulus generated in the brain by one or more sense mechanism.
5. Perception is a mental process in which sensory cues and relevant past experiences organize together to give us meaningfulness to the perceived object.

■ FACTORS INFLUENCING PERCEPTION (Fig. 10.1)

Sense organs: Perception depends upon sense impressions, which is related to the sense organ concerned with the specific stimulus. To perceive different auditory stimuli, auditory sense organ must be developed and should function properly.

Brain function: It provides various frames of references in organizing the past experiences and sensory information, which helps in perception.

Motive: Our perception often depends upon our motives working at the given moment, when we are hungry we perceive certain objects as eatables even though they are not eatables in reality.

Familiarity: Past experiences are required to associate the sensory information, which helps in apprehension.

Set or readiness: It has been observed that what we see is influenced by what we are set

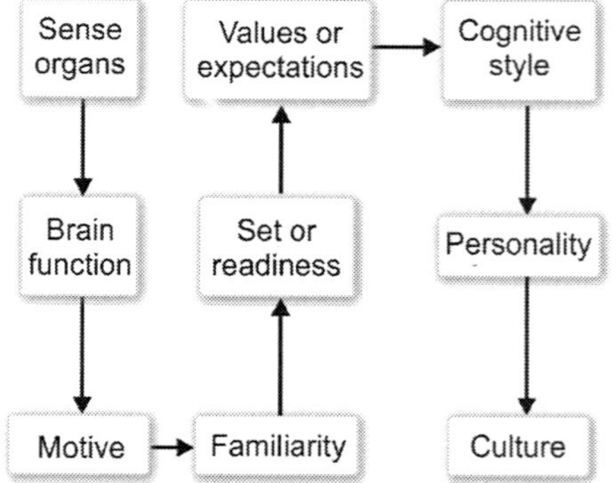

Figure 10.1: Factors influencing perception

to see. When we are in good mood we do not perceive the mistakes of others very easily.

Values: When a person places a high premium on a stimulus he/she tends to perceive it differently. In an experiment, children were asked to compare the size of a chip with the adjustable circle of a light. After a few trails the children were told that the chips could be exchanged for a candy. Thus, the children were taught to value the chips higher than before. Then they were rewarded with candy for chips. Subsequently, when the children were asked to compare the size of the chip with the circle of the light most of them perceived the chips as longer than size of the circle.

Expectations: Anticipation influences one's perception. Sometimes one has a tendency to see what we expect to see. Thus, when subjects were shown a red light and asked to report the sign on a cardboard, most of them reported as stop sign, even though it was spelt as top.

Cognitive style: As a person matures each one of us develops a way of dealing with the situation/environment, which is known as cognitive style. The cognitive styles could be viewed differently. In one approach, field dependent and field independent approach; in the former, the person sees the environment as a whole and does not delineate it into its parts. But in the later, the person perceives the elements of the environment with its parts.

Personality: A person's personality influences the way he/she perceives. In two studies, healthy colleagues were compared to depressed patients or students with eating disorder in terms of their ability to identify words related to food. Persons with depression were able to identify adjectives related to depressed traits.

Culture: The culture background of a person have influences on the perception of that person. The way in which a person uses the cues depend on one's culture.

■ DIFFERENCE BETWEEN SENSATION AND PERCEPTION (Table 10.1)

Normally, sensation and perception are two sides of a same coin. We can only think of them separately, but cannot experience them separately. It is rather difficult to understand the differences between sensation and perception, because the two are inseparable and always go together:

1. Sensation is an experience that an individual will have, when his/her sensory area is stimulated by coded neural impulses (message), which are transmitted by the given sense organ to the concerned sensory area through the sensory nerves as when the sense organ is stimulated by either external or internal environment. Whereas, perception is interpretation of the sensory experience

Table 10.1: Difference between sensation and perception

Sl No.	Concepts	Sensation	Perception
1.	Organization	Not organized	Organized
2.	Organs involved	Sense organs	Brain
3.	Meaningfulness	Meaningless	Meaningful
4.	Organs stimulated	Sense organs	It is selection, organization and interpretation of the sensory inputs
5.	Action	Rudimentary action	Perception is a much higher act

by the association area of the cortex in collaboration with sensory area; and in the background of the past experience, present mental and physical status of the individual.
2. A sensation begins with the stimulation of the sense organ and ends with the interpretation of the sense experiences or perception.
3. A sensation by itself cannot bring about the experience of an object, it is the psychological processes, which interprets the sensation, gives the knowledge of the object perception.
4. Pure sensation is a primary passive mental process, which is the resultant of the external stimulating energy, whereas perception is an active process of grouping and organizing the sensory experience and its interpretation in the background of past experience.
5. A sensation by itself cannot give us complete and meaningful experience, and it cannot independently lead to perception. In addition to sensation, a number of symbolic processes such as images, memories, revival of a past experiences, etc. together cause perception. In short, the activity of converting a sense impression into awareness of some meaningful situation is called perception.
6. The sensory information merely provides raw data. The data then combined with previous information and with thought processes to create the world we actually experience perception.

■ PRINCIPLES OF ORGANIZATION OF PERCEPTION

Gestalt Principles

Individuals tend to organize environmental stimuli into some meaningful patterns or wholes according to certain principles.

Principle of Figure-ground Relationship

According to this principle, a figure is perceived in relationship to its background. The perception of the object or figure in terms of color, size, shape and intensity, etc. depends upon the figure-ground relationship. We perceive a figure against a background or background against a figure depending upon the characteristics of the perceiver as well as the relative strength of the figure or ground. A proper figure-ground relationship is quite important from the angle of perception of the figure or the ground. In case where such relationship does not exist, we may witness ambiguity in terms of clear perception. Sensory experiences other than visual experiences may also be perceived as figure and ground. Sometimes, when there are various parts within the general field of awareness, having equally balanced qualities, there could be a conflict and two more figures may be formed. In such a case, there will be a shifting of the ground and the figure. One part may be the ground at one moment and at the next moment the ground may become the figure. In Figure 10.2 either the black faces or the white vase may become the figure. Moreover, it is impossible to perceive both figure and background at the same time.

Principle of Closure

According to this principle, while confronting an incomplete pattern, one tends to complete

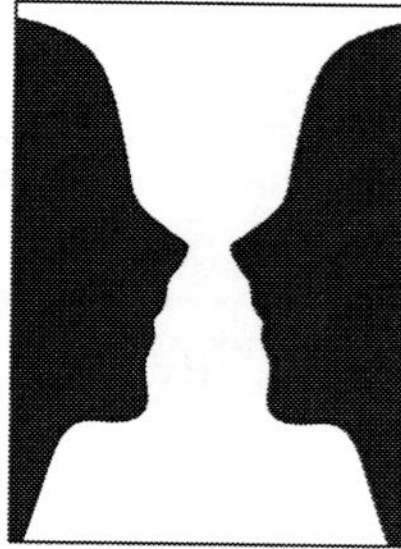

Figure 10.2: Figure-ground relationship

or close the pattern or fill in sensory gaps and perceive it as a meaningful whole. This type of organization is extremely helpful in making valuable interpretation of various incomplete objects, patterns or stimuli present in the environment. For example, the lines in the Figure 10.3 may be well perceived as letters W, M and D.

Principle of Grouping

Principle of grouping refers to the tendency to perceive stimuli in some organized meaningful patterns by grouping them on some solid basis such as similarity, proximity and continuity.

On the basis of similarity, objects or stimuli that look alike are usually perceived as a unit. For example, in the Figure 10.4A vertical rows of black dots and blank dots may be seen to form separate groups in terms of their perception.

On proximity basis, objects or stimuli that appear close to one another are likely to be perceived as belonging to the same group. For example, we see three sets of two lines each and not six separate lines (Fig. 10.4B).

The objects or stimuli are perceived as a unit or group on the basis of their continuity. Our attention is being held more by a continuous pattern rather than discontinuous ones. For example, we see a curved line and a straight line. We do not see a straight line with small semicircles above and below (Fig. 10.4C).

Principle of Simplicity

We perceive the simplest possible pattern because they enable the perceiver to perceive the whole from some of its parts.

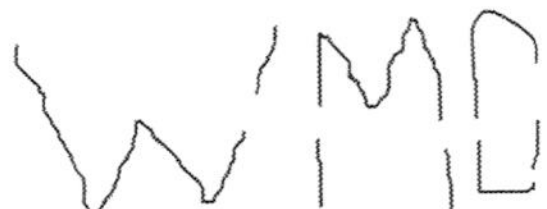

Figure 10.3: Principle of closure

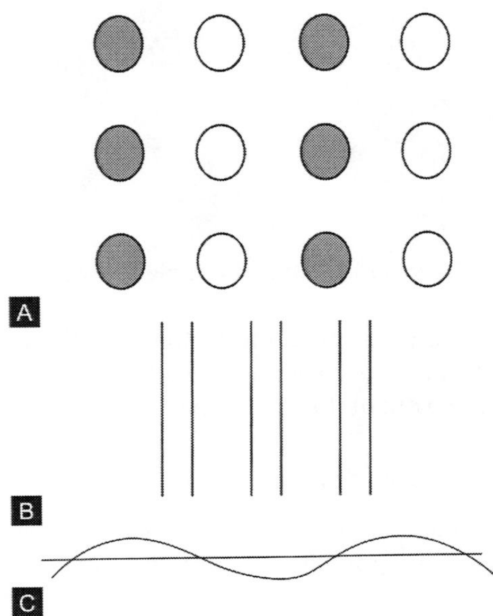

Figures 10.4A to C: Principle of grouping. **A.** Laws of similarity; **B.** Proximity; **C.** Continuity.

Principle of Contour

A contour is said to be a boundary between a figure and its ground. The degree of the quality of this contour separating the figure from the ground is responsible for enabling us to organize stimuli or objects into meaningful patterns.

Principle of Context

Perceptual organization is also governed by the principle of context, i.e. an examiner may award higher marks to the same answer book in a pleasant context than in an unpleasant one.

Principle of Contrast

Perceptual organization is very much affected through contrast effects, as the stimuli that are in sharp contrast to nearby stimuli may draw our maximum attention and carry different perceptual effects. For example, here the surrounding circles in Figure 10.5A

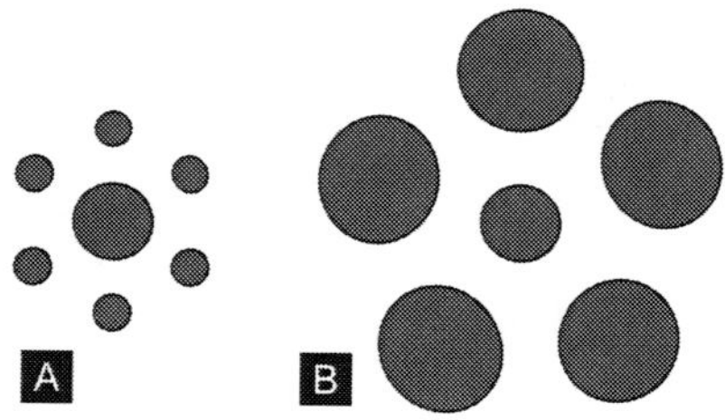

Figures 10.5A and B: Principle of contrast

make the central circle seem larger than the central circle in Figure 10.5B even though the two are of the same size.

Principle of Adaptability

The perceptual organization for some stimuli depends upon the adaptability of the perceiver to perceive similar stimuli. An individual who adapts himself to work before an intense bright light will perceive normal sunlight as quite dim.

■ PERCEPTION AND CONSTANCIES

A tendency to experience a stable perception in spite of changing sensory input or changes in sensory information is known as perceptual constancy. This may apply to shape, size and brightness or color (Fig. 10.6).

Shape Constancy

The tendency to see an object as the same shape irrespective of the angle in which it is viewed is known as shape constancy. For example, familiar objects are seen as having the same shape though the retinal images may change for different angles.

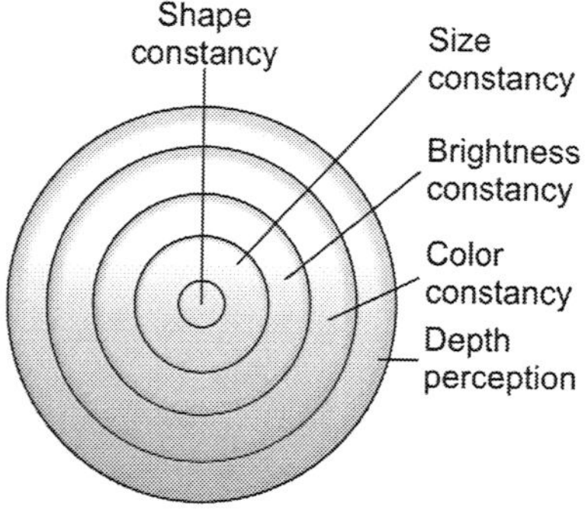

Figure 10.6: Perceptual constancy

Size Constancy

Size constancy is the tendency to perceive objects of the same size regardless of the distance from which it is viewed. For example, a beautiful lady standing at 20 feet distance looks the same, as she would be at 10 feet distance even though there is change in the retinal image.

Brightness Constancy

The perception of brightness is the same even though the amount of light reaching the retina changes. This is known as brightness constancy. For example, the brightness of white paper remains same in sunlight or candle light.

Color Constancy

The tendency to perceive objects, as retaining their color despite changes in sensory information is known as brightness constancy. For example, the red-colored car looks red under street light as well as in the dark garage.

Depth Perception

The process by which one interprets visual cues to know how near or far away objects are known as depth perception. There are two types of cues namely, monocular and binocular that helps in depth perception. Monocular cues are the visual cues requiring the use of one eye. Binocular cues are visual cues requiring both the eyes.

■ INACCURATE PERCEPTIONS

Sometimes our perceptions are inaccurate. We cannot make correct interpretations. The following may be the reasons:

1. We cannot perceive and observe correctly, sometimes our sense organs may be functioning defectively, e.g. we are suffering from myopia or deafness, or any other sensory defect.
2. Our receptors may not be stimulated adequately because the stimuli were not strong enough to stimulate them or the stimuli were rather vague and indefinite.
3. We may not perceive correctly because, we do not know what to perceive. In order that a student nurse should perceive correctly in the word for proper nursing care, she needs to be guided by her instructor.
4. Our span of apprehension and attention is limited. If we try to apprehend more things that we can at a time, we are liable to have inaccurate perceptions.
5. Sometimes objects or figures are perceived with difficulty because they resemble their surroundings. The figure merges in the ground. For example, a white patch is difficult to detect on a white wall.
6. We are liable to perceive things wrongly, if we are not in good health. Sick people's perceptions, at times are not correct for this reason. Our sense organs cannot function adequately and correctly as a result of ill ness. Sensory disturbances of perceptions are detailed in Table 10.2.

Sensory Abnormalities

Common sensory abnormalities and perceptual disorders are:

1. **Anesthesia:**
   a. It implies complete absence/inability to respond to sensory (touch) sensation. It means a loss is absence of sensitivity.
   b. Anesthesia may be caused by defective sense organs, effects or drugs, or also by some emotional or functional factors.
   c. For example, we sometime do not notice a pen or a bunch keys lying before us and make a frantic search of it. We are either emotionally disturbed or preoccupied with some other thoughts.
2. **Hyperesthesia:**
   a. It means excessive response to stimuli. Sick people often shows this in their behavior.
   b. They react violently to noises or bright lights. When we are fatigued, we become hypersensitive to lights, to sounds or to the weight of clothing and to odors.

■ ERRORS IN PERCEPTION

It has been observed that we get the experience of objective reality through our perception. But perceptions are at times descriptive. They do not always give us the correct experience of facts that exist. Some erroneous illusive experience is the result of such descriptive perceptions. False perceptions occur when perceptual stimulus fails to correspond with the real stimulus in the environment. Two frequently occurring errors in perceptions are discussed under two different phenomena, namely illusion and hallucinations.

Illusion

Actually, we always evaluate the world around us with our perceptual habits that help us to respond quickly and effectively to our normal environment. Sometimes our perceptual process may distort the images we receive, rather than correcting them with superficial changes in appearance.

An illusion is a mistaken perception of an object. In such cases the stimulus is, no doubt, present giving rise to definite sensory impulses. But, while interpreting the sensory impulses it is in the form of a meaningful experiences and fears or expectations.

Table 10.2: Sensory disturbances of perceptions

Sl No.	Sensory disturbances	Description
1.	Pain sensation: • Analgesia • Hypoalgesia • Hyperalgesia	 Absence of pain appreciation Decrease of pain appreciation Exaggeration of pain appreciation, which is often unpleasant
2.	Temperature sensation: • Thermanalgesia • Thermanesthesia • Thermhyperesthesia	 Absence of temperature appreciation Decrease of temperature appreciation Exaggeration of temperature sensation, which is often unpleasant
3.	Sensory abnormalities: • Paresthesia • Dysesthesia	 Abnormal sensation perceived without specific stimulation; they may be tactile, thermal or painful, episodic or constant Painful sensation elicited by and painful cutaneous stimulus such as a light touch or gentle stroking over affected areas of the body
4.	Proprioceptive sensation (deep sensation): • Joint position sense (arthresthesia) • Vibratory sense (pallesthesia) • Kinesthesia	 Absence of joint position sense Absence of vibratory sense Perception of muscular motion
5.	Cortical sensory function: • Astereognosis • Graph anesthesia • Topagnosia • Sensory extinction	 Inability to recognize and identify objects by feeling them Symbols written on the skin Inability to localize stimuli to parts of the body Inability to perceive a sensory stimulus, when corresponding areas on the opposite side of the body are stimulated simultaneously

Definition

1. Illusion is one such perceptual distortion. Illusions may create bias in us to distort reality; consequently we make faulty interpretation of the environment.
2. An illusion is a wrong or inaccurate or mistaken perception of an existing sensory stimulus.

Nature of Illusion

1. An illusion is a wrong perception, mistaking a rope for a snake, a tree for an animal and other things for something that is not really there.
2. Most of our illusions are visual and auditory, but others are also possible. Illusions are caused by inadequacies of our sense organs, which has to perceive it, misleading stimuli in the environment, our preconceived notions and expectancy.
3. These illusions are usually referred as any interpretation of sense in formations. Psychologists usually distinguish illusions into two groups.

Causes of Illusions (Fig. 10.7)

Optical illusions are caused by many factors; some causes are more predominant in some

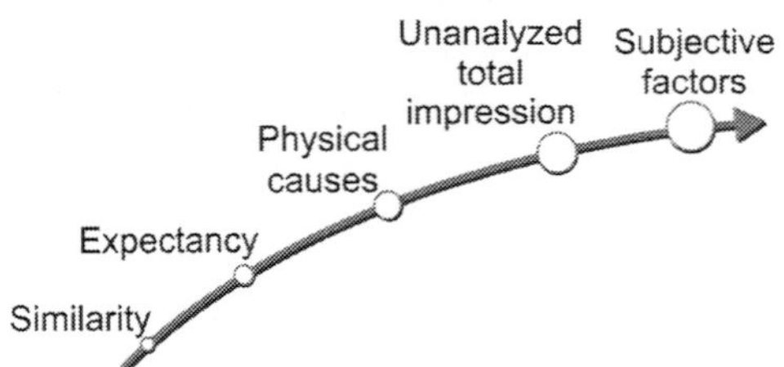

Figure 10.7: Causes of illusion

forms of illusions. In some other forms of illusion, some other causes are predominant; some illusion will have more than one cause. However, some of the causes of illusion are:

1. **Similarity:** If two objects are similar in appearance illusion occur more easily than others. For example, it is natural to mistake a curled rope for snake due to similarity.
2. **Expectancy:** If we are waiting for a friend, every individual at a distance will be mistaken for a friend. While searching for a coin lost every glittering is mistaken for the coin, which we are searching.
3. **Physical causes:** The mirror and the echo illusion are good examples for this. The former is due to reflection of light and the latter is due to echo of sound. The mirrored objects seem to be behind the mirror because the light reaches the eyes from that direction. In the echo illusion, the echo seems to come from somebody across the lake because the sound actually reaches the ears from that direction.
4. **Unanalyzed total impression:** This is clear from Müller-Lyer illusion. Here though we are supporting to perceive and estimate the actual length of the lines excluding the appendages we will be compelled to perceive the total figure and thus overestimate or underestimate the lines. Thus, this unanalyzed total impression cause's illusion.
5. **Subjective factors:** The factors such as habit and familiarity causes illusions. For example, cross two fingers and touch a marble or hold a pencil with the crossed part of both the fingers, that will feel two marbles or two pencils. Another example is proofreader's illusion.

Perceptual Illusions

1. Physical illusions occur because of the distortion of information. For example, when a portion of a stick is dipped in water, there appears a bent to the stick. Many physical illusions are created by our natural tendency to view two dimensional scenes as projections of three dimensional realities.
2. Perceptual illusions occur because when the stimulus contains misleading cues that cause perceptions that are inaccurate or impossible.

Classifications/Types of Illusions (Fig. 10.8)

1. **Moon illusion:** Moon appears large near the horizon than it does later at night, when it is directly overhead. One explanation says that moon illusion depends on visual constancy, i.e. when it is close to the horizon we have cues of distance and while it is overhead we do not get any cues to distance.

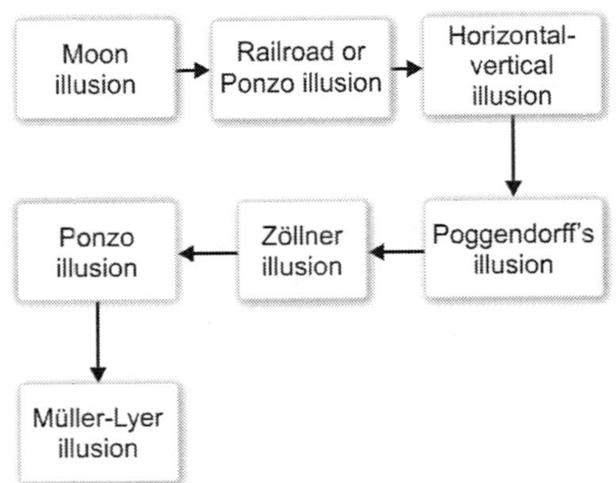

Figure 10.8: Classification of illusion

2. **Railroad or Ponzo illusion:** In simple forms Ponzo illusion, which consists of two gradually converging lines that give the impression of increasing depth in between two crosswise parallel lines.
3. **Horizontal-vertical illusion:** Though both the horizontal and vertical lines are equal in length, the vertical line is perceived as longer than the horizontal.
4. **Poggendorff's illusion:** A straight line should appear to become slightly displaced, as it passes through two parallel rectangles.
5. **Zöllner illusion:** When two parallel lines are intersected by numerous short diagonal lines slanting in opposite direction, then the parallel lines are perceived as diverging. All these illusions originate from our perceptual processes, creating an internal representation based on inaccurate and misleading information caused by visual illusions.
6. **Ponzo illusion:** The geometrical illusions that a horizontal line appearing within the smaller end of a pair of divergent vertical lines is longer than an equal length line located at a point at which the vertical lines are farther apart.
7. **Müller-Lyer illusion:** It is a geometrical illusion where one line is longer than another of equal length when the former has obtuse angles at both ends and the later has acute angles at both ends.

Hallucination

Hallucination is a false perception that is idiosyncratic, not shared by others in the same situation. It is generally seen in some mental disorder such as schizophrenia, alcoholic intoxication or drug abuse. Some people claim that their perceptions are quite vivid and lifelike, and they think them real. They may even become confused with reality. They are extreme forms of inaccurate observation. Such observations are usually associated with severe psychological disorders, but they occasionally occur among even non-mentally ill individuals as well.

Definitions

1. Hallucinations are vivid sensory experiences that occur in the absence of external stimulus.
2. Hallucination is the imaginary perceptions; it is a gross error of perception seeing objects that do not exist. They are an extreme form of inaccurate observation in which one sees or hear something that is not seen or heard by others around him.

Nature of Hallucinations

1. Hallucinations appear most frequently in the life of mentally disordered persons. The person hearing sounds seeing objects moving in a room and are false, are called hallucinations.
2. Hallucinations are deceptive perceptions at times caused purely because of the subjective makeup. The perception has no basis of a real sensory stimulus.
3. Hallucinations are found to be most common with auditory and visual perceptive. Hallucination is also caused due to certain organic condition such as damage of cerebral cortex or sense organs. Certain drugs and alcohol can also produce hallucination.
4. Hallucinations are directly related to sensation; they can be classified into visual hallucination, auditory hallucination, taste hallucination, smell hallucination and cutaneous hallucination.

Difference Between Illusion and Hallucination (Table 10.3)

Though illusions and hallucinations are common experiences, the incidence of hallucination is more severe. It is a serious form

Table 10.3: Difference between illusion and hallucination

Illusion	Hallucination
In illusion there will always be one or more stimuli	In hallucination, external stimulus is completely absent
Objective	Subjective
Stimulus is present	Stimulus is not present
Normal or universal	Abnormal
Mistaken perception	False perception

of mental illness. Illusion and hallucination shows us that our perception depends to a large extend on subjective factors such as set, attitudes and inner needs.

Hallucinations usually occur when individuals lose the capacity to differentiate between inner sensation and the outer environment. Both hallucination and illusion have impact on behavior and distort our knowledge leading to many personal, social and psychological problems.

■ EXTRASENSORY PERCEPTION

If there are so many influences upon perception other than those coming from the presented stimuli, perhaps there may be perceptions that require no sense organ stimulation what so ever. The answer to this question is the source of a major controversy within contemporary psychology over the status of extrasensory perception (ESP). Parapsychology is the search for paranormal phenomena, such as ESP and psychokinesis. Parapsychologists too observe unexplainable phenomena. All other sciences have led us away from superstition and magical thinking, while parapsychology has tried to find a scientific basis for magical power and spirits.

Definition

Extrasensory perception is perception occurring independently of sight, hearing or other sensory processes. EPS also refers to telepathy, clairvoyance and precognition. It influences the physical events by mental operations; is the source of controversy in contemporary psychology.

Characteristics of ESP

1. It is a most unstable ability, disappearing suddenly or gradually, often without recognized causes.
2. The ESP process is diametric in its function, encompassing more than a single object in its scope.
3. The ESP process is entirely unconscious, i.e. it is not thus far found reliability available to introspection in any way or degree. It is variable and undependable effect upon performance in the tests.
4. The ESP does not seem to subject to development through use as other specific capacities.

Nature of ESP

1. The experiments go at work in accordance with the usual Miles of science and generally disavow the connection between this work an d spiritualism, supernaturalism, mediumistic phenomena and other occult effects.
2. Many psychologists who are not convinced would find it congenital to accept evidence that they found satisfactory.
3. The case for ESP is based largely on experiments in card guessing in which under various conditions, the subject attempts to guess the symbols on cards randomly arranged in packs.

■ NURSING IMPLICATIONS OF PERCEPTION

1. Accurate perception and observation are very important for a nurse to provide quality care to a patient. All nursing

activities require accurate observation and perception. For example, checking vital signs, assessing patient, administering medications, etc.
2. If he/she is not a keen observer, then he/she will not be able to note some very critical or important symptoms with the result that sometimes the patient may die premature.
3. Accurate perception and observation will help the nurse to gather accurate information and knowledge, which will help the nurse to learn more easily, adjust more quickly to new situations. It also prevents accidents and incidents harmful to the patient.

■ NURSES' ROLE IN PERCEPTION (Table 10.4)

In caring the sick, nurse needs to remember the words of Plato, the treatments of a part should not be attempted without treatment of the entity. It emphasizes that wholeness of something is more than the sum of its parts, because a part is meaningful only in the context of the whole.

■ CONCLUSION

The physical and social environments with their inherent nature draw our attention to them. When any stimulus is attended by the

Table 10.4: Nurses' role in perception

Sl No.	Perception	Description
1.	Perception of outside world	Our perception of the world outside is greatly affected by current state of mind For example, we may feel particularly anxious when we tend to perceive our own different disturbed state of mind A nurse needs to understand the role of sensation and attention in acquiring knowledge of environment, which depends to larger extent on the sensation received by the sense organs
2.	Perception influences memory, thinking and emotions	Perception is essential to deal with the world around us as it influences our memory, thinking, reasoning and emotions, etc. A nurse should understand and try to interpret the whole environment, and apply different types of perceptual skills to understand his/her patients In caring the sick, nurse needs to remember the words of Plato, the treatment of a part should not be attempted without treatment of the entity It emphasizes that wholeness of something is more than the sum of its parts because a part is meaningful only in the context of the whole
3.	Provides positive outlook to sick	The perception of the nurse and that of the patient may be different in the hospital environment The nurse is familiar with the hospital environment and also well-accustomed The nurse being a healthy and energetic person is working with a positive outlook and enthusiasm to help the patient

Contd...

Contd...

Sl No.	Perception	Description
4.	Helps to reduce the anxiety	The hospital may seem an alien and frightening environment to the patient Because the new and unfamiliar hospital environment creates a lot of anxieties in the patient It may influence the thought, behaviors and perceptual set of the patient Emotional maturity is also another important factor influencing a person's perception of sensory data
5.	Promotes coping	A nurse should share the worries, fears and emotions of the sick and then help them to solve As a nursing student, he/she must learn to assess all factors with accuracy and efficiency

respective sense organ, it releases natural impulses. The encoded information in the form of natural impulses constitutes sensation. Interpretation of sense impression is perception. Thus, these functions are interrelated. They provide knowledge of the environment, so that the organism can act appropriately to adjust to the environment. So to understand behavior, we have to know their interrelated functions.

■ REVIEW QUESTIONS

Long Essays

1. Define perception. Discuss the factors that influence perception.
2. Explain the principles of organization of perception in detail.

Short Essays

3. Write the difference between sensation and perception.
4. Describe perception and constancies.
5. Explain about inaccurate perception.
6. Enumerate the perceptional errors.
7. Difference between illusion and hallucination.
8. Briefly discuss about extrasensory perception.
9. Explain the nurse's role in perception.

Short Answers

10. Gestalt principle.
11. Color constancies.
12. Illusions and hallucinations.
13. Moon illusions.
14. Sensory abnormalities.

CHAPTER 11

Learning

■ INTRODUCTION

An individual begins to learn soon after his/her birth and goes on learning throughout the lifetime. An infant is quite helpless at birth, suit slowly learns to adapt to the environment around. There are usually two factors involved in learning for adjustment to the environment; they are maturation and the ability to profit by experience. Learning occupies an important position in the life of an individual. Most of one's behavior shows evidence of some type of learning or the other. It is learning that makes an adequate adjustment of life situations possible. Learning implies cumulative improvement. The nature of improvement can be clearly gauged by the changes, which take place while learning is progress.

■ MEANINGS OF LEARNING

1. Learning is a change in behavior; it is a change that takes place through practice or experience.
2. Learning is not a reflex action, it means that winking or withdrawal of leg when knee is struck, is not learning.
3. Learning may be for conscious purpose or it may be for biological and social adjustments.
4. Through learning, in a person permanent or temporary changes are produced.
5. It can be for adjustment or maladjustment. It can create a socially adjusted individual or it may give rise to antisocial behavior.
6. Learning is a self-active process, which takes place in a social setup or environment.
7. Learning is a process that is purposeful and goal directed. It also consists in establishing the right stimulus-response (S-R) connections.
8. Learning is universal and continuous; it is a continuous never-ending process that goes from womb to tomb.
9. Learning prepares an individual for the necessary adjustments and adaptation.

■ DEFINITION

1. The more or less permanent modification of an individual's activity in a given situation, due to the practice in attempts to achieve some goal or solve some problem. —*Bernhardt*
2. Learning is a change in the individual following upon changes in his environment. —*Peel*
3. Learning is the process by which behavior is originated or changes through practice or training. —*Kingsley and Garry*

4. The term learning covers every modification in behavior to meet environmental requirements. —*Gardener Murphy*
5. Learning is the process by which an activity originates or is changed through reacting to an encountered situation, provided that the characteristics of the changes in activity cannot be explained on the basis of native response, tendencies, maturation or temporary states of organism. —*Hilgard*
6. Learning defined as an expected and permanent change in the behavior, brought about as a result of practice. —*Hilgard and Atkinson.*
7. Learning is acquiring new activities or enhancing or improving the old activities. —*Underwood*
8. Comparatively, learning is the serial or gradual change of the behavior. This is a special process, which takes place as a result of observation or training. —*Mann ML*

■ DETERMINANTS OF LEARNING (Fig. 11.1)

Kind of Material

It is observed that certain type of material is more easily mastered than some other type. The meaningful material is more easily learned than the matters that lacks meaning. Verbal learning takes place at an ideational level. When one tries to understand the concept of specific gravity, he/she learns with the help of ideas.

Method of Learning

There are certain methods of learning, which are found to be effective than certain others. These methods are related to the way they breaks up the learning material and the time spent in learning.

Practice

Repetition in terms of trials is necessary for all learning activities. All learning is based up on some amount of practice.

Motivation

Effective learning is directly related to the strength of the motives. Educationist try to utilize different motives to make the pupil's learn better. Out of all the external goals with which motives can be connected, the inner goals such as interest and curiosity are bound to be strong motivating forces.

Intelligence

Learning cannot take place effectively without intelligence. Intelligence enables to understand things, to see relationships between things, to reason and judge correctly and critically.

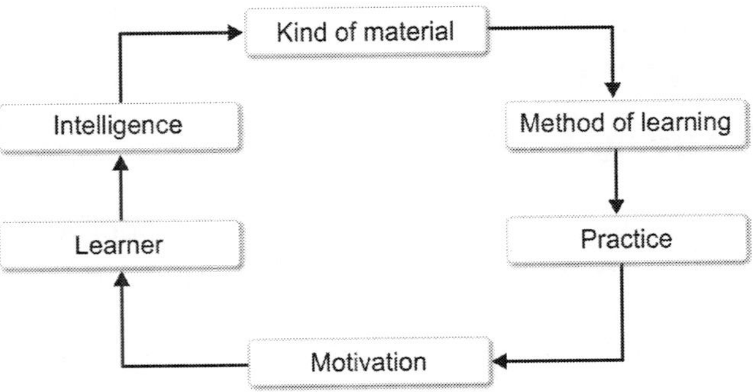

Figure 11.1: Determinants of learning

Maturation

Learning and maturation contribute to the development of the person. Those two actually are so interlinked that any line of separation is hardly visible. Maturation is growth, which takes place regularly in an individual without special condition of stimulation, such as training and practice.

Learner

Besides these situational factors, the learner is the most vital factor in deciding the efficiency of learning. The learner's intelligence, their age and experience make considerable difference in learning effectiveness.

▪ STEPS IN LEARNING PROCESS

1. Motivation within the learner.
2. Goal or goals become related to the motivation.
3. Barriers or difficulties are perceived and experienced and tension arises. Strong barriers may cause excessive tension, which may altogether discourage and confuse the learner.
4. The search for an appropriate solution to the problem or an appropriate line of action to reach the goal.
5. The most appropriate line of action is selected and practiced, and inappropriate behaviors dropped.

▪ LAWS OF EFFECTIVE LEARNING (THORNDIKE)

Major Laws of Learning

Law of Readiness

1. Learning takes place best when a person is ready to learn. If a person is ready to act, acting gives satisfaction.
2. Some sort of preparatory attitude or the mindset is necessary. The learner should be stimulated to learn new things in such a way that he/she obtains satisfaction out of learning.

Law of Exercise, Use and Disuse or Practice

1. Learning takes place through exercise and repetition. We learn skills in games, music, craft, typing or in nursing by constant exercise and practice.
2. An activity, which is not used or practiced, or exercised for some time tends to be forgotten by disuse.
3. The learner should be provided with opportunities of practicing and repetition. But repetition should be continual rather than continuous.
4. Most of the nursing skills and procedures are learned through practice on the wards and in the public health field.

Law of Effect or Satisfaction and Dissatisfaction

1. We learn things and to do things that give us satisfaction and we learn not to do things, which annoy us.
2. The connections between stimuli and response become strong when we derive satisfaction from those responses, but remain weak or are unformed when we are annoyed.
3. Activities, which are accompanied by a feeling of pleasure or satisfaction, are more readily and effectively learnt than activities that are unpleasant or annoying.

Minor Laws

- Law of maturation
- Law of purpose
- Law of selection
- Law of association
- Law of recency
- Law of multiple learning.

■ TYPES OF LEARNING (Fig. 11.2)

Verbal Learning

1. Learning of this type helps in the acquisition of verbal behavior.
2. Language we speak, the communication devices we use, are the result of such learning.
3. Rote learning and rote memorization, which is a type of school learning, is also included in verbal learning.
4. Sign, pictures, symbols, words, figures, sounds and voices, etc. are employed by the individual as an essential instrument for engaging him/her in the process of verbal learning.

Motor Learning

1. The learning of all types of motor skills may be included in such type of learning.
2. Learning—how to swim, riding a horse, driving a car, flying a plane, playing piano and handling various instruments are the example of such learning.
3. The art of these skills can be acquired through a systematic and planned way of the acquisition and fixation of a series of organized actions or responses by making use of some appropriate learning methods and devices.

Concept Learning

1. A concept in the form of a mental image denotes a generalized idea about the things, persons or events.
2. The formation of such concepts on accounts of previous experiences, training or cognitive process is called concept learning.
3. Such type of concept learning proves very useful in recognizing, naming and identifying the things. All of our behaviors such as verbal, symbolic, motor as well as cognitive are influenced by our concepts.

Problem-solving Learning

1. In the ladder of learning and acquisition of behavior, problem-solving denotes a higher type of learning.
2. Problem-solving learning requires the use of the cognitive abilities such as reasoning, power of observation, discrimination, generalization, imagination, ability to infer and draw conclusions, trying out novel ways and experimenting, etc.
3. Problem-solving learning has essentially caused human being to contribute significantly to the process and improvement of society.

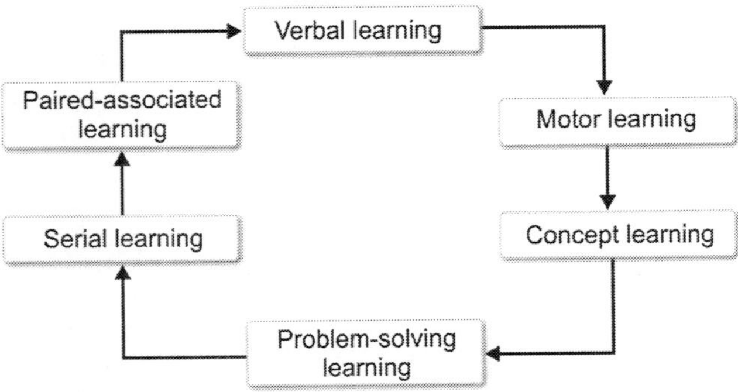

Figure 11.2: Types of learning

Serial Learning

1. Serial learning consists of such learning in which the learner is presented with such type of learning material that exhibits some sequential or serial order.
2. Children often encounter such a learning situation in schools where they are expected to master lists of material such as the alphabet, multiplication tables, the names of all the states in their country, etc.

Paired-associated Learning

1. In this learning, learning tasks are presented in such a way that they may be learned on account of their associations.
2. The name of a village such as Krishnapur is remembered on its association with the name of Lord Krishna or a girl's name Ganga by learning it in the form of making paired association with the river Ganges.
3. The practice with such procedure then helps in building what is known as associate learning.

■ GOALS OF LEARNING

1. The goals of learning can be classified into two broad categories, i.e. the acquisition of knowledge and the acquisition of skill (Fig. 11.3).
2. The acquisition of knowledge means bringing up of intellectual and emotional modification, and control in the individual through learning.
3. The acquisition of skill refers to the sensory motor modification and control through learning.

Acquisition of Knowledge

Perception

1. Perception refers to the acquisition of specific knowledge about objects or events directly stimulating the sense at any particular moment.
2. A young child sees a women, in the past, the women has fed her. On the basis of that experience, he/she comprehends that a women is their nurse or mother. The type of learning at perceptual level is known as perceptual learning.

Conception

1. Conception means the acquisition of organized knowledge in the form of concepts or general ideas, which transcend any particular percept.
2. The child gets the perception of orange, apple, banana, etc. and is able to locate certain general qualities in them.

Associate Learning

1. Associate learning corresponds to memory both as the deliberate recall and recognition, past experience and a habit or automatic memory due to association.
2. Associate learning is fundamental to all other learning.

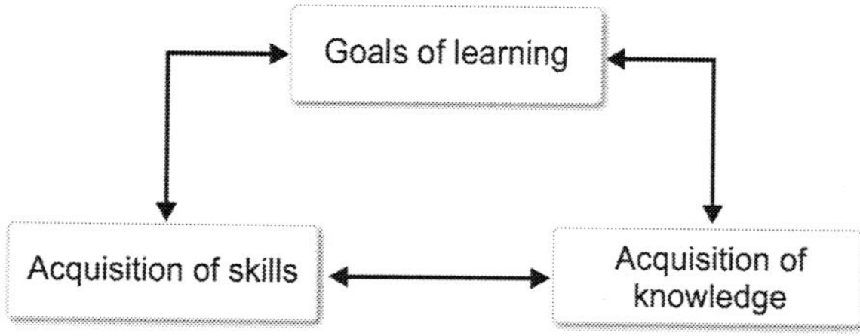

Figure 11.3: Goals of learning

Appreciation

1. Appreciation is the acquisition of ideas, attitudes or dispositions characterized by an emotional tone.
2. In our knowledge this factor is present as the effective or feeling element. When one talks about an ideal, one is talking about a concept, which is colored by appreciation.

Acquisition of Skills

1. Under skill are included the sensory motor process such as writing, reading, musical performance, language acquisition in its vocal aspect, drawing and the arts generally.
2. True learning is enrichment of experience it is because of this view of learning process that today we find an emphasis on activity programs, learning by doing the project method, self-activity, etc. rather than on book learning.

■ THEORIES OF LEARNING

Classical Conditioning (Table 11.1)

Classical conditioning gets its name from the fact that it is the kind of learning situation that existed in the early 'classical' experiments of Ivan P Pavlov (1849–1936). In the late 1890s, this famous Russian physiologist began to establish many of the basic principles of this form of conditioning. Classical conditioning is also called respondent conditioning or Pavlovian conditioning.

Concept of Classical Conditioning

1. The dog salivated not only upon actual eating, but also they saw the food, noticed the man who brings it.
2. In every animal and person, there is a number of innate S-R association connections wired in at birth, before any learning occurs.
3. The classical conditioning is constructed upon these inborn neurological connections.
4. Through learning, a pervious neutral stimulus can come to acquire some of the same properties as unconditional stimuli. In this case, the previously neutral stimulus is called conditioned stimulus (CS) and the response it produces is called conditioned response (CR).
5. Pavlov described the process by which associations are acquired and become the source for more general behavior or more complex ones, as well as the ways in which the learned responses could be unlearned or extinguished. These processes include acquisition, higher-order conditioning and extinction.

Table 11.1: Difference between classical and operant conditioning

Classical conditioning	Operant conditioning
It helps in the learning of respondent behavior	It helps in the learning of operant behavior
It is called type S conditioning because of the emphasize on the stimulus	It is called R conditioning because of the emphasis on the response
This beginning is being made with help of specific stimuli that bring certain response	Here, beginning is made with the responses as they occur naturally or unnaturally, shaping them into existence
Strength of conditioning is usually determined by the magnitude of the condition response	Here strength of conditioning is shown by the response rate

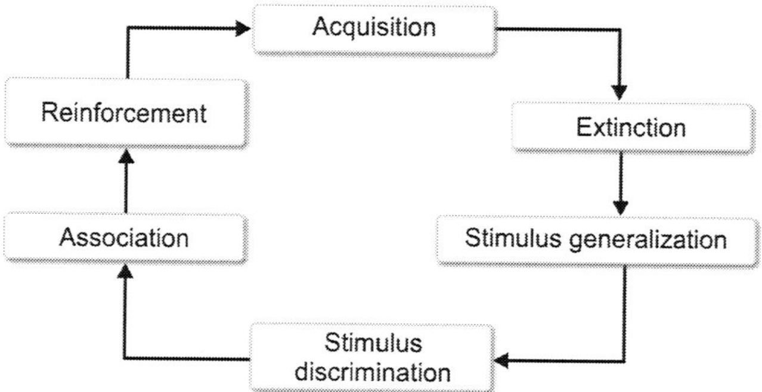

Figure 11.4: Principles of classical conditioning

Principles of Classical Conditioning (Fig. 11.4)

Acquisition: It is the process by which a stimulus comes to elicit a condition response. To see how this occur Pavlov performed an experiment to see whether he could produce salivation to previously neutral stimuli.

Extinction: This process related with the gradual disappearance of the conditioned response on disconnecting the S-R association is called extinction.

Stimulus generalization: It is referring to a particular state of learning behavior in which individual once condition to response to a specific stimulus is made to respond in the same in response to other stimuli of similar nature.

Stimulus discrimination: It is the opposite of stimulus generation. Here, in sharp contrast to response in a usual fashion the subject learns to react differently in different situations.

Association: Repetition of the conditioned stimulus, followed by the unconditioned stimulus and consequent response must occur without exception.

Reinforcement: It is not only the association of two stimuli and a response that is essential, but what works in conditioning is the effect of reinforcement. Food in this case, which has a reinforcing effect strengths and bond between the condition stimulus and the unconditioned response changing it ultimately in the form of a conditioned response.

Pavlov's Experimentation

1. Pavlov began to study this phenomenon, which he called 'conditioning'. Since the type of conditioning emphasizes was a classical one, which quite different from the conditioning emphasized by other psychologist; at the later stage, it has been renamed as classical conditioning.
2. Pavlov kept a dog hungry for a few days and the tried him on to the experimental table, which was made comfortable and distractions were excluded as far as it was possible to do.
3. The observer kept himself hidden from view of the dog, but was able to view the experiment by means of a set of mirrors. Arrangement was made to give food to the dog through automatic devices.
4. Every time the food was presented to the dog and the bell was rung, there was automatic secretion of saliva from the mouth of the dog. The activity of presenting the food accompanied with a ringing of the bell was repeated, several times and the amount of saliva secreted was measured.
5. After several trials, the dog was given no food, but the bell was rung. In this case also the amount of saliva secreted was recorded and measured. It was found that even in the absence of food (the natural stimulus), the ringing of the bell

(an artificial stimulus), caused the dog to secrete saliva (natural response).

6. The above experiment thus brings into the picture the four essential elements of conditioning process. They are natural or unconditioned stimulus, unconditional response, conditioned stimulus and condition response.
7. The theory of conditioning as advocated by Pavlov, thus considered learning as a habit formation and is based on the principle of association and substitution.

John Watson Theory of Conditioning

1. Watson (1878–1958), the Father of behaviorism, supported Pavlov's ideas on conditioned responses. Watson tried to demonstrate the role of conditioning in producing as well as eliminating the emotional response such as fear.
2. When a child receives there first injection at the doctor's dispensary, he/she cries when the needle is pricked. On receiving some more injections from the same doctor and at the same dispensary on following days, the child would start crying on seeing the doctor and later, even on passing by the dispensary along the road.
3. Most of our attitudes towards persons and situations early language responses, numerous components of complex skills and a number of emotional responses can be common place examples of conditioned responses.

Operant Conditioning

1. Operant conditioning refers to a kind of process whereby a response is made more probable or more frequent by reinforcement (refer Table 11.1).
2. Operant conditioning also known as instrumental conditioning, an action of the learner's instrumental in bringing about a change in the environment that makes the action more or likely to occur again in the future.
3. An environmental event that is the consequence of an instrumental response and that makes the response more likely to occur again is known as reinforcement.
4. A positive reinforce is a stimulus or event, which and when it is contingent on a response, increases the likelihood that the response will be made again.
5. A negative reinforcement is a stimulus of event, which and when its cessation or termination is contingent on a response, increases the likelihood that the response will occur again.
6. In instrumental or operant conditioning, the term shaping refers to the process of learning a complex response by first learning a number of simple responses leading up to the complex one.
7. Each step is learned by the application of contingent positive reinforcement and each step builds on the one before it until the complex response occurs and is reinforced.
8. In instrumental or operant conditioning, the procedure of not reinforcing a response is called extinction. If after learning, reinforcement is no longer contingent on a response, the response will become less likely to occur.
9. In instrumental or operant conditioning, reinforcement following every occurrence of a particular response is called continuous reinforcement.
10. But reinforcement in operant conditioning is often given according to certain schedules, not every occurrence of the response is reinforced. Fixed ratio (FR), fixed intervals (FI), variable ratio (VR) and variable-interval (VI) schedules are described to illustrate the concept of reinforcement schedules.

Skinner's Operant Experimentation

1. Operant conditioning experiments conducted by Skinner BF a specially devised box called Skinner box were used.
2. There was an iron bar inside the box. In order to get food, the rat had to press the iron bar. For every such pressing a food pills was dropped through a chute into the pallet.
3. Here, the rat after a few trails learns to press the bar and then run to the pallet to secure food.
4. Unless the animal presses the bar, it cannot get the reinforcement and habit cannot learn. But the basic factors involved in both these forms of learning are identical.

Schedules of Reinforcement

Continuous reinforcement schedule: It is 100% reinforcement schedules, where provision is made to reinforcement or rewards every correct response of the organism during acquisition of learning.

Fixed internal schedule: In this schedule, the reinforcement is given after a fixed number of responses.

Variable reinforcement schedule: When reinforcement is given at varying individuals of time or after a varying number of responses, it is called variable reinforcement schedule.

Implication of Operant Conditioning

1. The principle of operant conditioning may be successfully applied in the task of behavior modification.
2. The task of the development of human personality can be successfully manipulated through operant conditioning. According to Skinner, "we are what we have been rewarded for being".
3. The theory of operant conditioning does not attribute motivation to internal process within organism.
4. Operant conditioning lays stress on the importance of schedules in the process of reinforcement of the behavior.
5. The theory advocated the avoidance of punishment for unlearning the undesirable behavior and for shaping the desirable behavior.
6. In its most effective application, theory of operant conditioning has contributed a lot towards the development of teaching machines and programmed learning.

■ LAWS OF LEARNING BY THORNDIKE (Fig. 11.5)

Laws of frequency: When an activity is repeated a number of times; it requires a tendency to be permanently established. Any response that is repeated either some strength in its favor.

Laws of recency: In a series of activities, those at the close of the series would be more freshly retained in the repertoire of the animal so that when put to a similar situation it shows a tendency to respect them.

Law of effect: This is perhaps the most important among all the laws. It says that the response that gives the organism the satisfaction of success is the one that is most likely to be fixed. On the other hand, when the response does not lead to such a satisfaction is tends to be discarded.

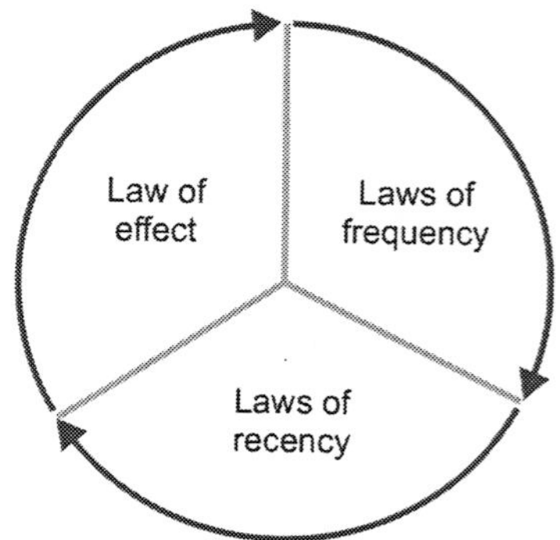

Figure 11.5: Laws of learning by Thorndike

■ TRIAL AND ERROR LEARNING

The theory of trial and error learning propagated by Thorndike emphasizes that we learn through a trial and error mechanism. In trying for a correct behavior, one tries hard in so many ways and may commit so many errors before a chance success. On subsequent trails he/she may learn to avoid erroneous ways, repeat the correct ones and finally learn the proper way.

Concept of Trial and Error

1. When we are placed in a new situation or face a new problem we have to seek solution, which we are not able to perceive in the beginning.
2. This made of learning is slow, wasteful and unintelligent. It requires more time and greater energy than higher types learning.
3. Learning implies establishment of new connections between the stimulus and response. These new connections are gradually established blind process of trial and error.
4. In this kind of learning, which is very common in animals, there is assumed to be at first nothing but random, aimless reaction, but in which there emerges after a time a chance correct response that finally is stamped into the neuromuscular system of the animal.
5. There are random movements in the beginning, gradually the number of random movements is reduced along with error and finally the goal is reached. Thus, improvement takes place through repetition.
6. The principle involved in the process by which the learner stabilizes the new response pattern gives the clue to the understanding of learning by trial and error.

Thorndike's Trial and Error Experiments

1. In the typical experiments of Thorndike, he made use of a puzzle box that could be opened by some mechanical contrivance, e.g. pressing a button on its floor.
2. When a hungry cat was placed inside this puzzle box and food, e.g. a fish, was placed outside the box within the sight of the animal, the cat would struggle hard to come out of the box.
3. In this process she went through a series as random activities that could not bring about the solution of her problem.
4. She may try to squeeze herself out of the bars, bite them, scratch the floor with her claws or run about. In the course of the new response pattern, her paw may accidentally fall on the button and the door is opened for her.
5. Out of all the series of responses given by the cat a single one proves to be the correct response, e.g. keeping her paw on the button and pressing it.
6. Immediately following this response she comes out and can take food that has a reinforcing effect. Her success during the first trial may be due to sheer chance.
7. But when the animal is put to the same situation next time there is a definite reduction of the random responses and the successful solution of the problem of the random responses and the successful solution of the problem requires less time than before.
8. This way with practice the errors or wrongs responds are gradually eliminated and the correct response is strengthened.
9. When a person learns to swim or to ride on a bicycle, the initial pattern of behavior display a large number of random responses. With practice, all the wrong movements are gradually eliminated.

Laws of Learning by Thorndike

Stages of Trial and Error Learning

Drive: In the present experiment it was hunger (Fig. 11.6), which was intensified with the sight of the food.

Goal: To get the food by getting out of the box.

Block: The cat was confined in the box with a closed door.

Random movements: The cat, persistently, tried to get out of the box.

Chance success: As a result of this striving and random movement the cat, by chance, succeeded in opening the door.

Selection: Gradually the cat recognized the correct manipulation of the latch. It selected the proper way of manipulating the latch out of its random movements.

Fixation: At least, the cat learned the proper way of opening the door by eliminating all the incorrect responses and fixing only the right responses. Now it was able to open the door without any error or, in other words, learned the way of opening the door.

Background of the Theorist

1. Edward L Thorndike a famous psychologist (1874–1949) is known as the propagator of the theory of trial and error learning.
2. Thorndike has written "learning is connecting. The mind is man's connection system."
3. Thorndike named the learning of his experimental cat as trial and error learning. He maintained that the learning is nothing, but the stamping in of the correct responses and stamping out of the incorrect responses through trial and error.

Implication of Trial and Error Learning

1. Whatever we want to learn or teach, we must first try to identify the things that are to be remembered or forgotten.
2. What is being thought or learnt at one time should be linked with past experiences and learning on the one hand and with the future learning on the other for utilizing the benefits of the mechanism of association, connection or bonds in the process of learning.
3. The learner should try to see similarities and dissimilarities between the different kinds of responses to stimuli and with the help of comparison and contrast should try to apply the learning of something in one situation to other similar situations.
4. The learner should be encouraged to do his task independently. He must try various solutions of the problem before arriving at a correct one.

■ LEARNING BY INSIGHT

The Gestalt psychologist has offered an altogether different explanation of the learning process. They do not believe that learning is a process of blind habit formation.

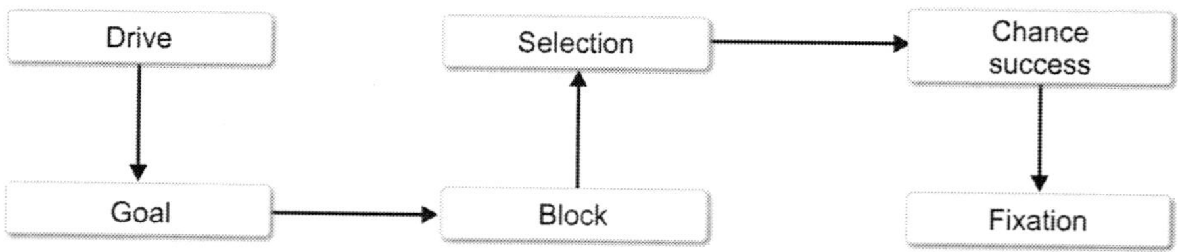

Figure 11.6: Stages of trial and learning

The learning process studied by Thorndike or the behaviorists occurs, according to Kohler, in a very unnatural and restricted situation, where the animal is denied all possibility of a clear perception of the whole situation.

Definition

Insight may be defined as sudden awareness of the relationships among various elements that had previously appeared to be independent of one another.

Background of the Theorist

1. Insight learning introduced by a group of German psychologist called Gestalts; Wolfgang Kohler in particular originated a learning theory known as insight learning.
2. The nearest English translation of gestalt is configuration or more simply an organized whole in contrast to a collection of parts. Gestalt psychologists consider the process of learning as a gestalt—an organized whole.
3. In practical sense, gestalt psychology is primarily concerned with the nature of perception.
4. Gestalt psychologists tried to interpret learning as a purposive, exploratory and creative enterprise instead of trial and error or simple S-R mechanism.

Concept of Insight Learning

1. It involves mental exploration and understanding of what is being learned. It implies some insight, some awareness of the consequences of performing an act.
2. The learner perceives the reactions, which the problem involves or the significant characteristics of the situation and connects the right response with the solution by using his intelligence.
3. He uses his past learning and his ability to generalize from one situation to another.
4. The principle involved in any learning process depends upon the nature of the learning situation.
5. Kohler in his experiments on learning offered different types of situation and eventually arrived at totally different conclusions regarding the principle involved in the learning process.
6. Insight involves a perceptual reorganization of elements in the environment such that new relationships among objects and events are suddenly seen.
7. It is goal directed and oriented towards the solution of a problem. When the organism is put to a problematic situation, it starts to tackle it. Such tackling involves the perception of the problem.

Kohler's Insight Learning Experimentation

1. Some of the well-known experiments of Kohler performed on chimpanzees had the following plan—the hungry chimpanzee was kept in a cage and a bunch of bananas was hung from the ceiling.
2. A number of wooden boxes were lying about. The chimpanzee tries to jump high to reach the bananas. When it was impossible to reach the highest he tries to jump from a ceiling.
3. When this too was found to be failure he gave up the efforts for some time. All of a sudden the chimpanzee got some new idea and started putting one box upon the other.
4. Finally by getting up on the topmost he could successfully grab the bananas.
5. In the situation described above, there was no evidence of a blind trial and error procedure where the corrected responses occurred gradually.

TRANSFER OF LEARNING

Learning one skill sometimes influences the acquisition of other skills. This influence may be positive that can facilitate the new learning. It can also be negative when it interferes with the acquisition of new learning. In the first case we have positive transfer of training, often referred to as merely 'transfer of training' or transfer of learning. In the second case we have what is commonly called habit interference.

Definition

According to Sorenson, transfer refers to the transfer of knowledge training and habits acquired in one situation to another situation.

Meaning of Transfer of Learning

1. Transfer of training or learning influences to carry over the learning from one task to another. The learning or skill acquired in one task is transferred or carried over to other tasks.
2. Transfer of training is the carry-over of habits of thinking, feeling or working of knowledge of skills from one learning area to another usually is referred to as the transfer of training.
3. One of the simplest examples of positive transfer is to be found in experiments showing improvement in performance with the left hand as a result of practice with the right hand. This is called bilateral transfer or cross education.

Types of Transfer

Positive transfer: Transfer is said to be positive when something previously learned benefits performance or learning in a new situation.

Negative transfer: When something previously learned hinders performance or learning in a new situation, we call negative transfer.

Zero transfer: In this case, the previous learning makes no difference at all to the performance or learning in a new situation, there is said to be zero transfer.

Principles of Transfer (Fig. 11.7)

Similarity of contents: A person familiar with several card games will learn the rules of new card game readily. This is possible as the rules are similar to those he already knows. Learning to drive one model of car a person any soon master the control of another, since many of the activities involved in driving cars are identical.

Similarity of techniques: When subjects were given practice to toss a ball in air and then catch it in a cup with their right hand, there was bilateral transfer when they performed the same task with their left hand.

Similarity of principles: Transfer of principles is not always different from transfer of techniques because the use of techniques may involve the application of principles.

Formal discipline: Transfer was once sought to be explained on the basis of the doctrine of formal discipline of mental faculties. The mind was supported to be a bundle of independent faculties of reasoning, memory imagination, etc. Transfer of training was thus supposed to be automatically achieved, through the exercise of mental faculty.

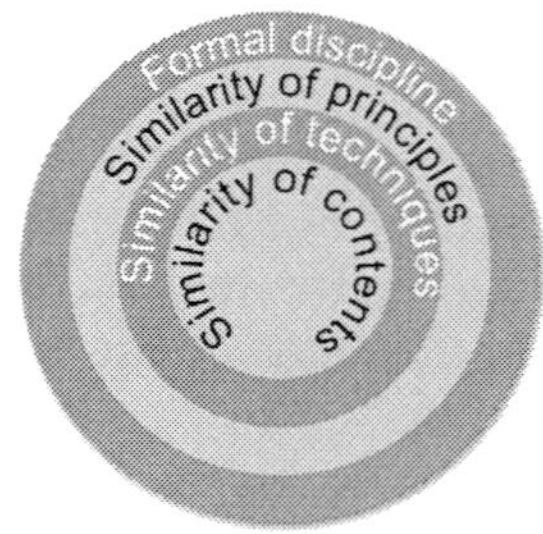

Figure 11.7: Principles of transfer

Characteristics of Transfer Learning

Transfer to a similar activity: Learning one activity sometimes easier the learning of another activity.

Transfer in verbal learning: Transfer is also evident for several verbal skills. When comparable lists of non-sense syllabus are learned one after the other, there is a gradual reduction in the trials required to learn successive list.

Bagley's Transfer of Training

1. The transfer of training or learning can also be explained on the basis of the theory of ideals put forward by Begley WC.
2. According to this theory, transfer of learning or training takes place in the form of ideals.
3. The experience we have, the generalization or conclusions we arrive at, all do transfer if they are imbibed as ideals of some value or desirable by the individual.
4. Bagley (1922), the ideals of neatness developed on the basis of stress laid on doing things quite neatly in school is likely to transfer in performing all other activities in a quite neat and clean way.
5. If we wish to seek positive transfer from one situation to another we must strive for the formation of general attitude for an ideal.

■ NURSES' ROLE IN LEARNING

1. Learning is fundamental to the development and modification of behavior, thus knowledge of the learning process may be usefully applied to many clinical situations and academic work.
2. Many of our subjective feelings, emotions and attitudes are probably conditioned responses. Through generalization it becomes difficult to identify the origin of our emotional responses. Both our adaptive emotional responses as well as unadaptive responses are learned and can be unlearned through principle of learning.
3. Learning methods have wide applications in educational setting. In programmed learning the material to be learned is broken up into small easy steps, so that the learner can accomplish without frustrations. Also with programmed learning, learner can master the task at his own pace; with versatile and flexible learning, the learner can improve learning style.
4. Applications of reinforcement principles can often increase productivity both in studies as well as in vocation.
5. A nurse should understand the nature of learning and the factors, which will affect learning. As learning modifies our behavior, it is necessary for a nurse to learn only the right things, so that modification takes place in the right direction.
6. They must have a well-defined purpose and goal in all learning situations.

■ CONCLUSION

One of the most important characteristics of human being is their capacity to learn. A person's personality, habits, skills, knowledge, attitudes, interests and character are largely the result of learning. Learning is central to all our behaviors as one learns to speak, write, think and perceive. One's attitudes and emotional expressions are also learned behaviors. Learning is the process by which an activity originates or is changed through training procedures, as is distinguished from changes by factors and attributable to training.

REVIEW QUESTIONS

Long Essays

1. Define learning. Describe the determinants of learning.
2. Describe the different types of learning.
3. Explain different theories of learning.

Short Essays

4. Discuss the methods of learning.
5. Enumerate the laws of learning.
6. Principles of classical learning.
7. Describe the Pavlov's experiment.
8. Enumerate Skinner's operant conditioning.
9. Trial and error learning.
10. Give a brief account about learning by insight.
11. Role of nurse in learning.

Short Answers

12. Briefly write about the steps in learning process.
13. Law of readiness.
14. Problem-solving learning.
15. Discuss the goals of learning.
16. Difference between classical and operant conditioning.
17. Transfer of learning.

CHAPTER 12

Memory

■ INTRODUCTION

The problem of retention is an important problem for a student of learning. He/She is curious to know as to how much amount of learning is retained by him/her. He/She also wants to know why he forgets, at times, certain common things. Remembering and forgetting are the opposite sides of the same coin. What can be directly measured is only the amount that is retained. But thus, it has a reference to the amount that is forgotten. Our concept of memory is somehow associated with verbal memory. No doubt, we have to memorize a majority of verbal facts; but in actual life situation, all forms of memory need not involve verbalization. Thus we remember someone's look, we remember places and we remember the taste of a particular food, which requires no verbalization, moreover, our concept of memory indicates that it is single function. Memory denotes the ability or a power of mind to retain and reproduce learning. This ability helps in the process of memorizing. Memory consists of remembering what has previously learned. Thus, the process begins with learning and ends with its retrieval and reproduction.

■ MEMORY

Memory is a general word, which includes several mental activities, such as recall, recognition. One see indications of memory all around as a person or animal experiences ease in relearning any activity, which he/she had learnt previously, but had forgotten. This proves very obviously that the previous learning had not been wiped out completely, but had left an impression on the mind or a change in the nerves, which facilitated relearning. People do not completely forget the story of any motive they have seen, but recount it with ease when they are requested to do so by a friend. Memory can be called structural mental process, in which the person brings the learned material to his/her conscious mind and then tries to recall it. To remember or memorize, it is essential to first learn the subject and then retain it. The meaning of memory in Latin and Greek words is 'to be mindful' or 'to remember'. Effective memory is not a function of how much time is spend on the material to be remembered, but is directly influenced by the kind of strategy and method of organization imposed on the material to be remembered.

Definition

1. Memory means showing the signs of earlier learned activities in present activities. *—Hillgard and Atkinson*
2. Memory is the capacity of a person to represent the information in response to the collection of previously learned activities and specific stimuli. *—Isenk HJ*
3. Memory defined as the power that we have to store our experiences and bring them into the field of unconscious sometimes after the experiences have occurred. *—Ryburn*
4. Memory is the ideal revival so far as ideal revival is merely reproductive. This productive aspect of ideal revival requires the object of past experiences to be reinstated as far as possible in the order and manner in their original occurrence. *—Stout*
5. Memory consists in remembering what has previously been learned. *—Woodworth and Marquis*

Qualities of Good Memory

1. Good retention power of the person.
2. Representing the facts quickly.
3. Quick and clear recognition.
4. Learning the subject matter quickly and immediately.
5. Using the facts and thoughts at the suitable time.

Components of Memory

Memory operates through four important components, which are registration, retention, recall and recognition (Fig. 12.1).

Registration

Registration is the short-term storage of the sensory input. Most of the information briefly held in the sensory register is lost.

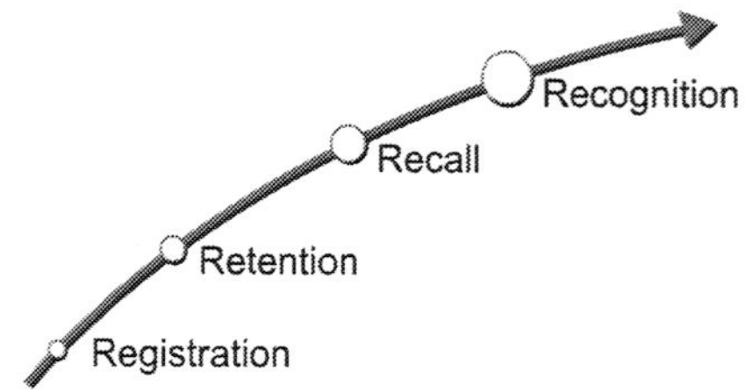

Figure 12.1: Components of memory

However, one should pay special attention to some of the information in the sensory register. When we do this, the attended information is passed on to the short-term store. The sensory register holds information for such a brief time that some psychologist prepares to discuss it as related to perception rather than memory.

Retention

Retention refers a performance of what was learnt. When the active process of learning ceases, then a comparatively passive process of retaining takes place. The material is retained when we are not thinking about it. People differ in their retentive capacity, which is largely due to genetic constitution.

Recall

Recall is the third aspect of memory. Things are learned in order to recall them whenever need arises. Recall is affected by a number of conditions as interference, set, attitude, etc. Failure to recall does not necessarily indicate the absence of retention. Without retention there cannot be recall. But there can be retention without recall.

Recognition

Recognition is closely related to recall. It is the act of affirming that a particular object or situation has been seen or experienced before. During the process of recalling, our cognitive effort is more obvious and hence one may think that recalling is an active process, whereas recognition is a passive state. But in fact recognition also is an active phenomenon.

Factors of Memory

One feels that a certain person has good memory whereas some other person has a bad memory. Experiments in memory show that although there is a general factor of memory, the actual functioning of memorizing is seen through specific operation that differ from person to person. People may differ in their visual memory, auditory memory or olfactory memory. The following factors are influencing on memory (Fig. 12.2).

Learning

Learning will be quite in keeping with the context to give a brief description of each of these activities. It has been mentioned above, the first step or activity is learning. If the learning is good, memory will also be good. Thus the methods, which assist learning, do the same for memory. Learning creates memory traces on the mind on the basis of which recollection is affected.

Retention

Retention means making permanent, the remains of experience. The remains of experiences are left on the mind in the form of memory traces where they are safe though they are acted upon the interest and other mental states. The proofs of retention are recollection, recognition and relearning.

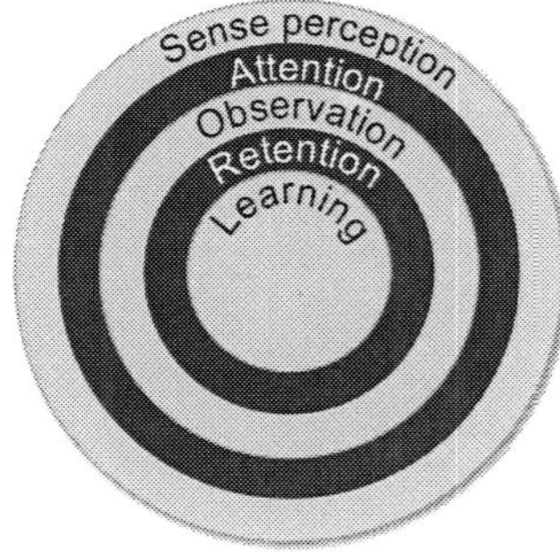

Figure 12.2: Factors of memory

Favorable conditions in retention

Duration: A sensation, which continues for a longer time can be retained for a longer time in mind. A sensation of a shorter duration will be, correspondingly, retained for a shorter duration.

Amount of material: The subject being pursued is long. It will be retained for a longer time, while a shorter subject will take less time before it is forgotten. The amount of material to be learnt has favorable effect on its retention.

Nature of material: Intensity, distinctness and meaning help in its retention to a large extent.

Amount of learning: The extent of retention is directly proportional to the amount of learning, i.e. to say that retention will be more, if the amount of learning is large. A subject studied more stays longer in the mind, while subject studied less will remain in the mind for a shorter period. Over learning has a favorable effect on the retention.

Methods of learning: Learning by the whole method instead of the part method spaced and active method instead of the passive method result in better and longer retention.

Speed of learning: The faster the learning, the better the retention. This is the principle in accordance with which people learning faster seem to retain the subject learned for longer period as compared to the slow learners.

Feeling: Freud and other psychologist assert that one retain pleasant experiences for a longer time whereas we forget painful experiences quickly.

Attention: While studying a subject, if greater attention is paid to the subject, the retention will be better. On the contrary, the retention will be weakened by inattention.

Sleep: Sometimes elapsed after study, before the subject is retained in the mind and if this time of strengthening and retention is used for sleep, the memory traces get a good opportunity to be etched upon the memory.

Mental review: If some experiences is incessantly contemplated upon its retention, it is better than one about which the mind does not trouble itself. Really speaking by mental review a repetition of the subject is caused, which strengthen retention.

Mental set: A person retains those things for a longer period, which coincide with his/her mental inclinations. A religious person remembers ideas relating to religion for long time and a sensuous man remembers things of sexual interest.

Apperception: It means the assimilating of learned subjects with the knowledge already present. The retention of a newly learned subject is greatly facilitated, if it is assimilated with the present store of knowledge to start with and on the other time is needed for retention, if this assimilation is not effected.

Intention: If the subject is learned with the express intention of being retained, the aim will be fulfilled with extraordinary success. But if there is no such retention, the subject removes itself from the memory of the person after sometimes. Learning gathered with a view to appear in the examinations is remembered better and things picked up here and there in ordinary course are easily forgotten unless the person has a special inclination towards them.

Massive experience: The retention will be more, if the experience is massive. If a person has ever loved, he/she never forgets it because it affects their whole personality and it is a fact that one remembers that thing longer, which affects them more.

Observation

Correct observation gives us correct and accurate information. Observation keeps us alert and informed of latest events happening, which helps in remembering.

Attention

Attention here denotes concentrating our mind on the purpose, which helps in collecting information. Therefore, if one pays attention it will help in retaining.

Sense Perception

Sense perception is the process by means of which one becomes aware of the environment. Sense perception is necessary for accurate observation of object, event, thing, person, etc.

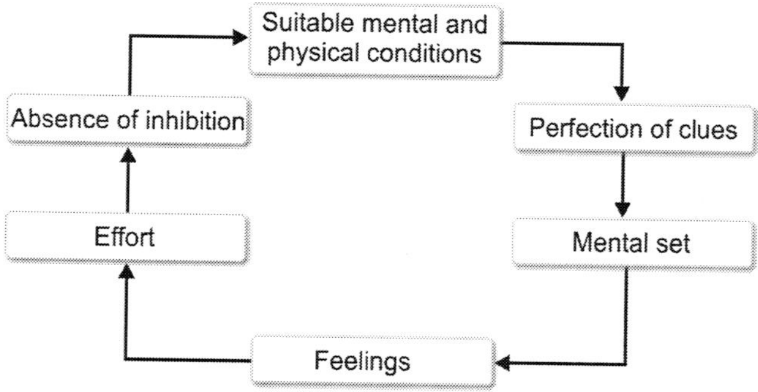

Figure 12.3: Favorable conditions in recall

Other Factors (Recall/Recognition)

Favorable conditions in recall (Fig. 12.3)

Suitable mental and physical conditions: Recall is comparatively easy, when both the mind and the body are healthy and fresh. Adverse and indifferent physical and mental conditions hinder recollection.

Perfection of clues: Recall is done with the help of clues, which are stimulators of recall. For example, if one learns a poem, one cannot recall it without the help of the title, the first line or the clue to some part of it and clue are necessary for the recall of anything in mind.

Mental set: The mental set of the individual too affect recall. A religious minded person remembers religious subjects easily, while sensuous person will find it easy to remember things associated with sex.

Motives: When a person is under the extreme influence of a motive, person has such clear recollection of related incidents that person sometimes has hallucination.

Feelings: Recollection is not immune to feelings of pleasure and pain. These feelings and experiences of pain and pleasure are recollected easily than indifferent feelings, while pleasurable experiences are comparatively easily recollected.

Effort: This has a very significant effect on recollection. Unless the extreme limit of effect has been passed, recollection generally increases with the effort.

Absence of inhibition: Recollection is better in the absence of any inhibition, because inhibition obstructs recollection and it may be caused by the conflict of the simultaneous arising of two activities or by repression and again by fear or other emotions.

Favorable conditions in recognition

Mental set: Recognition is helped by the mental set, in the manner in which other factors assists memory. Recognition is the correct, when the mental set is favorable and it is incorrect when the mental set is unfavorable.

Confidence: It is an indispensable element in recognition. In its absence even correct recognition, becomes infested with doubt and mistake is the outcome.

Types of Memory (Fig. 12.4)

Immediate Memory

Immediate memory or sensory memory is that memory, which helps an individual to recall something a split second after having perceived it. Immediate memory is needed when one wants to remember a thing for a shorter time and then forget it. One enters the cinema hall; see the seat number given on the ticket. After occupying the seat, one forgets the seat number. We look up a telephone number from the directory and remember it. But after making the call, one usually forgets it. In such type of memory retentive time is extremely brief, generally from a fraction of a second to several seconds.

Short-term Memory

Short-term memory can hold items fairly well for the first few seconds. After 12 seconds however, recall is poor and after 20 seconds the information has disappeared entirely unless one keeps repeating the material to themselves. A phone number that one looks up and dial is often forgotten by the time the call is answered. Short-term memory can also be called working memory.

Short-term memory is the immediate memory, which refers to storage of learning for a few seconds. The limited storage capacity of short-term memory is seen from the fact that our memory span for a single repetition is not more than seven items. Whenever it appears that one has a longer span, it is because of recording the material in convenient chunks. Most of us learn to break the material

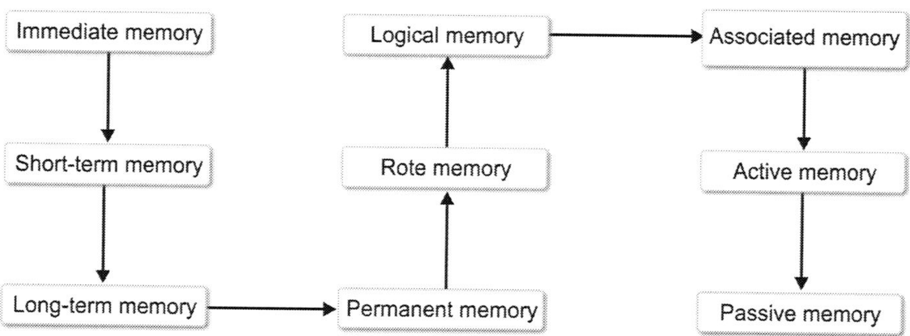

Figure 12.4: Types of memory

and organize it in groups. Thus even though the material retained is longer the units retained are fewer. The six or seven digit telephone numbers have a reference to span of immediate memory.

Long-term Memory

Long-term memory is relatively permanent in which information is stored for us at a longer time. Material enters a storehouse of almost unlimited capacity. Long-term memory seems to be much more complex, for it stores many different aspects of one's experiences. Remembering or identifying data such as the name, father's name, date of birth, date of marriage, etc. is the simplest example of long-term memory. The long-term memory differs (Table 12.1) from short-term memory in which the information is stored for a long duration.

Permanent Memory

Under permanent memory it is possible to remember a thing permanently. Remembering of our name is the simplest example of our permanent memory. It may or may not involve understanding and insight.

Rote Memory

Under rote memory, the things are learnt without understanding their meaning. Some students have a good rote memory. They can mug up material and reproduce it at the time of examination. Although rote memory can serve the purpose well, when it is need to remember a thing for the time being and for a specific purpose yet it is unreliable and fails to bring an enduring and lasting remembrance.

Table 12.1: Differences between short- and long-term memories

Sl No.	Short-term memory	Long-term memory
1.	The memory is carried by active neural process	This memory on the other hand is carried by permanent structural changes in nervous system
2.	The memory traces decay spontaneously	This memory traces show resistance to such spontaneous decay
3.	The memory storage capacity is limited; it is easily subjected to interference	A single exposure to stimuli is not seen to produce long-term retention in human verbal learning; many trials are usually required for long-term retention

Logical Memory

Logical memory is based on logical thinking. It takes into consideration, the purposeful and insightful learning. Here instead of mechanical memorization, the learner tries to understand what one learns and why one is learning.

Associated Memory

The individual having this type of memory is able to associate the previously learned things with so many related things and then establish multiple connections. It demands that the learning or memorization of a particular thing should not be in isolation. One must try to connect or associate it with as many other things as one can. It will help the memory to maintain multiple relationships. One can have a memory of so many things at a time by adopting the principle of association of ideas and images, and make maximum use of the memory.

Active Memory

In active memory, one has to remain active or make deliberate attempts for recollecting past experiences. In answering the question in examination hall we are required to make use of this type of memory.

Passive Memory

In passive memory, the past experiences are recalled spontaneously with or without any serious attempt, e.g. when somebody comes from the native village, the mere sight of him/her is enough to remind us about the fields, neighbors and other so many things.

■ MEASUREMENTS OF SHORT- AND LONG-TERM RETENTION

Short-term Retention

The subject is presented as a stimulus in the form of non-sense syllable by a three digit number. He/She is given some task such as counting the number in reverse or something similar to prevent further rehearsal on his/her part. He/She is then asked to reproduce the stimulus, when a signal is given. Thus recall was elicited after every 3 seconds. The recall was seen to drop down considerably till it was almost nonexistent after 18 seconds. This effect of reduction becomes more permanent after first few trials. This shows that previous activity interferes with retention. It is known as proactive interference.

Long-term Memory (Fig. 12.5)

There are several ways in which long-term retention is measured.

Recall

The method of recall is used in studying retention of verbal material, e.g. a poem or paragraph from a book. The subject then has to reproduce what has learnt without any cues. It is either estimated in terms of the amount that was initially assimilated or in terms of saving of learning in a relearning situation. This former type of examinations with essay type questions utilizes recall method for measuring retention.

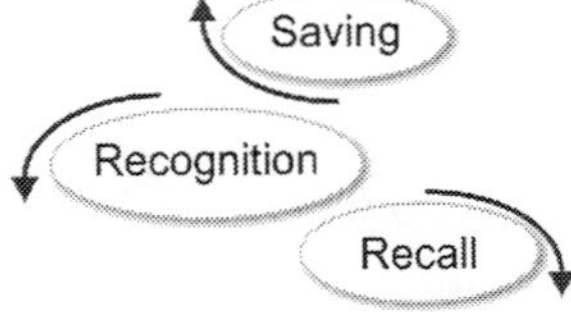

Figure 12.5: Long-term memory

Recognition

Another method of measuring retention is recognition. Recall and recognition are measured as two independent entities. One may fail to recall the face of the person one meets at a certain social function. But if one happens to see him/her, one may easily recognize him/her.

Between recognition and recall, the former is considered to be a more reliable criterion of retention. In most of the memory experiments retention is measured by recognition rather than recall. After presenting a list of non-sense syllables, they are intermingled with new and unfamiliar non-sense syllables. The subject has to recognize from among this bigger list, which were presented to them. Similar experiments are conducted by using photographs of persons or sceneries instead of non-sense syllables. The modern trend of examination with objective questions in place of the essay type questions is mainly based upon the belief that recognition is a better indication of memory than recall. In the essay type questions, where the pupil has to be recalled, it may happen that one with adequate retention may fail to recall due to a number of emotional and situational factors. If one is asked to recognize, as is done by the objective questions there are less chances of the above mentioned factors affecting the expression of the level of retention. Actually, so far as the experience in life is concerned, one are more often required to recognize than recall.

Saving

Saving method is frequently used in psychological experiments. The subject is made to learn a certain task. The trials required to master the task are noted. He/She is again made to relearn the task after a lapse of sometime interval. The measure of retention is the difference in number of trails required in the original learning and relearning situations. Such a method is sensitive and reliable. The saving method can show the retention long after other methods have caused to show any degree of it.

Theories of Memory

Fading of Memory

The theory regards the memory trace as resembling the marks of a pencil on a piece of paper, or a path worn into a plot of grass. It can be kept functioning through use as a pencil mark, can be emphasized by tracing and retracing, and a pathway can be kept clear by continuing to walk over it. But without use, the memory trace may vanish, as a pencil mark fades with time and pathway becomes over grown when abandoned. Memory theorists continue to believe that memory trace has some physical quality that changes with passage of time, thus reducing, the likelihood that it can be retraced or reactivated. Indeed they think of it as having two qualities. The first is its strength—meaning how likely it is to pop into mind. This quality the strength of the memory trace is at its peak immediately after learning and declines with the passage of time. The second quality is resistance to extinction, meaning how well the trace can manage to survive and become immune to fade.

Failure in Retrieval Theory

Failure in retrieval theory believes that memory trace, once it has been established as part of long-term memory, probably persists for as long as one lives. But information held in memory is of no use to us unless it remains not only stored, but available. To remember it, one must be able to find it and call upon it when needed, a process called retrieval. If one cannot call upon then one has forgotten it. Thus forgetting may be not a failure in memory, but rather a failure in retrieval.

As one psychologist has put it in this respect memory is similar to a huge ware house in which all sorts of things are stored, but which less than perfectly organized is. So that it is not always easy to find a given item upon demand, there is evidence that forgetting may be a failure in retrieval.

Interference Theory

Interference theory holds that the memory for what one learns today is often adversely affected by what one have learned in the past and also by what one will learn in the future. The various pieces of information complete for attention and survival, and not all of them can prevail. When old information causes us to forget new information, this process is called proactive interference; the phenomenon of proactive interference can be demonstrated very strikingly through simple laboratory procedures, such as asking subjects to try to learn and remember several lists of words. A steady decline in the ability to remember new material was caused by more and more proactive interference from prior learning. In proactive interference, old information gets in the way of remembering new information. The opposite situation—when new information causes us to forget old information is called retroactive interference.

■ MOTIVATED FORGETTING

The fact that one seems to forget something deliberately has already been mentioned in connection with the processes that take place in short-term memory. Motivated forgetting has been widely studied by psychoanalysis, who has found it often plays a part in certain forms of abnormal or neurotic behavior.

■ FORGETTING

The term forgetting seems to be a part of our day-to-day speech. Forgetting is a spontaneous or gradual process in which old memories are unable to recall from memory storage, it is called forgetting. In other words it refers to inability to recall.

Definition

1. Forgetting is the loss, permanent or temporary of the ability to recall or recognize learned earlier. —*Munn*
2. Forgetting means failure at any time to recall an experience, when attempting to do so or to perform an action previously learned. —*Drever*
3. Forgetting is the failure of the individual to revive in consciousness an idea or group of ideas without the help of the original stimulus. —*Bhatia*

Curve of Forgetting (Table 12.2)

The studies made by the psychologist Ebbinghaus (1885) present the earliest systematic works in studying the phenomenon of forgetting. He memorized a list of non-sense syllables and then test himself at intervals from 20 minutes to a month to see how much of the list he remembered. The results in terms of the percentage of material forgotten with the lapse of time found in the following order.

Table 12.2: Curve of forgetting

Sl No.	Time elapsed	Amount forgotten
1.	20 minute	47%
2.	1 day	66%
3.	2 day	72%
4.	6 day	75%
5.	31 day	79%

He tried to plot the above data on a piece of graph paper. The curve obtained on the graph paper by plotting the amount forgotten against a function of time was named by him as curve of forgetting. Ebbingghaus concluded the following:

1. The amount of learnt material forgotten depends upon the time lapsed after learning.

2. The rate of forgetting is very rapid at first and then gradually diminishes proportionately as the interval lengthens.

Causes of Forgetting

Interpolated Activity

As far as behaviorists are concerned, it is the interpolated activity after learning which causes forgetting, the extend of forgetting depends upon the divergence of these activities from the material learnt.

Disuse

The theory of disuse postulates that any learnt activity or accumulated knowledge will be gradually forgotten, if it is not regularly practiced.

Retroactive Inhibition

Some learning tends to contradict some previous learning, a tendency entitled retroactive inhibition, meaning the fatal effect of interpolated activity on learning.

Repression

The psychologists believe that the major cause of forgetting is repression, i.e. the pushing of the experience or thoughts into the unconsciousness.

Deficiency of Thinking and Repetition

Mental thinking and repetition assist retention and recollection, and in the same manner these factors also affect forgetting, i.e. in absence of these factors forgetting increases.

Deficiency of the Mental Set

Mental set is factor assistance in the retention and recollection of a subject so that its greater concurrences will reduce forgetting.

Brain Injury

Often when a person suffers a brain injury, he/she forgets many incidents and experiences, and the extent of the forgetting depends upon the seriousness of the injury.

Uses of Stimulants

Wine and other stimulants have a detrimental effect on the brain, because they weaken the memory traces. Thus forgetting will be increased, if such intoxicants are used.

Altered Stimulus Condition

If there is an association between the stimulus and situation, then forgetting is facilitated by any change in the situation or condition of the stimulus. People who stay abroad for long forget their correct dialect.

Zeigarnik Effect

According to Zeigarnik, completed tasks are forgotten more than the uncompleted task. Her theory is based on Lewin's field theory. According to this theory, when the individual undertakes a task, tension develops within a person and it persists until the task is completed that motivates the learner. This enables the learner to remember the task. In case of completed task, the tension disappears and forgetting will be more.

Lack of Rest and Sleep

Continuous learning without rest and sleep may lead to greater forgetting due to inefficient consolidation. Experimental studies have shown that sleep following learning favors retention; it also has been found that saving (retention) is definitely greater after sleep especially with 8 hours interval. Forgetting may slow during sleep.

Raise in Emotion

Emotions play an important role in learning and forgetting. Sudden rise of emotions blocks the recall. During the high emotional state blood sugar level is impaired to maintain the balance of adrenal gland that produces cortisol, which disturbs memory cells.

Types of Forgetting (Fig. 12.6)

Passive or Natural Forgetting

The kind of forgetting in which there is no intention of forgetting on the part of individual is known passive or natural forgetting. In this kind of forgetting one has not to make any deliberate efforts. In a quite normal way, with the lapse of time, one gradually forgets so many things experienced and learned earlier.

Active or Morbid Forgetting

Active or morbid forgetting is also known as abnormal forgetting. In this forgetting one deliberately tries to forget something. Freud explains this kind of forgetfulness, originates from expression. Under this process, the painful experience and bitter memories are deliberately pushed into the unconscious layer of the mind and are left there for forgetting.

Abnormal Forgetting

Abnormal forgetting is seen that forgetting is a function of times as shown in the curve of retention. The other explanation of forgetting is also discussed. But the cause of forgetting frequently has an emotional background. One has already referred to the affective nature of memory. Overexcitement or nervousness is often seen to prevent recall. One facing a big audience for the first time may be well-prepared with the speech, but also may not be able to utter a word on the stage.

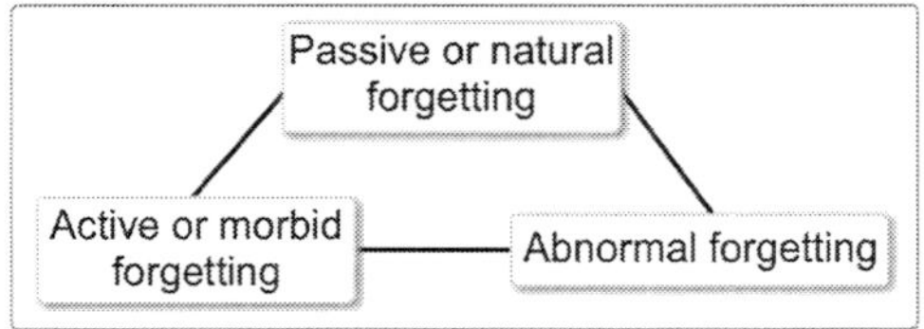

Figure 12.6: Types of forgetting

Emotional blocking also results from repression. The defense mechanism or repression has already been discussed by us. It shows how the experiences that bring disgrace or a feeling of guilt to us are pushed to the unconscious. Facts that are in keeping with our attitudes or those that support our view better remembered than those of a contrary nature. Similarly memories of happy events are seen to be more lasting than those of unhappy events.

When experiences are forgetting as a result of repression not only that the said experience is forgotten, but also any associated idea likely to call back the repressed experience to consciousness will be also be clamped down. Sigmund Freud in his book psychopathology of everyday life has discussed the events of such forgetting at length. He has analyzed a number of memory lapsed of this kind showing how recent events too can be easily forgotten due to emotional blocking.

One interesting thing to know about the process of forgetting is that it is not simply a passive progress involving gradual elimination of the facts retained. It is partly active too. While the originally retained facts are eliminated, the gaps are filled up by entirely new details. So whatever portion that is remembered goes through constant distortion. Our needs, interests, attitudes and prejudices play an active role in filling up the gaps of memory. Sir Frederic C Bartlett has shown by has interesting experiments how is reproducing by memory, though the outline is maintained, the details go through a number of changes. In his experiments, on memory for form, the subject were shown some drawing and asked to reproduce them out of memory. A number of details were either seen to be changed or omitted in the reproductions.

It is this quality of memory that really facilitates the spreading of rumors. Since rumors are circulated from person to person, at every juncture some of the details are omitted and some new filled in that is why there is a world of difference between the actual event and the rumor concerning it. The distortion is not intentional. It is the outcome of the nature of the memory process.

Theories of Forgetting (Fig. 12.7)

Trace Decay Theory

According to many psychologists, time is the cause of much forgetting, what is learnt or experienced is forgotten with the lapse of time. The cause of such natural forgetting can be explained through a process known as decay of the memory trace. It says that learning results in neurological changes leaving certain types of memory traces or engrams in the brain. With the passage of time through disuse, these memory traces of learning impressions get weaker and weaker, and finally fade away. It leads us to conclude that the older an experience, the weaker its memory and as time passes, the amount of forgetting goes on increasing.

This theory has proved a failure in many instances of forgetting. In long-term memory, such as learning to ride a bicycle, forgetting does not occur even after years of neglect. However, this theory has provided good results in explaining forgetfulness in the case of short-term memory. Drill, practice, rehearsal or repetition of learning always results in preventing decay.

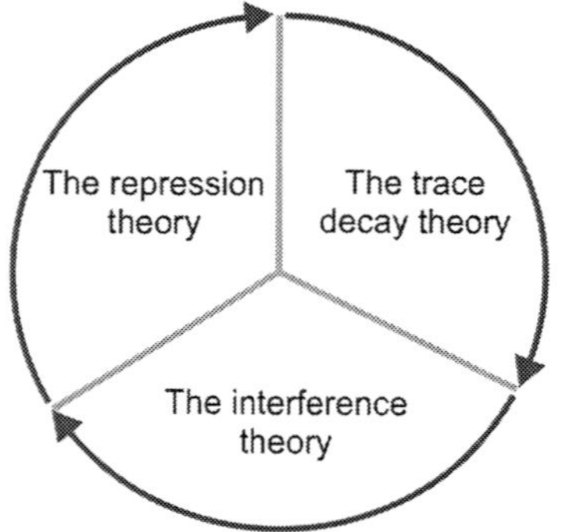

Figure 12.7: Theories of forgetting

Interference Theory

Mechanism of interference is responsible for forgetting. Interference is caused on account of the negative inhibiting effects of one learning experience on another. One forgets things because of such interference. The interfering effects of things previously learnt and retained in our memory with the things of our recent memory can work both ways, backward and forward. The psychological term used for these types of interference is retroactive inhibition and proactive inhibition.

In retroactive inhibition, the acquisition of new learning works backward to impair the retention of the previously learned material. For example, a second list of words, formulations or equations may impair the retention of a first list.

Proactive inhibition is just the reverse of retroactive inhibition. Here the old learning or experiences retained in the memory works forward to disrupt the memory of what one acquires or learn afterwards. For example, learning a new formula may be hampered on account of the previously learned formulae in one's memory.

In both types of the above inhibitions, it can be easily seen that similar experiences, when follow each other produce more interference than dissimilar experiences. Because in this case all experiences are so intermingled that a state of utter confusion prevails in the mind of an individual and consequently one faces a difficulty in retention and recall. Interference theory on the whole has been proved quite successful in providing adequate explanation for natural and normal forgetting for both the short- and long-term memory.

Repression Theory

The 'repression theory' is put forward by Freud's psychoanalytic school of psychology. Repression according to this school is a mental function that safeguards the mind from, the impact of painful experiences. As a result of this function one actually pushes the unpleasant and painful memories into the unconscious and thus try to avoid at least consciously the conflicts that bother us. As a result of the repression one forgets the things, which one do not want to remember.

People under a heavy emotional shock tend to forget even their names, homes, spouse and children. Apart from causing abnormal forgetting, an impaired emotional behavior of an individual does also play its part in disrupting their normal memory process. For example, a sudden rise of emotions in excess may completely block the process of recall. When one is taken over by emotions such as fear, anger or love, one may forget all one has experienced, learned or thought beforehand. During these emotions one becomes so self-conscious that his/her thinking is paralyzed. That is why a child fails to recall the answer to a question in the presence of a teacher whom he/she fears very much.

Economical Methods of Memorization or Remembering

The problem of having economy in memorizing something has persuaded many psychologists to devise various methods of memorization (Fig. 12.8).

Recitation Method

In this method the learner first reads the matter once or twice and then tries to recite, and recall without looking at that material. In this way, the recitation method provides continuous self-appraisal. Learner evaluates himself/herself from time to time and notes the points, which he/she has been unable to recall. To these points attention can be paid and thus he/she is saved of unnecessarily repeating the already memorized material. Moreover the recitation method is more stimulating than the continued and avoids them by close attention.

Whole and Part Method

There are two methods of memorizing a thing, e.g. poem. One is to read the poem again and again from the beginning till the end as a whole. This is called whole method of memorization. In other method—part method, the poem is divided into parts and each part is memorized separately.

Spaced or Unspaced Method

In the spaced or distributed practice method of memorization, the subject is not required to memorize the assigned material in one continuous sitting. After memorizing for some time, some rest is provided and in this

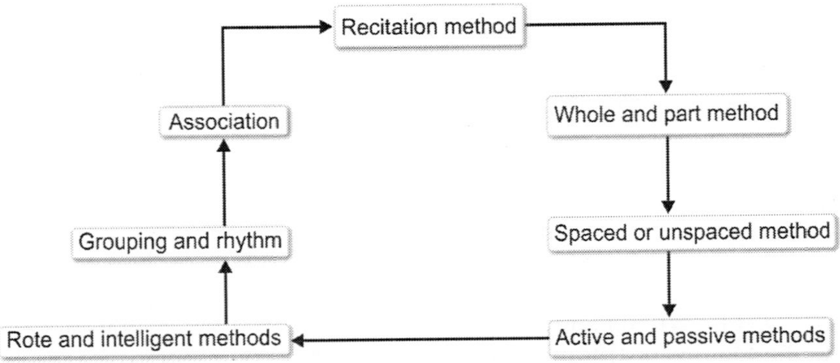

Figure 12.8: Economical methods of memorization

way the principle of work and rest is followed in this method. For example, if one has to memorize a piece of poetry by this method, then in beginning one will be advised to go repeating it. After some time one will be given some rest again one will memorize it and take rest. In this way with repeated intervals of work and rest one will be able to have mastery over the assigned piece.

Active and Passive Methods

Memorizing by utterance is the active method, while mental repetition is the passive method. Many experiments have been carried out to measure the economy, which this method may affect.

Rote and Intelligent Methods

In rote and intelligent methods, a person is learning or memorizing something without understanding it, then the person is said to be using the rote or unintelligent method. This is no apperception in this. On the other hand, by the use of the intelligent method it involves the understanding of the subject and apperception does come about.

Grouping and Rhythm

Memorization is considerably facilitated by rhythm and grouping. It is easier to memorize poetry than prose, but by rhythm and grouping. It is easier to memorize poetry than prose, but by the rhythm scheme. One couplet contains enough meaning to be spread over several pages, but the rhythm makes their memorization easier.

Association

Association as a factor, which keeps memorization is no less important than the other, suppose that one have to remember that the first step in the solution of arithmetical problems is the bracket and successive step are of division, multiplication, subtraction and addition, and in order to facilitate it.

Improvement of Memory or Memory Training

One at time is worried that the capacity for memory is being deteriorated. One may be considered with the consideration whether their ability to memorize can be improved. The answer to such question is that memory is not single faculty and moreover, it does not improve nor does it deteriorate. Psychology deals with process of memorizing and not with a composite faculty of memory. Experiments on the process of memorizing show that whatever assimilation is superior, retention is more durable and eventually recall or recognition is prompt. Since assimilation is more closely connected with the process of learning, a thing better learned has more chances of being better memorized.

Hence to facilitate memory, that entire one can do happens to be in the field of learning. All devices that promote learning are seen to help memory. Nothing can be independently done in the field of memory alone since memory is a counterpart of learning. The factors bringing about more permanent learning are obviously contributory for superior memory.

Will to Learn

There must be firm determination (strong will) to learn for achieving desired success in learning. Where there is a will there is a way. Materials read, heard or seen without intention or mood are difficult to be remembered at later times.

Interest and Attention

Interest as well as close attention is essential for effective learning and memorization. One who has no interest in what one learns, cannot give due attention to it and consequently, will not be able to learn it. Therefore, every care should be taken to create the desired interest in the material by making its purpose clear and link it with one's natural instincts and urges.

Adopting Proper Methods of Memorization

There are so many economical methods of memorization but all are not suitable on all occasions for all individuals. Therefore a judicious selection should be made in choosing a particular method in a given situation.

Principle of Association to Follow

Principle of association is always good to follow the principle of association in learning. A thing should never be learnt in a complete water tight compartment. Attempts should be made to connect it with one's previous learning on one hand and with so many related things on the other. Sometimes for association of ideas special techniques and devices are used that facilitate learning and recalling.

Grouping and Rhythm

Grouping and rhythm also facilitate learning and help in remembering. Rhythms also prove as an aid in learning and memorizing. Children learn effectively the multiplication tables in the sing-song fashion.

Utilizing as Many Senses as Possible

Senses are said to be the gateway of knowledge and it has also been found that the things are better learned and remembered when presented though more than one senses. Therefore attempts should be made to take the help for audio-visual aid material and receive impressions through as many senses as possible.

Arranging Better Learning Situation

Environmental factor also affect the learning process. Therefore care should be taken to arrange better learning situation and environment. A calm and quite atmosphere and stimulating environment proves an effective aid to learning.

Internal Factors Within the Learner

Besides the external factors there are things within the learner, which affect his/her learning and reproduction, his/her physical and mental health, and state of the mind at the time of learning as well as reproduction counts a lot to memory.

Provision for Change and Proper Rest

Adequate provision for change of work, rest and sleep should be made as it helps in removing fatigue and monotony. A fresh mind is necessarily able to learn more and retain it for a long time than a tried and dull one.

Repetition and Practice

An intelligent repetition with full understanding always helps in making the learning effective and enduring. The things repeated and practiced frequently learning effective and enduring. The things repeated and practiced frequently, and remembered for a long time. Therefore due care should be taken for drill work, practice and review, etc. in the process of memorization and learning.

Pulling it all Together

Organizing and ordering information can significantly improve memory. As learning a large amount of unconnected and unorganized information from various classes can be very challenging. By organizing and adding meaning to the material prior to learning it, you can facilitate both storage and retrieval.

Funnel Approach

Funnel approach means learning general concepts before moving on to specific details. When one understands the general concepts first, the details make more sense.

Vivid Associations

While learning something new and unfamiliar, try pairing it with something one knows very well such as images, puns, music, etc.

Active Learning

Active learning facilitates the memory by helping to attend to the process information. All of the memory techniques require active learning.

Talk it Out

Repeat ideas verbatim, repeat the ideas in the own words, repeating information aloud can help to encode the information and identify how well one have learned it.

Mnemonic

Mnemonic is a memory aid and most serve as a learning purpose. It is a powerful technique helps in remembering some specific things. One common mnemonic for remembering lists consists of an easily remembered word, phrase or rhyme whose first letter is associated with the list items. Mnemonic rely not only on repetition to remember facts but also on associations between easy to remember constructs and lists of data, based on principle that the human mind is much more easily remembers data attached to spatial, personal or otherwise meaningful information that occurring in meaningless sequences. The sequences must make sense.

■ AMNESIA

Amnesia is a condition in which memory is disturbed. The cause of amnesia is organic or functional. Organic causes include damage to the brain, through trauma or disease, or use of certain drugs. Functional causes are psychological factors, such as defense mechanisms. Hysterical post-traumatic amnesia is an example of functional amnesia. Amnesia may also be spontaneous, in the case of transient global amnesia.

Types of Amnesia

Anterograde Amnesia

New events are not transferred to long-term memory, so the sufferer will not be able to remember anything, this occurs after the onset of this type of amnesia for more than few moments. The complement of this is retrograde amnesia, where someone will be unable to recall events that occurred before the onset of amnesia.

Dissociative Amnesia

Dissociative amnesia is used to refer inability to recall information, usually about stressful or traumatic events in person's lives. A common form of dissociative amnesia involves amnesia for a person's identity, but intact memory of general information.

Long-term Alcoholism

Long-term alcoholism can cause a type of memory loss known Korsakoff's syndrome. This is caused by brain damage due to a vitamin

B_1 deficiency and will be progressive, if alcohol intake and nutrition pattern are not modified.

Lacunar Amnesia

Lacunar amnesia is the loss of memory about one specific event.

Childhood Amnesia

Childhood amnesia also known infantile amnesia is the common inability to remember events from one's own childhood.

Global Amnesia

Global amnesia is total memory loss. This may be a defense mechanism, which occurs after a traumatic event. This global type of amnesia is more common in middle aged to elderly people, particularly males and usually lasts less than 24 hours. Post-traumatic stress disorder can also involve the spontaneous, vivid retrieval of unwanted traumatic memories.

Posthypnotic Amnesia

Posthypnotic amnesia is where events during hypnosis are forgotten or where past memories are unable to be recalled.

Psychogenetic Amnesia

Psychogenetic amnesia results from a psychological cause as opposed to direct damage to the brain caused by head injury, physical trauma or disease, which is known organic amnesia.

Source Amnesia

Source amnesia is a memory disorder in which someone can recall certain information, but they do not know where or how they obtained it.

■ CONCLUSION

In psychology, an organism's ability to store, retain and subsequently retrieve information is known memory. The process of memory begins with learning or experiencing something and ends with its revival and reproduction. Therefore memory is said to involve four stages—learning or experiencing something, its retention and finally its recognition, and recall. Learning occupies a significant place in one's life. Whatever is learned need to be stored in the mind, so that it can be utilized whenever required in the future. Memory denotes the ability or a power of mind to retain and produce learning. Thus, this process begins with learning and ends with its retrieval and reproduction. Forgetting has positive and negative values of life. It is a great blessing to mankind. Forgetting is the temporary or long-term loss in our ability to reproduce the thing that has been previously learned.

■ REVIEW QUESTIONS

Long Essays

1. Define memory. Describe the components of memory.
2. Explain the factors that influence memory in detail.
3. Discuss various theories of memory.

Short Essays

4. Describe various types of memory.
5. List out the difference between long- and short-term memory.
6. Describe the measurement of long- and short-term memory.
7. Define forgetting. Explain the causes of forgetting.
8. Explain different types and theories of forgetting.
9. Describe various methods of improving memory.
10. Define amnesia. Explain different types of amnesia.

Short Answers

11. Qualities of memory.
12. Enumerate the favorable conditions of retaining.
13. Logical memory.
14. Rote memory.
15. Curve of forgetting.
16. Mnemonic.
17. Anterograde amnesia.

CHAPTER 13

Thinking and Reasoning

■ INTRODUCTION

The primary basis of man's progress is thinking. Many problems can be solved with the help of thinking. Various processes of teaching are accomplished due to thinking only. It is possible to change the attitudes and thoughts of a person through thinking. Perception, memory, imagination and reason are included in thinking; therefore thinking is considered to be a complex process. Thinking is an incredibly complex process and a most difficult concept in psychology to define or explain. Thinking the mental solution of problems, makes use of the symbols of objects instead of the objects. Thinking attempts the solution of problems by employing the trial and error method. There is a kind of flow in the activity of thinking, one problem leading to the thinking of another by reminding the person of that other problem.

■ NATURE OF THINKING

Thinking is the process of mentally solving the problems. It includes a flow of thoughts. Thoughts continue to come one after the other and this internal process continues till they are expressed. Here, attempts are made to solve the problems through trial and error method. If the person arises, its solution is sought through thinking or any new thought is evolved. Along with analysis, thinking also involves synthesis, foresight and hindsight. Here, one thinks about tangible objects through intangible signs and symbols, here thinking is a symbolic behavior. The main form of thinking is reason and this is a process of mental research health saves time and behaviors are given below:

1. Thinking is essentially a cognitive activity.
2. It is always directed to achieve some end or purpose. In genuine thinking one cannot let our thoughts wonder on without any definite end in mind as happens in the case of day dreaming and imagination.
3. Thinking is described as a problem-solving behavior. From the beginning to the end, there is some problem around which the whole process of thinking revolves. But every problem-solving behavior is not thinking. It is only related to the inner cognitive behavior.
4. In thinking there is mental exploration instead of motor exploration. One has to suspend immediately one's overt or motor activities, while engaging in thinking through some or other types of mental exploration.
5. Thinking is a symbolic activity. In thinking there is a mental solution of the problem, which is carried out through some signs, symbols and mental images.

6. Thinking can shift very rapidly, covering an expanse of time and space almost instantaneously.

■ DEFINITION

1. Thinking is the cognitive process that begins with the problem or work facing the person. It includes trial and error, but is affected by the readiness of person and ultimately it ends at the solution of problem or conclusion. —*Warren*
2. In strict psychological discussion it is well to keep the thinking for an activity, which consists essentially of a connected flow of ideas, which are directed towards some end or purpose. —*Valentine*
3. Thinking is mental activity in its cognitive aspect or mental activity with regard to psychological objects. —*Ross*
4. Thinking is behavior, which is often implicit and hidden, and in which symbols (images, ideas and concepts) are ordinarily employed. —*Garrett*
5. Thinking is an implicit problem-solving behavior. —*Mohsin*
6. Thinking is a problem-solving process in which we use or symbols in place of overt activity. —*Gilmer*
7. Thinking is the organization and reorganization of current learning in the present circumstances with the help of learning and past experiences.—*Vinake*
8. Thinking is a perceptual relationship, which provides for the solution of the problem. —*Maier*
9. Thinking is a complex cognitive form of behavior, which occurs only at a relatively advanced stage of development, when simpler and more direct methods of dealing with environment have proven ineffective and simple memory is adequate to solve problem. —*Whittaker*

■ TYPES OF THINKING (Fig. 13.1)

Imaginative Thinking

Here, thinking takes place without any basic sensory stimulus. Daydreaming and only being aware of future plans are major examples of imaginative thinking.

Creative Thinking

Creative thinking is related to creative activities; it is the basis of adopting new thoughts and attitudes in life, inventions, research and other creative activities. Creative thinking is chiefly aimed at creating something new. It is in search of new relationship and associations to describe and interpret the nature of things, events and situations. It is not bounded by any pre-established rules.

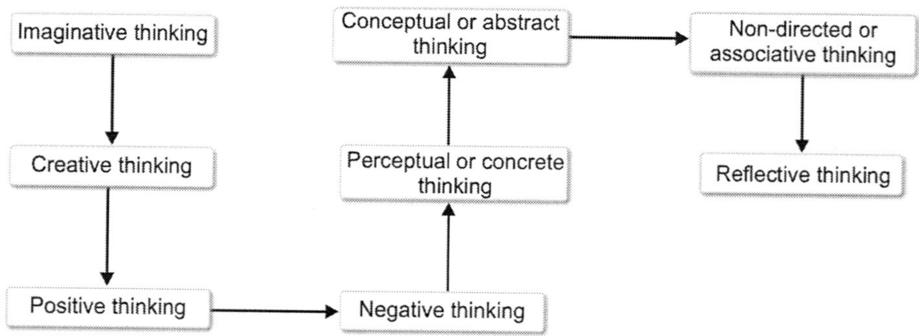

Figure 13.1: Types of thinking

Creative thinkers are great boons to the society as they enrich the knowledge of mankind.

Positive Thinking

Here, the thoughts of person are of optimistic and positive point of view. This thinking identifies the good mental health.

Negative Thinking

Here, person gives more important to negative thoughts. Negative thinking is not good for health.

Perceptual or Concrete Thinking

Perceptual or concrete thinking is the simple form of thinking. The basis of this type of thinking is perception, i.e. interpretation of sensation according to one's experience. It is also named as concrete thinking as it is carried over the perception of actual or concrete objects and events.

Conceptual or Abstract Thinking

Conceptual or abstract thinking does not require the perception of actual objects or events. It is also called abstract thinking as it makes the use of concepts or abstract ideas. It is superior to perceptual thinking as it economizes efforts in understanding and helps in discovery and invention. It is an abstract thinking where one makes use of concepts; the generalized ideas and languages. It is economizes effects in understanding and problem solving.

Non-directed or Associative Thinking

In strict psychological sense, what we have discussed above in terms of the types of categories of thinking constitutes real or genuine thinking. It is essentially a directed thinking, which pertains to reasoning and problem-solving procedure aimed at meeting specific goals.

Reflective Thinking

Reflective thinking is somewhat of a higher form of thinking. It can be distinguish from simple thinking in the following ways:

1. It aims at solving complex problems rather than simple problems.
2. It requires reorganization of all the relevant experiences and finding new ways of reacting to a situation or of removing an obstacle instead of simple association of experiences or ideas. Mental activity in reflective thinking does not undergo any mechanical trial and error type of effort. There is an insightful cognitive approach in reflective thinking. It takes logic into account in which all the relevant facts are arranged in a logical order, in order to get the solution of the problem in hand.

■ CHARACTERISTICS OF THINKING

A number of mental processes are included in thinking:

1. Thinking is affected by motives.
2. Thinking begins from general to speciality or specificity.
3. Analysis and synthesis have an important role in thinking.
4. Thought and language are very important in thinking.
5. Thinking begins with the beginning of problem.
6. Thinking can solve problem.
7. Brain remains active during thinking process.
8. Thinking enjoys challenges.
9. Thinking able us to suspend judgments.
10. Thinking challenges assumptions.
11. Thinking seeks the problems as opportunities.

■ TOOLS OF THINKING (Fig. 13.2)

Images

Images, as mind pictures, consist of personal experiences of objects, people or scenes once actually seen, heard or felt. These mind pictures symbolize the actual objects, experiences and activities. In thinking, one usually manipulates the images instead of actual objects, experiences and activities. The uses of images in thinking depends in no small measure upon the method of thinking, which the individual employs. Some people use other symbols in their thinking instead of images.

Concepts

Concepts are the abstract forms of past experiences. Humanity is the quality of the human species, found equally in all human beings. A concept is a general idea that stands for a general class and represents the common property of all the objects or events of this general class. The concepts is a tool that economies our efforts in thinking. Concept formed with the help of abstraction is mental. Concepts extend the limits of thinking to include both the past and future. Reasoning cannot be done without concepts, which are both the past and future.

Signs and Symbols

Signs and symbols represent and stand as substitutes for actual objects, experiences and activities. In this sense they cannot be confined to words and mathematical numerals and terms. Traffic lights, railway signals, school bells, badges, songs, flags and slogans all stand for the symbolic expression. These signs and symbols stimulate and economies thinking.

Language

Language is the most efficient and developed vehicle used for carrying out the process of thinking. When one listens or reads, or writes words, phrases or sentences or observes gesture in any language, one is stimulated to think. Reading and writing of the written documents and literature also help in stimulating and promoting the thinking process.

Muscle Activities

Thinking in one way or the other shows evidence of the involvement of a slight incipient movement of groups of our muscles. It can be easily noticed that there are slight muscular responses, when one thinks of a word, resembling the movements used when one utters the word aloud. A high-positive correlation has been found to exist between the thinking

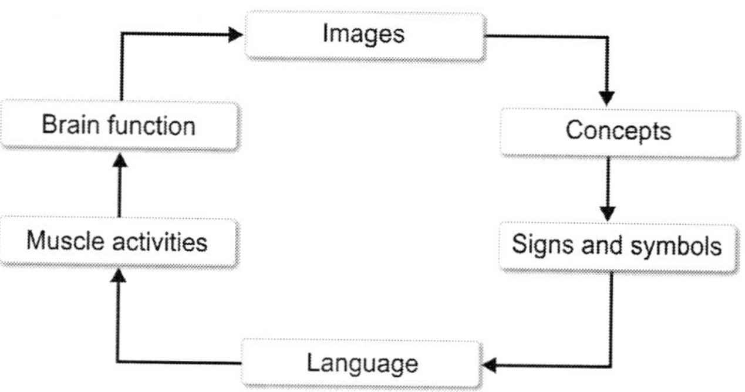

Figure 13.2: Tools of thinking

and muscular activities of an individual. The more one engages in thought, the greater is the general muscular tension and conversely as one proceeds toward muscular relaxation, our thought processes gradually diminish.

Brain Function

Whatever may be the role of muscles, thinking is a primarily function of the brain. Mind or brain is said to be the chief instrument or reservoir for carrying out the process of thinking. The mental picture of images can be stored, formed, reconstructed or put to some use only through the functioning of the brain.

■ STAGES OF THINKING

John Dewey says that there are distinct stages in thinking.

Awareness of the Problem

According to John Dewey reason for thinking is confusion or doubt and hence whenever one is aware or confronted with a problem one starts thinking. Therefore, being aware of the existing problem is essential, if one has to think. For instance the student who is not aware that his/her behavior would lead to problem may not think before showing the behavior.

Defining the Difficulty

Following the awareness of the problem, one should be able to understand the kind of problem he/she has. This is important to find out the root cause of the problem.

Discovering the Relationships and Formulating the Possible Solutions

This is problems of the third step. This helps in manipulating the information or as we have discussed in insight learning, this is helps in perceptual reorganization assisting in problem solving.

Evaluation

Evaluation is testing the solution. This helps in taking the effective steps to solve a problem. Applying the solution is the last stage where one shows the problem-solving behavior that is the result of thinking.

■ ELEMENTS IN THINKING

Favorable Elements in Thinking (Fig. 13.3)

Interest and Attention

Both interest and attention favor the thinking. Conclusive or authoritative thinking is

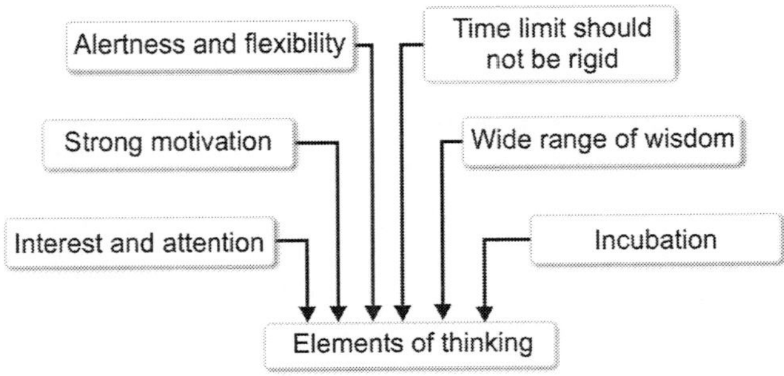

Figure 13.3: Favorable elements in thinking

extremely difficult, if not impossible when the subject is such as does not interest us. Too much attention is difficult in the absence of any interest. On the contrary, both attention and thinking are natural in a subject, which does interest us.

Strong Motivation

Strong motivation is needed in valid thinking, the latter being impossible in the absence of motivation. Organized and controlled thinking needs strong motivation. Thinking involves the solution of problems. The effort of the mind in thinking corresponds to the strength of motivation for the solution of problems. Motivation maintains enthusiasm and postpones fatigue.

Alertness and Flexibility

Alertness and flexibility also favor valid thinking, because they serve to keep external faults, from containing thinking. Alertness checks mistakes and fallacies from creeping into thinking. Flexibility keeps thinking free from conservation and blind beliefs. An alert person has new methods, ways and views, and makes use of them in thinking whenever necessary.

Time Limit Should Not be Rigid

When a solution to some problem is being sought, the time limit provided should not be too rigid because 'id' it so, then, normal thinking is hampered and our mental facilities become invalid. Very inflexible and short time limit cannot admit of valid thinking. Time limit for any interesting problem is superfluous because it is every person exerts himself/herself to the maximum.

Wide Range of Wisdom

The wide range of wisdom is also a favorable factor in thinking. Thinking needs insight, which is constituted of hindsight and foresight. A proper development of the faculties of the mind is essential for these activities.

Incubation

Another factor, which favors thinking, is incubation. If the solution of some problem proves elusive despite strenuous and persistent effort, it is advisable to lay aside the problem and to involve oneself in some other activity. While one is engaged in this work, the mind ponders over the earlier problem and just as eggs are hatched by incubation, a solution is evolved through pondering in this manner.

Unfavorable Elements in Thinking (Fig. 13.4)

Emotion

Emotion hinders thinking because strong emotion disturbs the mental equilibrium and thereby obstructs thinking. Even if thinking is pursued in an emotional state it will be extremely one sided and biased. If the emotion is very faint, the speed of thinking will be augmented instead of being hindered. But, for correct thinking it is better to have control over the emotions.

Suggestion

Suggestion also obstructs thinking, because it makes it one-sided. Thinking moves along

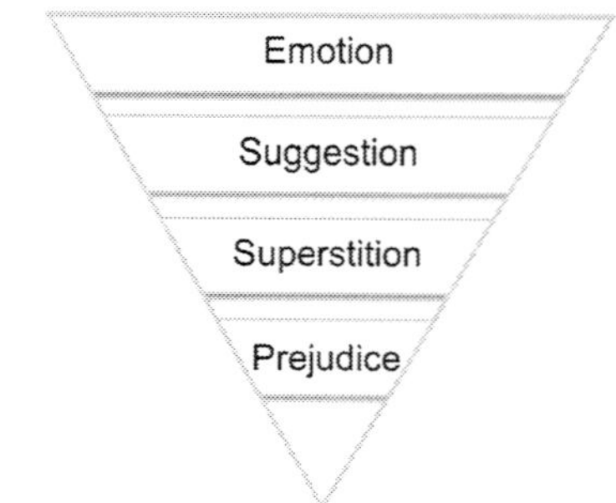

Figure 13.4: Unfavorable elements in thinking

the path suggested. For example, someone is told that 'he will not live for any length of time'; his thinking will be very badly affected, making him a pessimist. But, it is not essential that suggestions be invariably harmful to thinking because healthy suggestions assist thinking.

Superstition

Superstition is just as harmful as a prejudice. It contradicts the reasoning; superstition is belief in something without any thinking or reasoning. Superstition is unreasoned belief. For example, we superstitiously believe some theory, opinion or person, one always think in favor of him/her and never see his/her faults. The people who are superstitious in a certain religion believe mutually contradictory things, but never mentally reason them out.

Prejudice

Prejudice, a foreside factor, has a detrimental effect on thinking; the only point of distinction being the extent of damage, which is more in this case than in the two cases discussed earlier. The word prejudice suggests the meaning namely some preconceived idea. If one is going to start thinking on some problems with an inclination in a particular direction all our thinking will be colored by our bias and will not be impartial.

■ REASONING

Reasoning plays a significant role in adjusting to one's environment. It is not only controls one's abilities, but also the total behavior and personality is affected by the proper or improper development of one's reasoning ability. Reasoning depicts a higher type of thinking, which is quite careful, systematic and organized in its functioning. Reasoning is solving a problem by putting two or more elements of past experience together in a logical sequence to arrive at something new. Most human reasoning makes use of symbols—especially the verbal symbols. The process of reasoning follows some standard rules are rigid in nature and can be used as standards for reasoning. The rules are called logic. They prescribe what kind of implication statements can have and what kinds of conclusions it is permissible to draw from them.

Meaning of Reasoning

Reasoning is a form of thinking itself. When thinking process is guided by some logical principles, it is called reasoning. Good thinking and reasoning are clearly related. One facilitates the other. Reasoning is goal directed as is thinking in general. But in reasoning, the goal imposed upon the process at every step. Every step weighs the advancement of the process in terms of the accuracy in inaccuracy of the condition. When facts of data are put together according to the logical principles, reasoning is correct. Reasoning is mostly directed toward getting at certain definite conclusions and inferences. In this process the facts relevant to the particular problem.

Definitions

1. Reasoning is step-wise thinking with a purpose or goal in mind. —*Garrett*
2. Reasoning is the term, which is applied to highly purposeful controlled selective thinking. —*Gates*
3. In reasoning, items (facts or principles) furnished by recall present, observation or both are combined and examined to see what conclusion can be drawn from the combination. —*Woodworth*
4. Reasoning is the word used to describe the mental recognition of cause and effect relationships. It may be the prediction of an event from an observed cause or the inference of a cause from an observed event. —*Skinner*

5. Reasoning is combining past experiences in order to solve a problem, which cannot be solved by mere reproduction of earlier solutions. —*Munn*

Characteristics of Reasoning

1. It is genuine thinking; it involves a definite purpose or goal.
2. It is also an implicit act and involves problem-solving behavior.
3. Similar to thinking here one makes use of one's previous knowledge and experience.
4. Similar to thinking there is mental exploration instead of motor exploration in reasoning as one tries to explore mentally the reason or cause of the event or happening.
5. Similar to thinking, reasoning is a highly symbolic function. The ability to interpret various symbols, development of concepts and linguistic ability helps much in reasoning.

Steps of Reasoning

1. Identification of the goal or purpose for which reasoning is to be directed.
2. The mental exploration or search for the various possibilities, causes and effects relationships or solutions for releasing the set goals or purposes based on previous learning or experiences and present observation or attempts.
3. Selection of the most appropriate possibility or solution by careful mental analysis of all the available alternatives.
4. Testing the validity of the selected possibility or solution, purely through mental exercise and thus finally accepted or reject it for actual solution of the problem.

Types of Reasoning (Fig. 13.5)

Inductive Reasoning

In this type of reasoning one usually follows the process of induction. Induction is a way of proving a statement or generalizing a rule or principle by proving or showing that if a statement or a rule is true in one particular case, it will be true in cases, which appear in some serial order and thus it may be applied generally to all such type of cases.

Deductive Reasoning

Deductive reasoning is just opposite to inductive reasoning. Here, one starts completely agreeing with some already discovered or pre-established generalized fact or principle and tries to apply it to particular cases.

Assessment of Reasoning and Problem Solving

Wisconsin Card Sorting Test

Wisconsin card sorting test assesses abstract reasoning and flexibility in problem-solving stimulus cards of different color, form and number are presented to patients to sort into groups according to the principle established by the examiner, but unknown to the patient (e.g. to sort by color, ignoring form and number).

As the patient sots the cards, he/she is told whether the responses are correct or incorrect and the number of trials required to achieve 10 consecutive correct responses is recorded. When the patient has mastered the task, the examiner changes the principle of sorting and the number of trials required to achieve correct sorting is recorded.

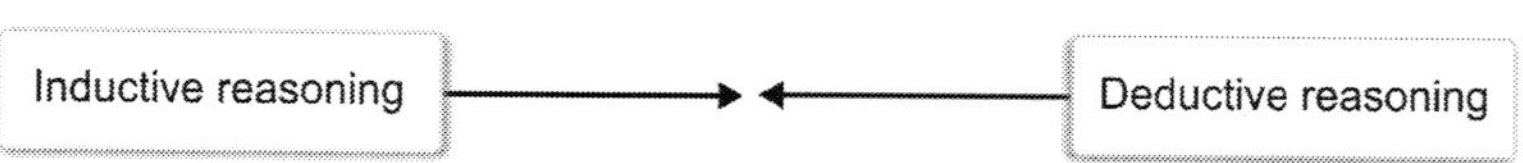

Figure 13.5: Types of reasoning

The procedure, repeated several times, measures the capacity for abstract thinking (i.e. the number of trials required to achieve a solution) and flexibility (perseverated error on successive sorting trials).

Persons with damage to the frontal lobes or to the caudate and some person with schizophrenia give abnormal response.

Patients with cerebral disease are likely to lose the capacity to reason abstractly and to lack flexibility in problem solving or adopting to change situations.

■ CREATIVE THINKING

At times, thinking leads to fertile results. Such thinking that brings about novel results is known creative thinking. The creative thinkers such as artists, writers or scientists try to create something new and non-existent in the world. In contrast with ordinary problems solving creating solutions are new ones that other people have not thought of before. Creative thinking results in offering new and unique ways of conceptualizing the world around us. The word new is of importance in creative thinking. Usually it appears that a creative thinker becomes aware of a new idea suddenly. The sudden appearance of new ideas is called insight. In fact, instead of being sudden such an insight is based on unconscious deliberations. All the discoveries or inventions of the scientists are instances of creative thinking.

Steps Involved in Creative Thinking (Fig. 13.6)

Preparation

In a way, all education is a preparation for creating thinking in general. But specific problems require special training and preparation in that particular field. The creative results in such thinking are mostly the results of insightful inspiration. But this inspiration

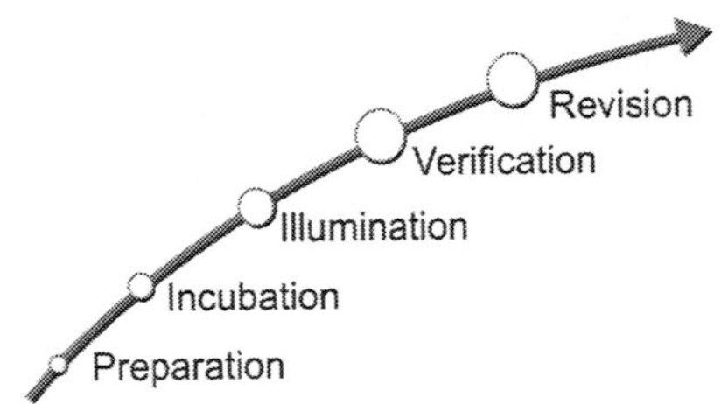

Figure 13.6: Steps involved in creative thinking

is possible within the relevant field of training and experience. It cannot take place in a vacuum. Much emphasis is, therefore, placed on training for creative thinking in the field of modern day educational psychology.

Incubation

The new ideas take some time to ripen or to get mature. They are to be hatched. The productive solution does not occur in the movement as it is started upon. Often the thinker has to struggle hard for the solution. Sometimes he/she may even give up thinking about it in despair.

Illumination

When the solution occurs after the period of incubation, it occurs all of a sudden in the form of illuminating insight. Naturally, the thinker feels that something similar to inspiration is at work. He/She cannot explain it in terms of his/her own attempts. He/She feels that the solution occurs by a sudden flash. But illumination can be well explained, taking the incubation period into account.

Verification

The solution of idea that results from illumination cannot be the final stage of creative thinking. The idea should well fit in the system of existing knowledge. Hence, evaluation of the solution is the essential stage following the solution. Especially, for the scientific invention, it is necessary to get idea verified and see whatever it is correct and workable.

Revision

The final stage is that of revision where the new solutions are further tested by applying them to other situations. Many thinkers find it necessary to get their ideas revised and modified before the results of their thinking are satisfactory.

■ PROBLEM SOLVING

Problem solving is an important characteristic of thinking, i.e. problem-solving behavior. It is always directed toward the solution of a problem. Whenever a need arises, man tries to satisfy it by some already established pattern of behavior. A problematic situation arises, when this fixed pattern fails to satisfy the need. Man is constantly faced by some problems or the other, as his/her needs are numerous. Even when the needs necessary for his/her physical and social well-being are satisfied, he/she may still have a number of intellectual or spiritual needs, which has to get satisfied. Being thus constantly confronted with problems, man has to keep on thinking all the time. If he/she stops thinking, the problems due to the unsatisfied needs may affect his/her adjustment to life. He/She has to think in the most diverse possible manner.

Definition

1. Problem-solving behavior occurs in novel or difficult situations in which a solution is not obtainable by the habitual methods of applying concepts and principles derived from past experience in very familiar situations.
   —*Woodworth and Marquis*
2. Problem solving is a process of overcoming difficulties that appear to interfere with the attainment of a goal. It is a procedure of making adjustment in spite of interferences. —*Skinner*

Scientific Methods of Problem Solving

Problem Awareness

The first step in the problem-solving behavior of an individual concerns his/her awareness of the difficulty or problem that needs a solution. He/She must be confronted with some obstacle or interference in the path of the realization of his/her needs or motives and consequently they must be conscious of the felt difficulty or problem.

Problem Understanding

The difficulty or problem felt by the individual should be properly identified by a careful analysis. He/She should be clear about what exactly is his/her problem. The problem then should be pin pointed in terms of the specific goals and objectives.

Collection of the Relevant Information

In this step, the individual is required to collect all the relevant information about the problem through all possible sources. He/She may consult experienced persons, read the available literature, revive his/her old experiences, think of possible solutions and put in all relevant efforts for widening the scope of knowledge concerning the problem in hand.

Formulation of Hypothesis or Hunch for Possible Solutions

In the light of the collected relevant information and nature of his/her problem, one may engage in some serious cognitive activities to think of the various possibilities for the solution of one's problem.

Selection of a Proper Solution

In this important step, all the possible solutions thought in the previous step are closely analyzed and evaluated. Gates and others (1946) have suggested the following activities in the evaluation of the assumed hypotheses or solution:

1. One should determine the conclusion that completely satisfies the demand of the problem.
2. One should find out whether the solution is consistent with other facts and principles, which have been well established.
3. One should make a deliberate search for negative instances, which might cast doubts on the conclusion.

Verification of the Concluded Solutions or Hypothesis

The solution arrived at or conclusion drawn must be further verified by utilizing it in the solution of the various likewise problem. In case, the derived solution helps in solving these likewise problems, then only one is free to agree with his/her findings regarding the solution of his/her problem.

An important step in problem solving is the direction or set. A wrong direction may interfere with the correct solution of the problem. A flexibility of mental set is often helpful in giving the proper direction to problem solving. The thinking, which is done in problem solving, is goal directed and is motivated by the need to reduce discrepancy between one state of affairs and another. The direction required for problem solving is given by the rules associated with the solutions of most of the problem. In everyday problems, these rules are supplied by our social experience. In some formal problems they are the part of the problem itself. Some of these rules when followed correctly, guarantee a solution to a problem. In most problems where such rules are not supplied one falls back on the past experiences with problems, which are likely to lead to a solution. The problem at hand is broken down in smaller such problems, each of which is a little closer to the end goal. However, there is no guarantee of correct solutions. Hence, thinking may be described as an implicit problem-solving behavior.

■ ATTRIBUTION

Social perception is the process through which one seeks to know and understand others. It is the most basic aspect of social life. One always try to understand others current or present feelings, moods, emotions, etc. The process through which one seeks to determine the causes behind others behavior is known attribution. In other words attribute refers to the effects to understand causes behind behavior and on some occasions, the causes behind one's own behavior. Attribute are influences that people draw about causes of events, others and their own behavior. Attribution is necessary to understand the experiences. If one can attribute other's behavior, it will help in making adjustments with others and to maintain self-image.

Theories of Attribution (Fig. 13.7)

Kelly's Covariation Model

Kelly's covariation model is based on assumption that people attribute behavior to factors that are present when the behavior takes place and absent when it does not. According to Kelly, when people attempt to infer the cause of an actor's behavior they usually consider three types of behavior.

Consensus: At first, one considers to the extent to which an individual responds in the same manner to different stimuli or situation.

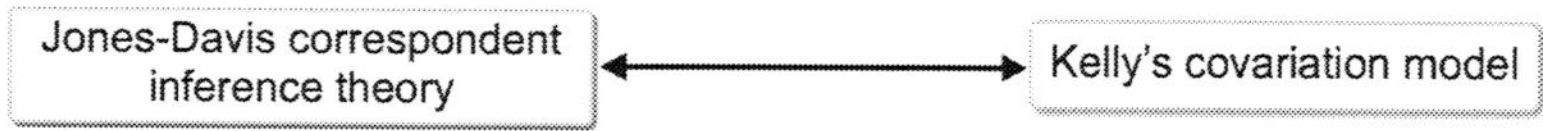

Figure 13.7: Theories of attribution

Consistency: One considers constancy, the extent to which this reacts to stimulus or event in the same way on other occasions.

Distinctiveness: The extent to which the person reacts in the same manner for other different stimulus and events.

According to Kelly, low consistency favors an external attribution, but high consistency is compatible with either an internal or external attribution.

Jones-Davis Correspondent Inference Theory

Jones-Davis correspondent inference theory describes how with information about others behavior is used as a basis for inferring their stable traits and hence when one is making attributions about the people, one compares their action with alternative actions, evaluating the choices they have made. Information about five factors is sought to make their inferences:

1. Whether the behavior being considered is voluntary and freely chosen?
2. What is unexpected about the behavior (rare effects)?
3. Whether the behavior is socially desirable?
4. Whether the behavior impacts the person?

■ WAYS TO IMPROVE THINKING

Keeping oneself only with current project; clutters create confusion. Getting organized and working with fresh canvas. On an average, one spends about 45 minutes a day looking for things. Dedicating an hour of focus time to the most important task, multitasking is highly over-rated and cause a loss of up to 40% efficiency. Get 1 hour of focused seclusion to work on the most important task. Stir up the visual sense and creative talents with exposure to the arts, go to a gallery picking up an art book or spending time with nature. Some of the ways are:

1. Learn how to mind map: This is a best practice that allows one to visualize and map the projects and strategies. It is also a life-saving memory device that will help to remember more and organize the thinking.
2. Give rest for thinking: When one has been working on something for more than an hour, one starts losing concentration and focus. So stop, get up and walk around and go back to the work.

Alterations in Thinking

Psychosis

Psychosis is a major psychiatric disorder in which reality testing is not intact; behavior may violate gross social norm. It is just opposite to nervous in which reality testing is intact and behavior may not violate social norms. Many psychiatric disorders such as schizophrenia, mania, depression, etc. come under psychosis. It includes various disturbances in thinking.

Delusion

Delusion is a false, persistent, irrational belief not shared by persons of some age, race, education and standard, which cannot be altered by logical arguments (Table 13.1).

Table 13.1: Types of delusions

Sl No.	Types	Descriptions
1	Persecutory delusions	The individuals feel interfered, discriminates against threatened or mistreated, e.g. the patient says, my family members wants to kill me
2.	Delusion of reference	The individual feels that others are talking about him/her, other's remarks/actions have special significance for him/her
3.	Delusions of influence/passivity	The individual believes that he/she is influenced by and controlled by others, e.g. the cardiologist puts transmitter near heart that controls my feelings and thoughts
4.	Delusion of sin and guilt	The individual has a belief that he/she has committed unforgivable sin/some wickedness in past leads to calamity to others; so he/she is evil and worthless
5.	Hypochondriacal delusions	These are delusions of some bodily diseases
6.	Delusion of grandeur	The individual has an exaggerated feeling of importance, power, knowledge or identity

■ CONCLUSION

Thinking starts with a problem and concludes with its solution. This activity of thinking continuous till either the solution is found or till the person becomes fatigued by the effort. There cannot be any thinking in the absence of some problem. Problems in human life come in an incessant stream and they have to be solved by thinking. Thinking the mental solution of problem, makes use of the symbols of objects instead of the objects. Thinking attempts the solution of problems by employing the trial and error method. There is a kind of flow in the activity of thinking, one problem leads to thinking of another by reminding the person another problem.

■ REVIEW QUESTIONS

Long Essays

1. Define thinking. Explain the nature and types of thinking. Describe various ways to improve thinking.
2. Describe the favorable and unfavorable elements of thinking.
3. Define problem solving. Explain various steps involved in problem solving.

Short Essays

4. Describe the tools used for measurement of thinking.
5. Explain various types of thinking.
6. Define reasoning. Explain characteristics of reasoning.
7. Enumerate the assessment of reasoning and problem solving.
8. Discuss the steps involved in creative thinking.
9. Discuss attribution. Explain various theories of attribution.
10. Briefly explain alternations in thinking.

Short Answers

11. Creative thinking.
12. Abstract thinking.
13. Deductive reasoning.
14. Steps of reasoning.
15. Formation of hypothesis.
16. Types of delusions.

CHAPTER 14

Intelligence

■ INTRODUCTION

The term intelligence is derived from Latin word 'intelligence' coined by Cicero, used to cover all mental process. The individuals differ from one another in their ability to understand complex ideas, to adapt effectively to the environment, to learn from experience, to engage in various forms of reasoning and to overcome obstacles by taking thought. Owning to their intelligence, they are to be considered better than other animals. Some people are very intelligent, while others do not have that ability. Intelligence is not a single trait or character, rather it is a combination of many triads. Intelligence is a composition of capabilities that make a person rational, able to think correctly and act purposefully. Persons can learn through signs and symbols, and can adjust effectively with their environment. Most of the people have an intuitive notion of what intelligence is and many words in English language distinguish between different levels of intellectual skills, i.e. bright, dull, smart, stupid, clever, slow and so on. It is necessary for a nurse to learn about intelligence, because difference in the amount and quality of intelligence bring and in their ability to make adjustments to situations around them. Intelligent patients want more explanations for their treatment they are getting, whereas less intelligent patients will be satisfied with a little or no explanations.

■ MEANING OF INTELLIGENCE

Intelligence is one of the most studied and debated personal qualities of the human being. It is invisible, cannot be directly seen, yet it is studied at greater length and is considered to be one of our most important qualities. The study of intelligence has made psychology a more interesting subject, but still psychologists are not unanimous about the nature of intelligence. Many aspects of intelligence are included in intelligent behavior because intelligence is a conceptual structure with many characteristics. It is difficult to perceive intelligence in physical form, but intelligent behavior can be assessed by the practicality, success in examinations and objectives, mental maturity and ability to adjust, etc. other than these ability to express himself/herself, sharpness of memory, ability to perceive, foresight, ability to forecast results, etc. also help in determining the intelligent behavior of person. Potential to accept challenges and passing the examination with good division, behaving as per one's age, position, prestige and social status are also the indicators of intelligent behavior.

■ DEFINITIONS

1. Intelligence is the potential or ability of a person to adjust to new conditions. *—William Stern*
2. Intelligence can be defined as the ability of a person to act purposefully, think rationally and deal effectively with his environment. *—DL Wechsler*
3. Intelligence can be described as the ability to learn quickly at a given time and to remember the learned material. *—Harbour and Freud*
4. Intelligence is organized around an ideal portiere. One's intelligence is defined by the degree of resemblance to this prototype. Since, there exist multiple prototypes; there would be no validated concept of intelligence. *—Nesser*
5. One's adaptation to the environment is called intelligence. *—Piaget*
6. Intelligence defined as a biological mechanism by which the effects of the complexity of stimuli are brought together and given a somewhat unified effect in behavior. *—Peterson*
7. Intelligence is the capacity to learn and adjust to relatively new and changing conditions. *—Wagnon*
8. An individual is intelligent in proportion as he/she is able to carry on abstract thinking. *—Terman*
9. Intelligence means intellect put to use. It is the use of intellectual abilities for handling a situation or accomplishing any task. *—Woodworth and Marquis*
10. Intelligence is defined as a mental activity consisting of grasping the essentials in a situation and responding appropriately to them. *—Heim*
11. Intelligence is defined as the effective all-round cognitive abilities to comprehend, to grasp relations and reasons. *—Vernon*
12. Intelligence is the capacity to learn and adjust to relatively new and changing conditions. *—Wagnon*
13. Intelligence is the property of recombining our behavior patterns so as to act better in a novel situation. *—Wells*
14. Intelligence is an ability demand in the solution of problems, which require the comprehension and use of symbols. *—Garret*
15. An intelligent person uses past experience effectively, is able to concentrate and keep his attention focused for longer periods of times, adjusts his/her to a new and unaccustomed situation rapidly, with less confusion and with fewer false moves. Variability of responses is able to see distinct relationships, can carry on abstract thinking, has a great capacity of inhibition or delay and is capable of exercising self-criticism. *—Husband*
16. Intelligence may be defined as the power of good responses from the point of view of truth or facts. *—Thorndike*

■ NATURE OF INTELLIGENCE

1. Intelligence is an innate mental ability, which grows and is influenced by the environment.
2. It shows the capacity to adapt to new or changed situations quickly and correctly.
3. It consists of the ability to carry on the higher mental processes each as reasoning, criticism, application and judgment.
4. It implies the capacity to learn difficult tasks and the ability to solve increasing difficult problems.
5. It shows the capacity to observe relationships and detect absurdities.
6. Intelligence may be regarded as a sort of mental energy (in the form of mental or cognitive abilities) available with an individual to enable him/her to handle his/her environment in terms of adaptation and facing novel situations as effectively as possible.

TYPES OF INTELLIGENCE

According to Sternberg's Triarchic Theory of Human Intelligence (1995), it is of three types (Fig. 14.1):

1. Analytical intelligence.
2. Creative intelligence.
3. Practical intelligence.

Analytical Intelligence

Analytical intelligence is academic problem-solving skills, based on combined operations of execution, performance and knowledge. These three operations will enable us to encode stimuli, hold information in short-term memory, make calculations, perform mental calculations and mentally compare different stimuli and retrieve information from long-term memory.

Creative Intelligence

Creative intelligence involves insights, synthesis and the ability to react to novel situations and stimuli. It consists of ability, which allows people to think creatively and adjust creatively and effectively to new situations. Novel task or situations are good measure of intellectual ability, because they assess an individual's ability to apply existing knowledge to new problems.

Practical Intelligence

Practical intelligence is the intelligence, which operates in the real world. People with this type of intelligence can adapt to or shape their environment. It is not only influenced by mental skills but also to attitudes and emotional factors. Gardner (1999) proposes eight type of intelligence:

1. **Linguistic intelligence:** Involved in reading, writing, listening and talking.
2. **Logical (mathematic) intelligence:** Involved in solving logical puzzles, deriving proofs and performing calculations.
3. **Musical intelligence:** Involved in playing, composing, singing and conducting, furthermore. Gardner believes that auto mechanics and cardiologists may have this kind of intelligence in abundance.
4. **Spatial intelligence:** Involved in moving from one location to another or determine one's orientation in space.
5. **Intrapersonal intelligence:** Involved in understanding oneself and having insight into one's own thoughts, actions and emotions, e.g. self-understanding.
6. **Bodily-kinesthetic intelligence:** Involved in using one's own body (or parts of it) to perform skillful and purposeful movements, e.g. dancer, athletes and surgeons.
7. **Naturalistic intelligence:** It involves the ability to understand and work effectively in the natural world, e.g. biologists and zoologists.
8. **Interpersonal intelligence:** Involved in understanding of others and one's reaction to others. Being high in social skills; psychologists, teacher and politicians are supposed to be high in this type of intelligence.

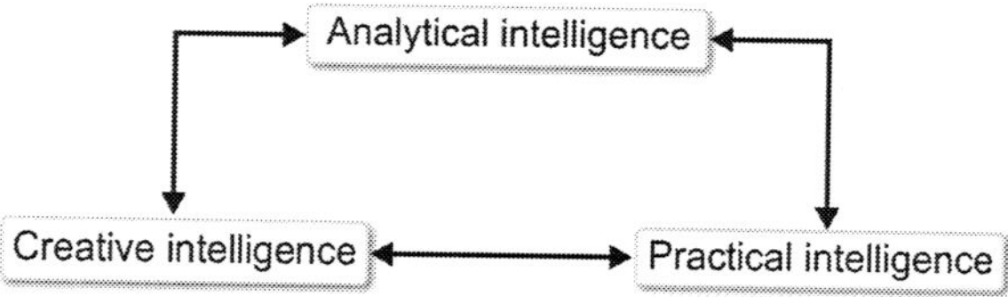

Figure 14.1: Types of intelligence

■ FACTORS INFLUENCING INTELLIGENCE

Biochemical Factors

1. From the recent studies it is found that the disturbances of biochemical balances of the body may underlie various disorders of learning and intelligence.
2. For optimum functioning of the nervous system, sufficient supply of oxygen and various nutrients are necessary. Apart from these, body temperature, pH balance and hormones also influence neural activities and thereby affect intellectual performances.
3. It is found that the defective genes may lead to defective enzyme functioning and this in turn produces a rare condition known as phenylpyruvic oligophrenia a type of feeble mindedness.
4. Cretinism is another type of mental deficiency caused by underactivity of the thyroid gland in childhood.
5. Mongolian idiocy is caused by defective cerebral metabolism. If the mother becomes pregnant nearing to menopause, the biochemical imbalances during pregnant may cause mongolian idiocy. Thus, various factors affect the growth of intelligence.

Sociocultural Factors (Fig. 14.2)

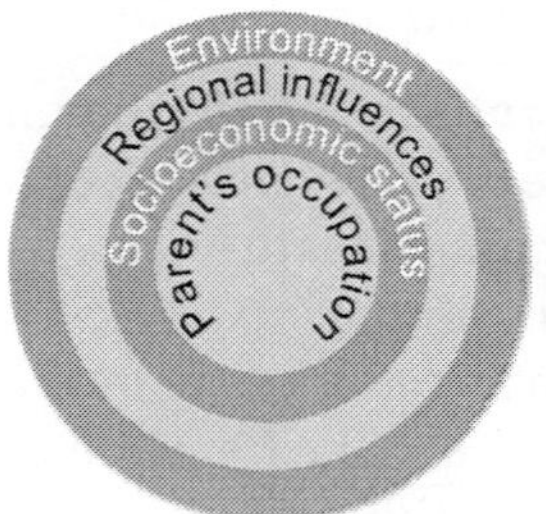

Figure 14.2: Sociocultural factors

All the intelligence tests to some extent or the other are subjected to the influence of sociocultural factors, because the test items are drawn from the culture from whom the test is developed. The tests reflect the cultural experiences and reveal how well an individual deals with cultural factors.

Parent's Occupation

It is found from the studies that there are pronounced difference in the intelligence quotient (IQ) of children, whose parents belong to different occupational groups. The children of professional parents have a mean IQ of about 115, children of laborers have a mean IQ of 94 and of intermediate occupational groups range between these two extremes. The rationale behind this is that only higher intellectual ability can reach higher occupation.

Socioeconomic Status

Socioeconomic status is more comprehensive factor than occupation. It includes factors such as education, source and level of income, ethnic and residential area, etc. The socioeconomic differences in IQ are attributed to the factors, which account for occupational differences. In any society, more intelligent man tend to rise up in the socioeconomic scale and remains there, while the less intelligent man comes down and remains in the lower strata.

Regional Influences

Regional location is correlated with performance on intelligence tests. According to McNemar, the mean IQ was 108 for urban children, 107 for suburban children and 96 for rural children. Cities offer better schools, better educational facilities, affords wide variety of extracurricular and recreational facilities, and thus provides a greater challenge to the growing child.

Environment

The environment wherein the educational facilities are poor and outside contacts are rare, will reduce the IQ as they grow older. In short, the poor environment will have progressively adverse effect as the age increases. On the other hand enriched environment are provided to the children. But it will have more beneficial effect it provided very early in life. If it is provided after 7 years of life, it will have no effect. Thus, various biochemical and environmental factors contribute their share to the intellectual growth of the individual.

■ INTELLIGENCE QUOTIENT

The intellectual capacity of the person can be accessed through IQ. This works as a guide in the future, but it is essential to know the stability and limits of IQ. The IQ of 80% of people is either 100 or around 100. According to modern concept, IQ is a measurement of quality and assessment of intelligence. Stanford-Binet had invented the method of quantifying and measuring intelligence. IQ can be obtained by multiplying the ratio of mental age and chronological age by 100. This can be explained by following formula:

$$IQ = \frac{\text{Mental age}}{\text{Chronological age}} \times 100$$

Mental Age

Mental age represents the development of performance level of a child at certain age. In other words, if 5-year-old child is able to do the tests meant for 6 years old, his/her mental age would be counted as 6 years. Failures in the tests meant for a particular age group, reduces the mental age.

Chronological Age

Chronological age is the physical age of the child that is based on his/her date of birth.

Distribution of IQ

Psychologists have described level of intelligence in many ways. The normal levels of IQ is explained in Table 14.1.

Intelligence quotient is determined by both hereditary and the environment. Hence, level of intelligence may change as result of environment. Similarly, repeated tests and using different types of tests may show a change in intelligence level.

Table 14.1: Levels of intelligence

Sl No.	Intelligence quotients	Descriptions
1.	140 and above	Genius
2.	120–139	Very superior
3.	110–119	Superior
4.	90–109	Normal
5.	80–89	Low normal
6.	70–79	Borderline
7.	50–69	Moron
8.	25–49	Imbecile
9.	0–24	Idiot

■ INTELLIGENCE TESTS

History of Intelligence Tests

In the beginning, mental tests were devised to study individual differences among college students. These tests were used to measure the speed of reaction, sensory acuity and other simple psychological processes. The primary interest was to study the extent of individual differences and not to assess the level of intelligence of the individual.

In 1896, Binet, a French psychologist who was studying process of school suggested special classes for children showing poor progress in classwork. About 8 years later, the French government requested Binet to discover children in public school, who were not having sufficient intelligence to benefit themselves by usual instruction.

Measurement of Intelligence Tests

Measurement of intelligence tests (Fig. 14.3) can be classified into the following categories:

1. **Individual intelligence tests:** These tests measure the intelligence of one person at a time. These are used to measure the intelligence of retarded children or to provide treatment and guidance. Major limitations of these tests include the skills of examiner and problems of qualification. Financially, these tests are more expensive. These tests can be administered not only individually but also as a group at a time. For example, Alexander's Battery of performance test, Bhatia tests of intelligence, form board test, Stanford-Binet, Wechsler's test, etc.
2. **Group intelligence tests:** This method of measuring intelligence is used to measure the intelligence of more than one person. These tests are very popular. Group intelligence tests were also used in World War I to measure the intelligence of the literature and illiterate soldiers. These tests can be administered to be a large number of individuals at a time, e.g. army alpha, army beta and Raven's Progressive Matrices (RPM).
3. **Verbal intelligence test:** In this test, intelligence of a person is measured on the basis of his/her answer or reactions to the given questions. This is a reliable test and is useful for both the individuals and group, but the examinees should have the knowledge of language or words. Examiner should be highly skilled to get maximum results from these tests.
4. **Non-verbal performance tests:** It involves no language, but require duplication of block patterns, completion of jigsaw puzzle, arrangements of pictures, drawing, etc. For example, Goddard's from board, Link's from board, Alexander's battery of performance tests, RPM, etc.
5. **Verbal, non-verbal combined tests:** It include both verbal and non-verbal items. For example, Wechsler's test for children and adults, Bhatia's test of intelligence, Army alpha and beta test of performance, Army General Classifications Test (AGCT), Armed Force Qualification Test (AFQT), etc.
6. **Power tests:** These tests allow sufficient time to the subject to try most or all the items he/she can do. The score they obtain as an indicator of their achievement, e.g. RPM.

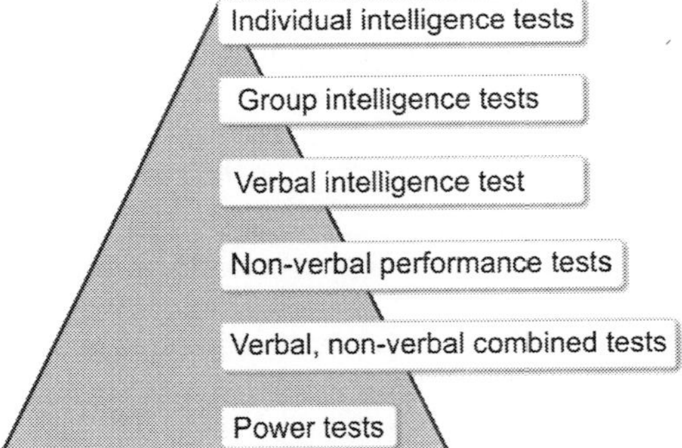

Figure 14.3: Measurement of intelligence tests

Uses of Intelligence Test

Intelligence tests are used in many walks of life to determine the levels of IQ of an individual, which is of utmost importance for success in any walk of life. Hence, innumerable tests have come into existence and this reveals its importance in life. Some of the areas in which intelligence tests are useful are:

1. Intelligence tests have helped us to understand fully the nature of the intelligence.
2. As intelligence plays a very significant role in the determination of personality; intelligence tests are used as a part of personality assessment.
3. Intelligence tests are useful to dispel the wrong notions of racial differences,

sex differences, caste differences, etc. These tests have ruled out the superiority of any race, sex or caste in intelligence over others.

4. Intelligence tests are useful in educational guidance of children. By determining the IQ, child may be guided to take up a particular course of study for which he/she studied.
5. Intelligence tests are used in many educational institutions to select the students for admission. If the student is found below the required level of intelligence for the courses they offer, they may be rejected.
6. Intelligence tests are also used as a part of vocational guidance. The success in any vocation partly depends upon intelligence in addition to aptitude and interest.

Other Uses

1. Studying the individual differences.
2. Identifying the retarded children and treating them.
3. Help in the field of education.
4. Finding the solution of disciplinary problems.
5. Use in business skills.
6. Use in armed forces.
7. Help in research work.

■ THEORIES OF INTELLIGENCE (Table 14.2)

Spearman's Two-factor Theory

Charles Spearman has proposed this two-factor theory of intelligence. According to Spearman, intelligence constitutes of two factors, they are:

1. General intelligence factor or G factor.
2. Specific intelligence or special factor called S factor.

He further said the G factor varies from person to person. Depending upon the amount of G they possess, people are described as generally brought bright or generally dull. Intelligence tests measure the amount of G factor, which individual possess.

Table 14.2: Theories of intelligence

Sl No.	Theories	Descriptions
1.	Monarchic theory or unitary theory	The theory holds that intelligence is one power or energy, which affects all the activities of the individual According to Victoria Hazlitt, intelligence is a general ability that determines the various specific abilities The theory has been proven to be fallacious Prominent people show a less than average ability in many activities, e.g. Darwin had a very bad handwriting
2.	Oligarchic theory	This theory postulates that intelligence is an aggregate of mutually independent powers Binet believed this theory Experiments disproved this theory by showing the mental powers are interdependent
3.	Multifactor or anarchic theory, or group factor theory (Thurstone, 1933)	Thorndike is the most prominent among those who believed this theory This theory holds that intelligence is the mean of undetermined independent rudimentary elements But Spearman has criticized this theory

Contd...

Contd...

Sl No.	Theories	Descriptions
4.	Two-factor theory (Spearman, 1927)	This theory was conceived by Spearman, who holds that intelligence has two parts such as general intelligence or G and specific intelligence or S Specific intelligence is confined to specific activities General intelligence is found in lesser or greater degree in everyone Specific intelligence is of various types, the several types being independent of each other They differ from individual to individual This intelligence of a person depends on his/her general intelligence
5.	Structure of intellect model (Guilford, 1959)	In structure of intellect model, he postulated many factors of intelligence He categorized these factors under three-board dimensions: • The process or operation performed • The kind of product involved • The kind of material or content involved. He then subclassified under each of these dimensions five operations, six types of products and four types of contents

The amount of S factor varies within the same individual. For example, a student may be very good in mathematics, but poor in spatial relations.

Louis Thurstone, another psychologist objected to Spearman's two-factor theory. Thurston said that human intelligence could break down into a number of primary abilities. His statistical studies lead to primary abilities (Table 14.3).

Group Factor Theory

Thurstone LL an American psychologist, while working on a trust of primary mental abilities, he came to the conclusion that certain mental operations have in common a primary factor, which gives them psychological and functional unity that differentiates them from other mental operations. These mental operations constitute a group factor. So, there are

Table 14.3: Primary abilities

Sl No.	Primary abilities	Descriptions
1.	Verbal comprehension	Ability to understand the meaning of words; vocabulary test intelligence measures this factor
2.	Word fluency	Ability to think words quickly
3.	Number	Ability to work with numbers and perform computations
4.	Space	Ability to visualize space from relationships, e.g. recognizing the same figure presentation in different orientation
5.	Memory	Ability to recall verbal stimulus such as pairs of words or sentences
6.	Perceptual speed	Ability to grasp visual details and to see similarities and differences between picture objects
7	Reasoning	Ability to find a general rule on the basis of presented instances

number of groups of mental abilities each of which has its own primary factor. Thurstone and his associates have differentiated nine such factors, which are detailed in Table 14.4.

The weakest link in the group factor theory was that it discarded the concept of common factor; it did not take much time for Thurstone to realize his mistake and to reveal a general factor in addition to group factors.

■ MENTALLY HANDICAPPED PERSON

Mentally handicapped person is one whose mental ability develops at a very slower rate than normal children of his/her age. They do not achieve the full intellectual functions of normal adult, finds difficulty in learning social adjustment and economic productivity. They will have physical and anatomical peculiarities and will be physically interior.

General Characteristics

1. Mentally handicapped person have difficulty in learning useful information and skills, poor in adaptation to new problems and conditions of life, profitless from experience, abstract and creative thinking is nil, critical judgment is absolutely poor. Reading, writing and arithmetic are so poor that are excluded from normal school. They forget soon unless reinforced by reviewing.
2. They are incapable of self-care, self-support or self-management in society. Need a lot of assistance during childhood. They must be fed, dressed, taken care against accidents and need supervision while playing, incapable of personal and social affairs even during adulthood. If not guided and controlled they may engage in delinquent acts. In short, they are incapable of adjusting to social environment by themselves.
3. It is difficult to draw and to hold their attention, interests are few, memory span is limited, and thinking is strenuous and hence avoids it.
4. The development of drives and emotions vary greatly with the degree of feeble mindedness. Laughing and giggling for no reason is common.
5. No two feeble minded are exactly alike in personality, but individual differences are less compared to normal. They are

Table 14.4: Factors of mental abilities

Sl No.	Factors	Descriptions
1.	Verbal factor (V)	Concerns comprehension of verbal relations, words and ideas
2.	Spatial factor (S)	Involved in any task in which the subject manipulates an object imaginatively in space
3.	Numerical factor (N)	Ability to do numerical calculations, rapidly and accurately
4.	Word fluency factor (W)	Involved whenever the subject is asked to think of the isolated words at rapid rate
5.	Inductive reasoning factor (RI)	Ability to draw inferences on conclusions on the basis of specific instances
6.	Memory factor (M)	Involving the ability to memorize quickly
7.	Deductive reasoning (DR)	Ability to make use of general results
8.	Perceptual factor (P)	Ability to perceive objects accurately
9.	Problem-solving ability factor (PS)	Ability to solve problems with independent efforts

rarely dynamic, charming, forceful, etc. they are submissive and easily subjected to influence, usually stable and apathetic.
6. They are very poor in physical resistance to illness and hence mortality is more.
7. They learn to walk and talk very much later than normal children. Their speech is defective, i.e. speeches are pedantic and walk with shuffling gait. Their visual and auditory defects are common at all levels. They are seemingly deaf, poor eye contact and unusual body language. These are some of the characteristic features of mentally handicapped persons.

Causes of Mental Retardation (Fig. 14.4)

There are more than 200 known causes and many more unknown causes. Some of the causes operate before birth, some during birth and some other after birth.

Prenatal Risk Factors

1. If the mother's age is under 15 years or over 40 years at the time of pregnancy, there is an increased risk of chromosomal abnormalities or prematurity.
2. History of difficult in previous pregnancy such as miscarriage, stillbirth, premature birth, etc.
3. Mother with chronic health disease such as diabetes mellitus, syphilis and hypertension.

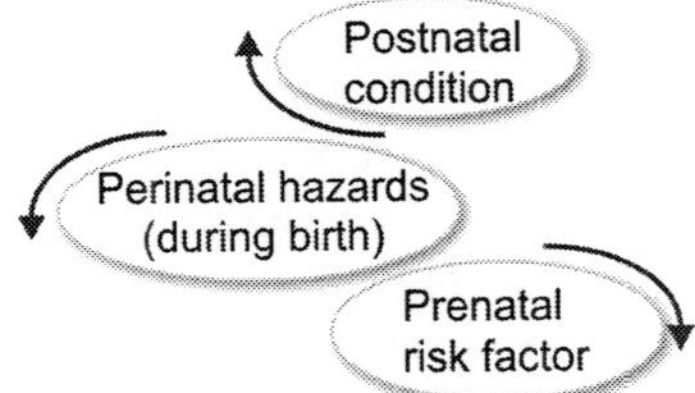

Figure 14.4: Causes of mental retardation

4. Parents with family history of congenital anomalies such as phenylketonuria (PKU) muscular dystrophy, etc.
5. Parental risk of biological origin, i.e. infections contacted during first 3 months of pregnancy, e.g. rubella, toxoplasmosis, cytomegalovirus (CMV), etc.
6. Subjecting pregnant lady (within 3 month) to frequent X-ray treatment.
7. Excessive drugging.
8. Taking certain drugs such as carbon monoxide, antitetanus serum, typhoid vaccine, etc. affect brain growth and development and cause mental efficiency.

Perinatal Hazards (During Birth)

1. Injury to head at the time of birth.
2. Anomalies (no respiration immediately after birth).
3. Deficiency of thiamine and glutamic acid.
4. Ineffective fevers such as encephalitis or meningitis and brain tumor.
5. Prematurely and low birth weight (intrauterine growth retardation) may cause congenital malformation and biological dysfunction.
6. Low blood pressure.
7. Premature separation of placenta.
8. Compression of cord.
9. Postmaturity, hypoglycemia and polycythemia.
10. Preeclampsia (toxemia of pregnancy).
11. Rh incompatibility along with the kernicterus.

Postnatal Condition

1. Meningitis.
2. Chronic lung diseases.
3. Meconium aspiration.
4. Persistent pulmonary hypertension.
5. Drugs.
6. Poisoning.
7. Poor nutrition or malnutrition.
8. Trauma during first 2 years of life.

9. Parent-child separation.
10. Very poor environment, which is not stimulating during babyhood and childhood.
11. Encephalitis affects the growth of intelligence and cause mental deficiency.

Classification of Mental Retardation (Fig. 14.5)

Borderline Mental Retardation

Borderline mental retardation people will have an IQ ranging between 68 and 83. These are slow learner and cannot understand complex ideas. Verbal training is slower than motor learning. They can make adequate adjustment to society and sometime they require help of others.

Mild Mental Retardation

Mild mental retardation people will have an IQ ranging between 52 and 67. They are equal to 8–11 years boys. They lack imagination, inventiveness and judgment. They need some supervision. With parental assistance and special attention, they can adjust socially, master simple skills and can become self-supporting.

Moderate Mental Retardation

Moderate mental retardation people will have an IQ ranging between 36 and 51, which is equal to 4–7 years old boys. They read and write a little, but very slow in learning. They look clumsy and suffer body deformities and motor coordination. With parental help and training, they can take care of themselves and be economically useful.

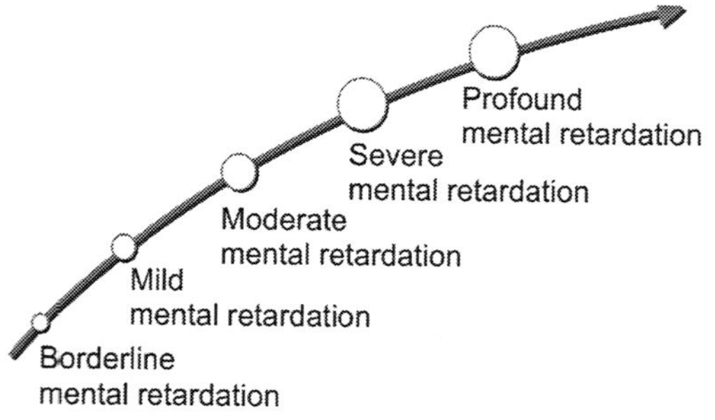

Figure 14.5: Classification of mental retardation

Severe Mental Retardation

Severe mental retardation people will have an IQ of 20–35, their motor and speech developments are severely retarded. Sensory defects and motor handicaps are common. They can develop limited personal hygiene and self-help skills. They can perform simple occupational tasks under supervision.

Profound Mental Retardation

Profound mental retardation people will have an IQ of 2 years child, absolutely deficits in adaptive behavior. Speech is very rudimentary, they will have severe physical deformities, retarded growth, convulsive seizures, mutism, deafness, etc. they largely depend on others. Resistance to disease is very low and short lived.

Clinical Types of Mental Retardation

Cretinism

Cretinism is a condition of mental deficiency and lack of physical and mental development caused by thyroid deficiency during prenatal and postnatal growth period.

Down Syndrome (Mongolism)

Down syndrome term is given to certain types of amentia, who have mongolian features; eyes are narrow slant and upward and poor muscular coordination. Mongoloids are particularly susceptible to circulatory, respiratory and gastrointestinal disorders.

Hydrocephalus

Hydrocephalus is a rare condition in which the accumulation of an abnormal amount of cerebrospinal fluid within cranium causes damage to the brain tissues and enlargement of the cranium. So, the skull looks very large. The head is either already enlarged at birth or begins to enlarge soon afterwards. This may be due to prenatal disturbances in the formation, absorption or circulation of the cerebrospinal fluid. The clinical picture depends on the extent of neural damage, this in turn, depends on the age at which the onset, duration and severity of the disorder. The degree of intellectual development varies depending upon the amount of pressure extorted on the brain tissue and damage caused to it.

Macrocephalus (Sclerotic Amentia)

Sclerotic amentia is a condition of enlarged head due to excessive development of glial cells or cells, which support the active nerves cells. Here, both skull and the face are grossly enlarged. On the basis of the shape of the head and skull, this can be differentiated from hydrocephalus. The main symptoms are pronounced mental defect, convulsions and fatty tumors of the face. Intelligence is below the level of imbecile. The mental age ranges between 3 and 7 years.

Microcephalus

The term microcephaly means small headedness. The head is usually small and cone shaped, and they are called pin-headed people. The circumference is usually less than 17 inch, as against normal 22 inch. The chin and forehead recede, hair is coarse, thick and wiry. The brain is small in size and less in weight. The convolutions are less and simpler than the normal. They are below average in stature and have a relatively short span of life. Microcephalics are uninhibited in their emotional expressions and restless, and hence quick in movement and repetition is much.

Phenylketonuria

Phenylketonuria is a rare metabolic disorder. They constitute about 1% of the mentally retarded population. The baby appears normal at birth, but lacks an enzyme needed to breakdown phenylalanine, which is an amino acid found in protein foods. If this condition is not detected, the phenylalanine accumulates in the blood and damages the brain. This appears between 6 and 12 months after birth with symptoms of vomiting, a peculiar odor, infantile eczema and seizures. The extent of retardation depends upon the degree of the disease progressed.

Congenital Syphilis

Children born to syphilitic mothers are sometimes infected with disease through placental circulation, while still in uterus. Many of these are terminated in abortion or stillbirth. Of those born alive many have normal mental development, but others are mentally retarded. These children will have generally physical handicaps such as paralysis of the limbs, epilepsy, blindness and deaf-mutism. Some children, who are infected show normal mental growth until puberty and then deteriorate, are diagnosed to have juvenile paresis.

Amaurotic Family Idiocy

Amaurotic family idiocy is also known as Tay-Sachs disease, which is very rare. This is essentially a neurological disorder characterized by diffused degeneration of brain cells, which leads to progressive blindness, wasting the limbs and mental enfeeblement. The mode of transmission is through mating of persons who are free of overt symptoms or carriers of the defective genes. This is more with the off spring of pedigrees of consanguineous mating.

Traumatic Amentia

Traumatic amentia brain injuries account for 5–10% of mental retardation. The cerebral damage may be inflicted before, during or after birth. Many cases are due to intracranial lesions and hemorrhages occurring during birth. In the later cases, there is always a history of difficult labor, with or without instrumental delivery. Severe head injuries occurring before or after birth sometimes result in mental deficiency. The degree of mental deficiency present in traumatic amentia ranges from idiocy to high-grade morality.

Pseudodementia

Pseudodementia, the ability is present but not used. He/She is an extreme introvert. External response is inadequate, because the patient is preoccupied with subjective problems. The mental ability is present, but is undeveloped because of inability to see or hear.

Treatment, Rehabilitation and Prevention

Mental retardation is not an illness and hence the question of treatment and cure do not arise when it sets in. It is a lifelong condition. No amount of training or medical care will transform a mentally retarded child into normal child. However, certain condition contributory to mental retardation can be improved or cured. For example, deafness, poor vision, emotional disturbances, poor living conditions, deficiency of nutrition and glandular imbalance makes the child to appear retarded. Early detection can help to lessen the degree of handicap. It is mainly a problem of education and rehabilitation. The treatment for mentally retarded lies in the stimulation and education from the earliest possible moment to develop their limited potentialities to the maximum possible extent. Mental ability grows when nourished by love and care.

Treatment Process (Fig. 14.6)

Parent education: The parents of the mentally retarded must be educated to accept the child's limitation and the permanency of mental retarded. Generally, parents refuse to admit that something is wrong with their child. Even when they realize that the child is subnormal, they believe that special education and good medical attention can make them normal, and hence spend a lot of money, but will be disappointed. So, it is essential to provide intensive parental counseling to enable family to provide love and security to the retarded child.

Home training: Home is the natural place for the beginning of training. Almost all mentally retarded remain at home during infancy and even during adulthood. Their mother's emotional attitude is of major importance. Some mothers reject and ignore their mentally retarded child and some are overprotective, even at the cost of normal children. In spite of the fact that a mentally retarded child is slow in learning and has poor memory. Some of the proper home training given by mother are:

1. The mother should make every effort to teach the child to feed and dress themselves, talk, walk and acquire habits of personal cleanliness.
2. As they grow up, they should be given responsibilities and duties to their mental abilities.
3. Special attention must be given for moral and personality training.
4. Misdeeds and temper outbursts should be checked and pleasant disposition must be encouraged.
5. The sibling and other children in the family should be encouraged to accept

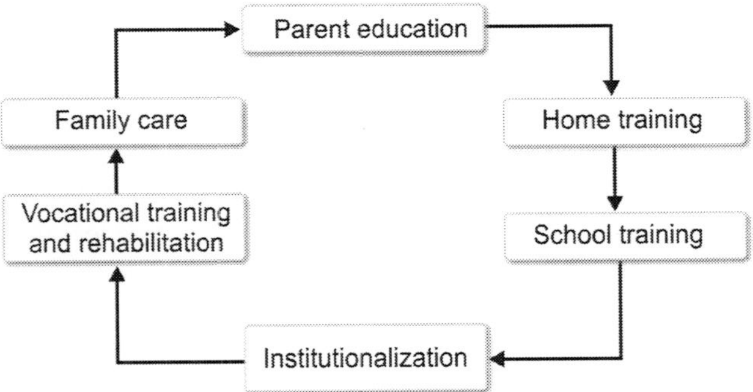

Figure 14.6: Treatment process

the sibling as less intelligent, but as an equal member of the family.

6. Opportunity to play with other children in the neighborhood should be permitted, but care must be taken to see that other children do not ridicule or exploit the defective child.

School training: Idiots and imbeciles cannot be sent to school, because they cannot be educated. Only morons can be sent to school at the age of 8 and not earlier, because of slow growth of mental ability. It is better to put them with other feeble minded of the same age to special classes. This has many advantages:

1. They need not have to compete with bright children and avoid ridicule and humiliation for failure.
2. In special classes, the competition will be with equals and hence, can experience some measure of achievement and success.
3. The curriculum of the special classes can be fitted to the capacity of the defective children.
4. The class can go slow with more emphasis on developing motor coordination, speech and desirable social traits.
5. The teacher can devote more time and attention to each pupil, which is very essential.

Institutionalization: Generally, these are overcrowded. Children sent to these schools are of two groups. One group is chiefly of idiots and imbeciles, who are generally handicapped. The parents are unwilling or unable to care for them at home. The second group consists of morons. These children (older) due to undesirable or delinquent behavior necessitate segregation from society. A large number of these are discharged after a period of social and occupational training, but the former group remains in the institution till their death.

Vocational training and rehabilitation: Higher grade defectives can be taught a variety of occupations, which will make them work in sheltered workshops or in open employment and can become self-supporting. Imbeciles can be trained for simple farming, laundry, dairy and kitchen work. Morons can be trained to assist carpenters, bakers, tailor, shoe maker, electricians, etc. They can also be trained to do complex farm work, poultry and livestock, and to operate many kind of machines, etc. thus they can be made self-supporting.

Family care: This is more economical and desirable way of segregating the mentally retards, by putting them under families in rural homes. This is better and keeping them in institution.

Legal facilities, insurance and trust schemes: For the retards must be provided, to make them economically independent.

Child guidance clinics: To help diagnosis the handicap and assess the children must be set up so that necessary action can be taken to improve their lots.

Home nursing and parent counseling program: Must be established to help the parents care for their children and to manage day-to-day problems.

Trained personnel: Like teachers, psychologists, occupational therapists and specialists in the concerned medical fields and social worker must be provided to cater to their special needs.

Specialized diagnostic facilities and special wards: These must be provided for them in all major hospitals and specialty in children's hospitals. The government should recognize their functional rights.

Prevention of Mental Retardation

1. Sterilization of all the imbeciles and morons on social ground is desirable, especially to girls. Defective boys rarely marry or produce children, because they cannot compete with normal boys for female attraction.
2. Institutionalization: If not sterilized, promiscuous defective girls must be institutionalized for the entire period of reproductive years. However, sterilization as a social measure is found to be useful.
3. Routine health measures: For the pregnant mother, precautions against possibility of intrauterine or birth damages and use of various diagnostic measures to detect and correct abnormalities early, can help prevent such births.
4. After detecting the defect early, if normal stimulating environment is provided, many kinds of mental retardation, which were once thought to be hereditary and inevitable, can be prevented to a great extent.
5. Genetic counseling: It is realized now that chromosomal anomalies lead to faculty development. Tests are developed to identify parents, who have these anomalies and to provide them genetic counseling, which will help prevention of such births.
6. Another way of prevention is alleviation of sociocultural conditions, which deprive children the necessary stimulation, motivation and opportunity for normal learning and mental development.

■ APPLICATIONS OF INTELLIGENCE IN NURSING

1. Hospitalized children, who are in the sensor motor stage have not achieved object permanence and therefore suffer from separation anxiety. They are best off if their mothers are allowed to stay with them overnight.
2. Children at the preoperational stage, who are unable to deal with concepts and abstractions, benefit more from role playing for medical procedures and situations than by having them verbally described in detail, e.g. a child who is to receive intravenous (IV) therapy is helped by acting out the procedure with a toy IV set and dolls.
3. As the children could not understand the cause and effect may interpret physical illness as punishment for bad thoughts or deeds.
4. Adolescent's thinking may appear abstract. Nurse can explain the procedure to an individual on the basis of his/her intellectual ability. They know to what extent, they can explain. Otherwise they educate the parents/relatives about necessary details of the patient. During any nursing procedure, the nurse must always understand the particular age and his/her cognitive ability.

NURSES' ROLE IN INTELLIGENCE

1. Knowledge about the nature of intelligence and its measurement is useful to the nurse in understanding themselves, their colleagues as well as their patients.
2. Nurse's explanations or guidance to the patient would be according to the patient's intellectual level.
3. As a student and later as a teacher the knowledge of intellectual function is useful for a nurse. Teaching method, content of the subject matter and expectations from students should be based on student's intellectual functioning.
4. Knowledge regarding intelligence helps the nurse in diagnosing a patient with mental subnormality or with very superior intelligence.
5. In diseases related to neuropsychiatry disorders, epilepsy, psychiatric disorders and some of the endocrinal disorders, assessment of intelligence is of great assistance in their management.
6. Knowledge about abnormalities in newborns and development of their intelligence helps the nurse in providing suitable care.
7. Ageing patients though physically slow, retain their levels of intelligence.
8. Respect and encouragement with the right mix of nursing care has to be ensured. Every individual is unique, especially when intelligence is the judging factor.
9. A nurse in the course of discharging his/her duties has to heavily rely on verbal and non-verbal communication patterns. They may have to interact with the patient, their family members, explain and clarify procedures and medications. The intelligence level of the patient and their family members decide how effectively the nurse is able to communicate and discharge their duties. Lower the levels of intelligence, more the time and patience the nurse will have to invest in caring for the patient.
10. The instructions may have to be simple and repeated more often. However, where the patient is more intelligent, they can be expected to take an active part in their own health care in the future.

CONCLUSION

The term intelligence is a very popular term used widely to mean many things such as quick understanding, fast learning, accuracy in learning, clever talking, quick doing, good memory, etc. Intelligence is generally mistaken for intellect. The concept of intelligence is defined by psychologists in different ways. There is little agreement regarding the suitability of the definition of intelligence. The most general definition stresses versatility or flexibility of adjustment. Alfred Binet, the pioneer in this field defines intelligence as something that is sensory acuity tests or reaction time experiments measure. As child grows older their intelligence also grows correspondingly. Under normal conditions, both chronological age and mental age increases proportionately up to 13 years. According to the studies, the growth of intelligence in the early childhood is rapid. It begins to slow down around the age of 12 or 13. The yearly increment becomes smaller and smaller until the growth ceases.

■ REVIEW QUESTIONS

Long Essays

1. Define intelligence. Explain the meaning and nature of intelligence.
2. Describe the various factors that influence intelligence.
3. Write about various theories of intelligence in detail.

Short Essays

4. Describe various types of intelligence.
5. Explain intelligence quotient. Describe measurement of intelligence.
6. List out the uses of intelligence tests.
7. Describe the general characteristics of mentally retarded children.
8. Discuss the clinical types of mental retardation.
9. Explain the nurse's role in improvement of intelligence.

Short Answers

10. Analytical intelligence.
11. Unitary theory.
12. Two-factor theory.
13. Causes of mental retardation.
14. Classifications of mental retardation.
15. Pseudodementia.
16. Prevention of mental retardation.

CHAPTER 15

Aptitude

■ INTRODUCTION

It is an observable fact that the people differ from one another and within themselves in their performance, in one or the other field of human activity such as leadership, music, art, mechanical work, teaching, etc. We usually come across the individuals who under similar circumstances excel the other persons in acquiring certain specific jobs. Such persons are said to possess certain specific abilities or aptitudes, besides general intellectual abilities or intelligence, which help them in achieving success in some specific occupations or activities. Therefore, in a simple way, aptitude may be considered a special ability or specific capacity besides the general ability, which helps an individual to acquire a required degree of proficiency or achievement in a specific field.

■ MEANING AND CONCEPTS OF APTITUDE

An aptitude is the capacity of a person to achieve along special lines. It is a special tendency, bent, fitness or aptness due to a special neural or muscular organization possessed by the individual. Aptitudes make for special abilities and our achievements in special areas. Some of the well-known aptitudes are the mechanical, artistic, musical, numerical or nursing aptitudes. Aptitude is to be distinguished from present ability. It shows that although a certain individual does not possess certain ability, he/she can acquire it or have it, provide the opportunities are available. Specific aptitudes can be assessed by means of specific aptitude tests. They can help us in knowing people who will be able to acquire a high degree of proficiency in fairly specific skills within minimum of training. The results of aptitude tests can be used for vocational guidance and adjustment.

An aptitude may be considered a special ability or specific capacity besides the general intellectual ability, which helps an individual to acquired degree of proficiency or achievement in a specific field. An aptitude is the interaction of heredity and environment. An individual is born with certain potentialities and begins to learn immediately. Therefore, everything they learn enables them to learn still more. It embraces any characteristics, which predisposes to learning including intelligence, achievements, personality, interests and special skills.

Intelligence is concerned with the general mental ability of an individual, but aptitude is related to specific abilities. Thus, the knowledge of intelligence of an individual predicts his/her success in a number of situations involving mental function or activity.

Usually, interest and aptitude go hand in hand. A person must have aptitude for activity and an interest in a given activity to desirable success. But interest and aptitude both are not one and same way. Aptitude is measured by tests of general mental activity, which are used to facilitate prediction of scholastic success.

■ DEFINITIONS

1. Aptitude refers to those qualities characterizing a person's ways of behavior, which serves to indicate how well he/she can learn to meet and solve certain specified kinds of problems. —*Bingham*
2. Aptitude is a condition, a quality or a set of qualities in an individual, which is indicative of the probable extent to which he/she will be able to acquire under suitable training, some knowledge, skill or composite of knowledge, understanding and skill, such as ability to contribute to art or music, mechanical ability, mathematical ability to read and speak a foreign language. —*Traxler*
3. An aptitude is a combination of characteristics indicative of an individual's capacity to acquire (with training) some specific knowledge, skill or set of organized responses, such as the ability to speak a language, to become a musicians and to do mechanical work. —*Freeman*

■ DIFFERENCES BETWEEN INTELLIGENCE AND APTITUDE

Differences between intelligence and aptitude are given in Table 15.1.

■ MEASUREMENT OF APTITUDE

The term intelligence, ability and aptitude are often used interchangeably to refer to behavior that is used to predict future learning or performance. However, subtle differences exist between the terms. Similar to intelligence tests, aptitude tests measure a student's overall performance across a broad range of mental capabilities. But aptitude tests also include items, which measure more specialized abilities, such as verbal and numerical skills that predict scholastic performance in educational programs (Fig. 15.1).

Specific Nature of Aptitude Tests

1. Mechanical aptitude tests.
2. Clerical aptitude tests.
3. Musical aptitude tests.
4. Art judgment tests.

Table 15.1: Differences between intelligence and aptitude

Area	Intelligence	Aptitude
Ability	They exist usually to test the general mental ability of an individual	Aptitudes are concerned with specific abilities
Knowledge	Through the knowledge of intelligence of an individual, one can predict his/her success in a number of situation involving mental function or activity	The knowledge of aptitudes acquaints us with those specific abilities and capacities of an individual, which give an indication of his/her ability or capacity to succeed in a special field or activity
Prediction	Predicting achievements of intelligence for general ability	Predicting achievement in some particular job, training, courses or specialized instruction we need to know more about one's aptitudes (specific abilities)

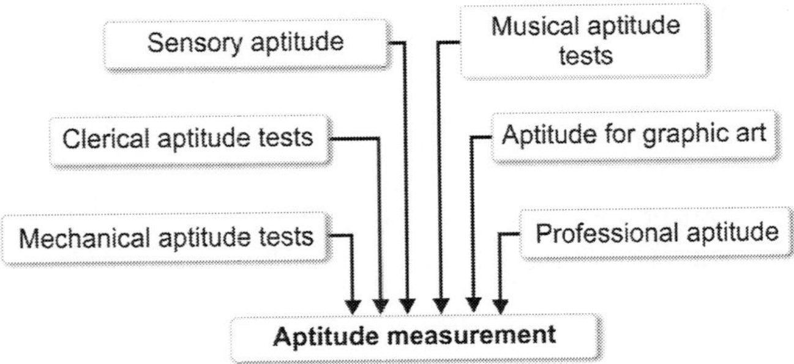

Figure 15.1: Measurement of aptitude

5. Professional aptitude tests, i.e. tests to measure the aptitudes for professionals such as teaching, salesmanship, research work, etc.
6. Scholastic aptitude tests, i.e. tests to measure the aptitude for different course of institution.

Mechanical Aptitude Test

Some persons have a specific bent of mind for the tasks related to the use of mechanical abilities and thus demonstrate their aptitude for all tasks and job that require the use of mechanical abilities. The term mechanical aptitude is not a single unitary function. It is a combination of sensory and motor capacities plus perception of spatial relations, the capacity to acquire information about mechanical matters and the capacity to comprehend mechanical relationships. Some of the well-known mechanical aptitude tests are:

1. Minnesota mechanical assembly test.
2. Minnesota spatial relation test.
3. The revised Minnesota power form board (1948).
4. Stenquist mechanical aptitude tests (part I and III).
5. LJO Rourke's mechanical aptitude tests (part I and III).
6. SRA mechanical aptitude test.
7. Bennett tests of mechanical aptitude tests (Hindi) prepared by Manovigyan Shala, Allahabad. Usually these tests contain the items of the following nature.
8. Asking the subject to put together the parts of mechanical devices.
9. Asking to replace cutouts of various shapes in their correct holes in the board.
10. Requiring the ability to solve problems in geometric terms.
11. Asking questions concerning the basic information about tools and their uses.
12. Questions relating to comprehension of physical and mechanical principles.

Clerical Aptitude Tests

Clerical aptitude is also a composite function. According to Bingham, it involves several specific abilities such as:

1. Perceptual ability: Ability to perceive words and numbers with speed and accuracy.
2. Intellectual ability: Ability to grasp the meaning of words and symbols.
3. Motor ability: Ability to use various types of machines and tools such as typewriter, duplicator, cyclostyle machine, punching machine, etc.

Some of the popular clerical aptitude tests are:

1. Detroit clerical aptitude examination.
2. Minnesota vocational test for clerical works.

3. The clerical ability test prepared by the Department of Psychology University of Mysore.
4. Clerical aptitude test Battery (English and Hindi), Bureau of Education and Vocational Guidance, Bihar.
5. Test of clerical aptitude prepared by the Parsee Panchayat Guidance Bureau, Mumbai.

Sensory Aptitude

In this category, we can include all those aptitude, which are related to the sensory capacities and abilities of the children. One may have aptitude in the task related to the use of his/her sense of hearing; other may have aptitude in the task related to the use of the sense of sight, sense of smell, sense of taste or sense of touch. Here depending upon their present ability concerning the particular sensory capacity, we can have an idea of their future success in the area or professions where the use of such sensory ability or capacity is most demanded.

Musical Aptitude Tests

Musical aptitude tests have been devised for discovering musical talent. One of these important musical aptitude tests is discovered below. Seashore measure of musical talent gives consideration to the following musical components:

1. Discrimination of pitch.
2. Discrimination of intensity of loudness.
3. Determination of time interval.
4. Discrimination of timber.
5. Judgment of rhythm.
6. Tonal memory.

The instruction in these tests is of following nature We will hear two tones, which differ in pitch and need to judge whether the second is higher or lower than the first. If the second is higher, then record H and if lower, record L.

Aptitude for Graphic Art

Aptitude for graphic art tests is devised to discover the talent for graphic art. The two important tests of this nature are:

1. The Meier art judgment test.
2. Horn art aptitude inventory.

In Meier art judgment test, there are 100 pairs of representational pictures in black and white. One member of each pair is an acknowledged art masterpiece, while the other is a slight distortion of the masterpiece. It is usually altered from the original, so as to violate some important principle of art. Tests are informed regarding, which aspect has been altered and are asked to choose from each pairs the one that is better such as more pleasing, more artistic and more satisfying. Another important test of measuring aptitude for graphic art is the horn art aptitude inventory. It requires the subject to produce sketches from given patterns to lines and figures. The created sketches of the subject are then evaluated according to the standard given by the author of this test.

Professional Aptitude

The aptitude related to the activities of various professions and occupations are included in this category. These aptitudes are able to predict the future success of an individual in the field or profession related to these aptitudes.

Tests for scholastic and professional aptitudes

This is for helping in the proper selection of students for the studies of specific courses of professions such as engineering, medicine, law, business, management, teaching, etc. The various specific aptitude tests have been designed, some of these aptitude tests are:

1. Stanford scientific aptitude test by DL Zyve.
2. Science aptitude test (after higher secondary stage), National Institute of Epidemiology (NIE), Delhi.

3. Moss scholastic aptitude test for medical students.
4. Ferguson and Stoddard's law aptitude examination.
5. Tale legal aptitude test.
6. Pre-engineering ability test (Education Testing Services, USA).
7. Minnesota engineering analogical test.
8. Coxe-Orleans prognosis test of teaching ability.
9. Teaching aptitude test by Jai Prakash and RP Shrivastava University of Saugar (MP).
10. Shah's teaching aptitude test.
11. Teaching aptitude test by Moss FA and others, George Washington University press.

■ CONTEMPORARY TRENDS IN APTITUDE TESTING

Instead of utilizing specific aptitude tests for measuring specific aptitude in very specific field or area, the trend at present, has now been changed towards multiple aptitude tests battery to find the suitability of people for different professions requiring different abilities on the basis of scores in the relevant aptitude tests in the battery. The examples of such tests are general aptitude test battery (GATB) and differential aptitude test (DAT).

General Aptitude Test Battery

The GATB, developed by the employment service bureau of USA, has 12 tests. Eight of which are paper-pencil tests as for name comparison, computation, vocabulary, arithmetic, reasoning form matching, test matching, three-dimensional spaces, etc. The other four require the use of simple equipment in the shape of moving pegs on boards, assembling and dissembling rivets and washers. From the scores obtained by the subject, the experimenter is able to draw inferences about the nine aptitude factors intelligence, verbal aptitude and numerical aptitude, spatial aptitude from perception, clerical perception, motor coordination, finger dexterity and manual dexterity. The GATB has proven to be one of the most successful multiple aptitude batteries particularly for the purposes of job classification.

Differential Aptitude Tests

The DAT is developed by USA psychological corporation. It has proved more successful in predicting academic success and found especially useful for providing educational and vocational guidance to secondary school children. The test induced in the battery of DAT is the following (Fig. 15.2):

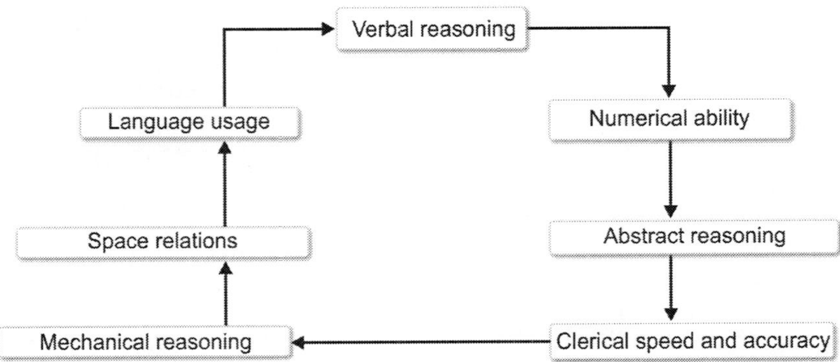

Figure 15.2: Types of differential aptitude tests

1. **Verbal reasoning:** It is a measure of ability to understand concepts framed in words. It is aimed at evaluation of the student's ability to abstract or generalize and to think constructively, rather than simple fluency or vocabulary recognition. The word used in these items may come from history, geography, literature, science or any other content area.
2. **Numerical ability:** These items are designed to test understanding of numerical relationships and facility in handling numerical concepts. This test is a measure of the student's ability to reason with numbers, to manipulate numerical relationships and to deal intelligently with quantitative materials. Educationally, it is important for prediction in such fields as mathematics, physics, chemistry, engineering and other curricula in which quantitative thinking is essential. Various amounts of numerical ability are required in occupations such as laboratory assistant, bookkeeper, statistical and shipping clerks as well as in professions related to the physical sciences.
3. **Abstract reasoning:** This test is intended as a verbal measure of the student's reasoning ability. It has many picture test yielding ambiguous scores, because they require the student to discriminate between lines are areas, which differ but slightly in size and shape. This test supplements the general intelligence aspects of the verbal and numerical tests.
4. **Clerical speed and accuracy:** This test is intended to measure speed of response in a simple perceptual task:
   a. Perceptual ability: Ability to perceive words and numbers with speed and accuracy.
   b. Intellectual ability: Ability to grasp the meaning of words and symbols.
   c. Motor ability: Ability to use various types machines and tools such as writer, duplicator, cyclostyle machine, punching machine, etc.
5. **Mechanical reasoning:** This tries to test mechanical aptitude, which is a combination of sensory and motor capacities plus perception of spatial relations, the capacity to acquire information about mechanical matters and the capacity to comprehend mechanical relationships.
6. **Space relations:** It is the ability to visualize a constructed object from a picture of a pattern and an ability to imagine how an object would appear if rotated in various ways for measurement of space perception. It means that these tests require mental manipulation of objects in three-dimensional spaces.
7. **Language usage:** This test has two sections:
   a. Language usage-1: Spelling.
   b. Language usage-2: Grammar.

■ VALUES OF APTITUDE TESTING

1. They are excellent predictors of future scholastic achievements.
2. They provide ways of comparing a child's performance with that of others children in the same situation.
3. They provide a profile of strength and weaknesses.
4. They assess differences among the individuals.
5. They have uncovered hidden talents in some children, thus improving their educational opportunities.
6. They are valuable tools for working with handicapped children.

■ USES OF APTITUDE TESTS (Fig. 15.3)

Instructional

Teacher can use aptitude test results to adopt their curricula to match the level of their students or to design assignments for students who differ orderly. Aptitude tests score can also help teachers from realistic expectations

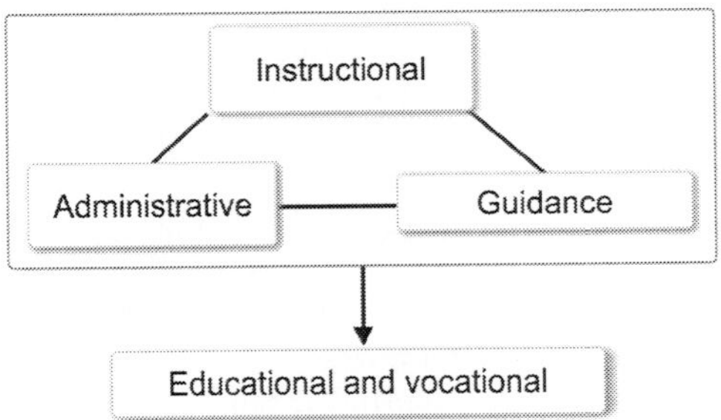

Figure 15.3: Uses of aptitude test

of students. Knowing something about the aptitude level of students in a given class can help a teacher identify, which students are not learning as much as could be predicted on the basis of aptitude scores. For instance, if a whole class were performing less will than would be predicted form aptitude test results, then curriculum, objectives, teaching methods or student characteristics might be investigated.

Administrative

Aptitude test scores can identify the general aptitude level of a high school. This can be helpful in determining how much emphasis should be given to college preparatory programs. Aptitude tests can be used to help identify students to be accelerated or given extra attention, for grouping and in predicting job training performance.

Guidance

Guidance counselors use aptitude tests to help parents develop realistic expectations for their child's school performance and to help students understand their own strengths and weakness. These tests are found to be very useful in helping the youngsters as well as youth in the selection of special courses of instruction, fields of activities and vocations.

Educational and Vocational

Aptitude tests can be safely used for the purpose of education and vocational selection. They help us in making scientific selection of the candidates for various educational and professional courses as well as specialized jobs as Munn puts it. The chief values of aptitude testing is, in fact that it enables us to pick out from those who do not yet have the ability to perform certain skills, those who, with a reasonable amount of training, will be most likely to acquire the skills in question and acquire them to a desirable level of proficiency.

■ APTITUDE AND NURSING

Aptitude is to be distinguished from present ability. A certain nurse may not at present have the ability to act as an operation theater nurse working with the surgeon, but they are clever and quick, able to think ahead and foresee what will be needed. They possess a high degree of aptitude for theater work and have good chances with proper training of becoming a very successful operation theater nurse. Nursing is an arts and science, which requires high degree of aptitude for being a good bedside nurse. The nurse needs to foresee the need and progress of the patient. The aptitude differs from one area to another based on their application of nursing.

■ CONCLUSION

Aptitude tests properly anticipate the future potentialities or capacities of an individual and thereby, help us in making selection of those individuals who are best fitted for a particular profession and course of instruction or those who are likely to be more benefited by the pre-professional training or experiences. Aptitude testing when combined with the other information received through interest inventory, personality tests, intelligence tests and cumulative record, etc. can help, to a greater extent, in avoiding the huge wastage of human as well as material resources by placing the individuals to their proper places and lines of work.

■ REVIEW QUESTIONS

Long Essays

1. Define aptitude. Explain the meaning and concepts of aptitude.
2. Discuss the various uses of aptitude testing.

Short Essays

3. Difference between intelligence and aptitude.
4. Measurement of aptitude.
5. Describe contemporary trends in aptitude test.
6. Values of aptitude test.
7. Describe the nurse's role in aptitude test.

Short Answers

8. Mechanical aptitude test.
9. Differential aptitude test.
10. General aptitude test battery.
11. Tests for scholastic and professional aptitudes.
12. Musical aptitude test.

■ BIBLIOGRAPHY

1. Arnold MB. The Nature of Emotion, Baltimore: Penguin; 1968.
2. Bandura A. Principles of Behavior Modifications, New York: Holt, Rinehart & Winston; 1969.
3. Bennett GK, Seashore HG, Wesman AG. Differential Aptitude Tests. New York: Psychological Corporation; 1947.
4. Bingham WV. Aptitude and Aptitude Testing. New York: Harper & Brothers; 1937.
5. Bizley JK, Walker KM. Sensitivity and selectivity of neurons in auditory cortex to the pitch, timbre, and location of sounds. Neuroscientist. 2010;16(4):453-69.
6. Boring EG. Sensation and Perception in the History of Experimental Psychology. New York, London; 1942.
7. Brubaker J. Modern Philosopher of Education. New York: McGraw-Hill; 1939.
8. Brynie FH. Brain Sense: The Science of the Senses and How We Process the World around US. American Management Association; 2009.
9. Carlson NR. Psychology of Behavior. Boston: Allyn and Bacon; 1977.
10. Crow LD, Crow A. Introduction to Guidance. New Delhi: Eurasia Publishing House; 1962.
11. Ferguson ED. Motivation: An Experimental Approach. New York: Holt, Rinehartt Winston; 1976.
12. Freeman FS. Theory and Practice of Psychological Testing (3rd Indian reprint). Bombay: Oxford and IBH; 1971.
13. Garrett HE, Mathew R Shneck. Psychological tests, methods and results. New York: Harper & Brothers; 1933.
14. Goddard FA. The Human Senses, 2nd edition. New York: Wiley; 1972.
15. Hawkins S. Phonological features, auditory objects, and illusions. J Phon. 2010;38(1):60-89.
16. Hickey C, Chelazzi L, Theeuwes J. Reward changes salience in human vision via the anterior Cingulate. J Neurosci. 2010;30(33):11096-103.
17. Hochberg JE. Perception, 2nd edition. Englewood Cliffs, New Jersey: Prentice Hall; 1978.
18. Hull CL. Aptitude Testing. New York, Yonkers: World Books Co; 1928.
19. Korman AK. The Psychology of Motivation, Englewood Cliffs, New Jersey: Prentice-Hall; 1974.
20. Li X. Acute central cord syndrome: injury mechanisms and stress features. Spine. 2010;35(19):E955-64.

21. Lindsay PH, Norman DA. Human Information Processing, 2nd edition. New York: Academic Press; 1977.
22. Macaluso E. Orienting of spatial attention and the interplay between the senses. Cortex. 2010;46(3):282-97.
23. Morgan CT. A Brief Introduction to Psychology, New Delhi: Tata McGraw-Hill; 1975.
24. Morgan T, King RA. Introduction to Psychology, 6th edition. New Delhi: Tata McGraw-Hill; 1982.
25. Mueller CG. Sensory Psychology. Englewood Cliffs, New Jersey: Prentice Hall; 1965.
26. Munn, Norman L. Introduction to Psychology. New Delhi: Oxford and IBH; 1973.
27. Purves Dale, et al. Neuroscience, 2nd edition. Sunderland, MA: Sinauer Associates Inc; 2008.
28. Robinson DN. An Intellectual History of Psychology, New York: Macmillan; 1976.
29. Stern W. Psychological Methods of Testing Intelligence. Baltimore: Warwick and York Inc; 1914.
30. Strongman KT. The Psychology of Emotion, New York: Wiley; 1973.
31. Terman LM. Symposium: Intelligence and its measurement. J Educ Psychol. 1921.
32. Thompson RF. Introduction to Psychological Psychology. New York: Harper and Row; 1975.
33. Wechsler D. The Measurement of Adult Intelligence, 3rd edition. New York: Williams & Wilkins Co; 1944.

Section IV

Motivational/Emotional Process and Personality

CHAPTER 16

Motivation

■ INTRODUCTION

The human behavior is controlled, directed and modified through certain motives. When a person is hungry and is searching for food or constructing a house or mating, or learning new skills, we will always be able to trace some such elements, which his/her activities guide them, and his/her behavior in the lights of his/her success or failures.

Motivation is that force, which impels or incites individual's action, determines the individual's direction of action and rate of action. When the individual gets any motives, he/she experiences a tension and disequilibrium and becomes restless. His/Her activities are then initiated. The individual feels a push to behave in a certain direction.

■ MEANING

1. Motivation is something, which prompts, compels and energizes an individual to act or behave in a particular fashion at a particular time for attaining some specific goal or purpose.
2. The term 'motivation' has been derived from the word 'motive'. A motive is an inner state that activities, energizes or moves an individual and channelizes his/her behavior towards goals.
3. Motivation is the art of understanding these motives and satisfying them to direct and sustain behavior towards the accomplishment of organizational goal.
4. Motivation is concerned with how behavior gets started, is energized, sustained, directed and stopped. As motivation is the process of inspiring and impelling people to take required actions by providing stimuli that satisfy their needs and motives.
5. Motivation is the complex of forces, which propel an individual into action and keep them at work. It reflects the will to work.
6. Motivation is defined as the process that initiates, guides and maintains goal-oriented behaviors. Motivation is what causes us to act, whether it is getting a glass of water to reduce thirst or reading a book to gain knowledge.

■ DEFINITION

1. Motivation means a process of stimulating people to action to accomplish desired goals. It refers to the way in which urges, drives, desires, aspirations, stirrings or needs direct, control or explain the behavior of human being. — *Scott*
2. Motivation is an inspirational process, which impels the members of the team

to pull their weight effectively, to give their loyalty to the group, to carry out properly the tasks that they have accepted and generally to play an effective part in the job that the group has undertaken. —*Breech*

3. Motivation is the willingness to exert high levels of effort toward organizational goals, conditioned by the effort's ability to satisfy some individual needs. —*Stephen P Robbins*
4. Motivation refers to the degree of readiness of an organism to pursue some designated goal and implies the determination of the nature, and laws of the focus including the degree of readiness. —*Encyclopedia*

▪ NATURE OF MOTIVATION

Motivation is the force that initiates, guides and maintains goal-oriented behaviors. It is what causes us to take action, whether to grab a snack to reduce hunger or enroll in college to earn a degree. The forces that lie beneath motivation can be biological, social, emotional or cognitive in nature:

1. Motivation is a psychological concept. It is concerned with the intrinsic forces operating within an individual, which impel him/her to act or not to act in a particular way.
2. Motivation is a dynamic and continuous process as it deals with human being, which is an ever-changing entity modifying itself every moment.
3. Motivation is a complex and difficult function. Every person adopts a different approach to satisfy their needs and one particular need may cause different behavior on the part of different people.
4. Motivation is a circular process. Feeling of an unsatisfied need causes tension and an individual takes action (drive) to reduce this tension.
5. Motivation is different from satisfaction. Motivation is the process of stimulating an individual or a group, to take desired action.
6. Motivation is the product of anticipated value from a given course of action and the perceived probability that the action will lead to these values.

▪ MOTIVATION PROCESS

The motivational process is the steps that you take to get motivated (Fig. 16.1). It is a process

Step 1: Need
Need to complete a report in 2 weeks
Step 2: Build up of tension
Worry that time will run out
Doubts about abilities
Fear of failure
Set aside other needs
Step 3: Focused activities
Research the topic
Take notes
Prepare the outlines
Write the report
Step 4: Achievement of goal
Turn in completed report
Step 5: Satisfaction and tension reduction
Feel freedom to satisfy other needs

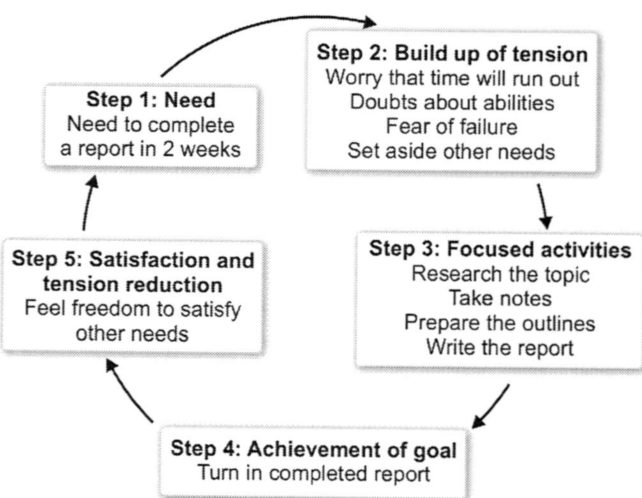

Figure 16.1: Steps of motivation process

that when followed produces incredible results. It is amazing what you can do if you are properly motivated and getting properly motivated is a matter of following the motivational process. As any other process it takes a little work and foresight, and planning on your part. However, the return on your investment of time is significant and it is important when needing extra motivation that you apply the motivational process:

1. An unsatisfied tension, which stimulates drives within the individual. This drives generate search behavior to find particular goals that if attained, will satisfy the need and lead to reduction of tension.
2. In order to relieve this tension, they engage in activity. The greater the tension, the more activity will be needed to bring about relief.
3. Therefore, when we see people working hard at some activity, we can conclude that they are driven by a desire to achieve some goal that they perceive as having value to them.

■ COMPONENTS OF MOTIVATION

There are three major components of motivation, i.e. activation, persistence and intensity. Activation involves the decision to initiate a behavior, such as enrolling in a psychology class. Persistence is the continued effort toward a goal even though obstacles may exist, such as taking more psychology courses in order to earn a degree, although it requires a significant investment of time, energy and resources. Finally, intensity can be seen in the concentration and vigor that goes into pursuing a goal. For example, one student might coast by without much effort, while another student will study regularly, participate in discussions and take advantage of research opportunities outside of class.

Extrinsic Versus Intrinsic Motivation

Different types of motivation are frequently described as being either extrinsic or intrinsic. Extrinsic motivations are those that arise from outside of the individual and often involve rewards such as trophies, money, social recognition or praise. Intrinsic motivations are those that arise from within the individual, such as doing a complicated crossword puzzle purely for the personal gratification of solving a problem.

■ MOTIVE

Meaning

1. Motive is a force that determines the activity of an individual. It energizes and directs his/her behavior along this or that channel.
2. When a motive is at work, it creates tension and these tensions arouse the individual towards an activity that will relieve the tension.
3. A motive is the force that initiates, sustains and directs the activity of an organism. A stimulus is an internal or external object, which excites the receptor or activates a sense organ.

Definitions

1. A need give rise to one or more motives. A motive is a rather specific process, which has been learned. It is directed towards a goal. —*Carroll*
2. A motive is an inclination or impulsion to action plus some degree of orientation or direction. —*Fisher*
3. A motive may be defined as a readiness or disposition to respond in some ways and not others to a variety of situations. —*Rosen, Fox and Gregory*

Classification (Fig. 16.2)

Physiological Motives (Fig. 16.3)

Temperature regulation: An organism is further active in maintaining a comfortable state of warmth and cold. This motivated activity is the result of the impulses sent to the brain by the skin receptors meant for the sensation of warmth and cold.

Pain: The sense receptors for pain are distributed in all the bodily organs such as skin, internal organs, blood vessels, etc. They are in the form of free nerve ending in these organs. Whenever, they are stimulated by some sort of injury to the body there is pain sensation. The organism puts in all possible efforts, consciously or at reflex level to avoid such pain.

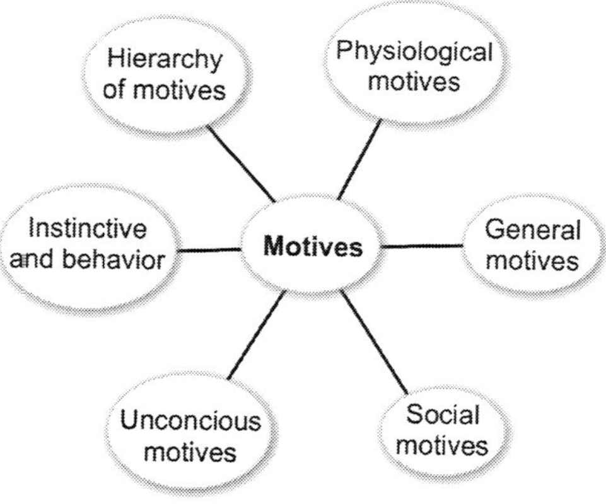

Figure 16.2: Classification of motives

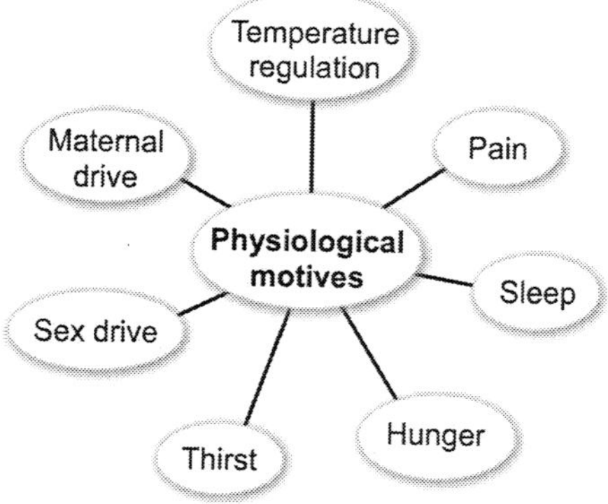

Figure 16.3: Physiological motives

Sleep: Need for sleep is one more physiological motive. Though, it curtails all activity of the organisms unlike other motives and make them assume an inactive position it can be observed, however, that the inactive position is the goal and the motive of sleep actually drives the individual to all possible efforts to go to sleep.

Hunger: When we feel emptiness in our stomach, we are hungry. When we are hungry, there occur two kinds of changes. One, if the change in our external behavior and other is the change in our internal conditions. The motive of hunger gives rise to the hunger pangs. The actual sensation a person gets in a type of acting sensation.

Thirst: When deprived of water over some period, the organism becomes excessively restless and needs intake of water. This drive for water comes from dryness of the mouth and thirst. However, the feeling of thirst is basically related to the degree of dehydration of the body tissue. Thirst is also a physiological need, which promotes activity. This need is very active when it is not immediately satisfied.

Sex drive: Sex is a very powerful drive, which influences the actions of the individual to a very great extent. According to general convention, this drive remains dormant during childhood. The Freudian theory shows evidence for sexual behavior right from infancy. With the onset of puberty the sex glands known as gonads start functioning and as a result, the sex drive is simulated.

Maternal drive: What has been said about the sex instinct applies equally well to maternal behavior. Prolactin, a hormone from the anterior pituitary gland plays an important role motivating maternal behavior. Human maternal motivation has several aspects. Child rearing practices and attitudes towards children differ from culture to culture, and from subculture to subculture.

General Motives (Fig. 16.4)

Activity: Men as well as animals are found to be spontaneously active. They enjoy it and spend considerable time in moving about. This innate motive for activity is visible even in a child's behavior. Activity also accompanies other physiological drives when these drives are stronger activity increases. Activity is closely related to sensors stimulations. More the stimulations in the environment, more active is the organism.

Exploratory drive: People like to explore new environments. We visit new places; mountaineers even risk their lives in exploratory expeditions. When animals are put into mazes, they are found to explore them without any specific aim to satisfying a physiological drive such as hunger. This drives of exploration in stronger, when the organism finds itself in a new situation.

Curiosity: This is a motive, which is close to exploration. Exploration is a drive that aids the satisfaction of curiosity. Animals as well as men including children are curious about the several things around them. A small child's curiosity tempts him/her even a break a new toy given to him/her.

Manipulation: This is one more motive, which is a related aspect of the two previously discussed. It is not so easy to differentiate clearly among the drive of exploration, curiosity and manipulation. All three seem to be different aspects of a single motivated activity. Curiosity leads to manipulation and manipulation in turn is a counterpart of exploration.

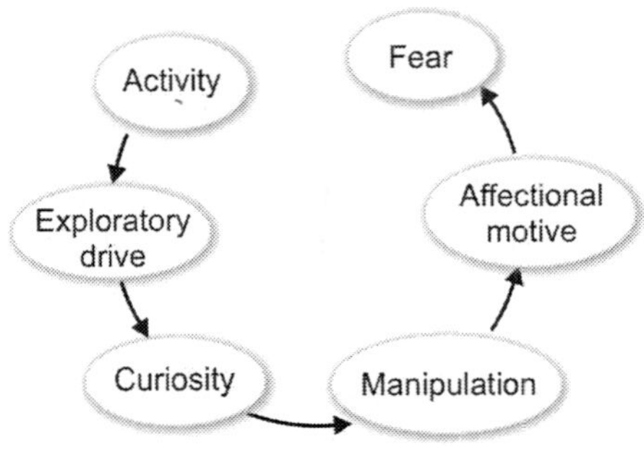

Figure 16.4: General motives

Affectional motive: Love is an important motive of human life; we love our parents, our brothers and sisters, children, friends, etc. The significant people in the environment become love objects through positive contact with him. There are enough reasons to believe that it is also an unlearned motive that emerges with maturation.

Fear: It is varying powerful motive. This motivates escape from fear-producing situation. Fear may also interfere with the satisfaction of other motives. Most of the fears are learned, but there is enough reason to believe that some fears are unlearned.

Social Motives (Fig. 16.5)

Affiliation: Our need for affiliation is well-expressed through our affiliation with clubs and other institutions. Though, marriage is partly a mean to satisfy many other needs including the need for affiliation. The motive of affiliation is usually seen in all human cultures. This motive perhaps has its roots in our childhood experiences when the helpless infant has to associate himself/herself with others for his/her basic need satisfaction.

Social approval: We seek social approval for all the things done similarly and try out best to avoid doing anything that may evoke social disapproval. We often show an almost compulsive tendency to confirm to the norms set by our social group. This may be the result of constant parental directions in childhood as to what is right and what is wrong for the child to do.

Status: All people are commonly motivated to achieve status among their fellowmen. This motive varies in strength from person to person. Some people show the minimum need for status in the form of the desire to be

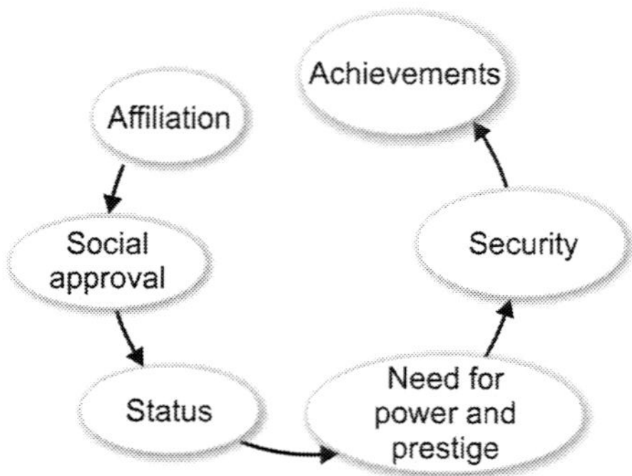

Figure 16.5: Social motives

taught well and have a respectable position in their professional field or in community.

Need for power and prestige: The need for prestige is expressed in the form of our striving to feel better than other persons with whom we compare ourselves. In daily life, there are many ways in which prestige is sought and achieved, such symbols as dress, money and other belongings are regarded as ways of feeling superior in comparison to others. The need of power is almost similar though, it differs slightly in its expression.

Security: An urge for feeling of security is also an important motive especially in complex modern societies. This feeling involves the ability to hold on to what one has and continue with the assurance to keep it up on the other hand. Insecurity is a haunting feeling that one may lose what he now has.

Achievements: It is a powerful motive in some societies. This is the motive to accomplish something, to succeed in one's undertaking and to avoid failure. The importance of this varies from culture to culture and from subculture to subculture. The strength of achievement motives depends partly on the past success of an individual.

Unconscious Motives

1. Not all our motives are conscious. A number of them are operating without our awareness. In our own behavior we come across instances of acts, the explanation of which cannot be found. All such instances of behavior can be explained with reference to unconscious motives.
2. Origin of unconscious motives can be found in the unconscious. The term unconscious should not be taken to mean that it is a part of mind separated from unconscious mind.
3. The repression itself is a function of the unconscious. Hence, constant repression enlarges the domain of the unconscious. Since, the material is related to our motives it is dynamic in nature and does not remain quiet in the unconscious.
4. According to Freud, the material of the unconscious is extremely difficult to top because a considerable part of it is originated in infantile preverbal ideas, which have never become conscious.

Instinctive and Behavior

1. McDougall defines an instinct as an inherited or innate psychophysical disposition, which determines its possessor to perceive and to pay attention to objects of a certain class, to experience an emotional excitement of a particular quality upon perceiving such an object, and to act in regard to it in a particular manner or at least to experience an impulse to such action.
2. According to McDougall, instincts are innate tendencies, which have a cognitive aspect, emotive aspect to feel certain emotion towards these objects, to act towards them in a particular way.
3. The human instincts sucking, crying, locomotion, curiosity, sociality, shyness, cleanliness, pressing downward on the feet, imitation, pugnacity, fear of dark places, acquisitiveness, love and jealousy.

Hierarchy of Motives

1. Hierarchy of motives helps us to understand the potency of different motives in understanding man's behavior.
2. According to White, motives at the lowest rung are those originating from homeostatic mechanism. Thus, all motives important for survival including the safely motives are included in this class. Affiliation motives are placed still higher. These motives include the need for social acceptance and belongingness.
3. According to Maslow, the highest type of needs, which he calls the need for self-actualization, the need for self-actualization is complicated concept, which needs some further explanation.

■ THEORIES OF MOTIVATION

Drive Reduction Theory

1. One of the earlier theories of motivation was the drive reduction theory. It was proposed by Clark Hull.
2. This theory proposes that organisms experiences the arousal of a drive when an important need is not satisfied. Hence, they engage in behavior to reduce the arousal and satisfy the need.
3. Primary drives are those that motivate the organism to fulfill some basic need necessary for its survival such as hunger, thirst or sex.
4. An important component of the drive reduction theory is homeostasis. The term homeostasis refers to a state of balance or equilibrium necessary in many physiological systems.
5. Primary drives are biological drives necessary for personal and species survival. Acquired drives develop through learning.
6. The drive is the force that motivates an organism to act. Which action the organism finally performs depends on the strength of the organism's habit.
7. A habit is a response to some stimulus. The strength of the habit depends on the connection between the stimulus and the response that influences what kind of behavior the drive will energize.

Optimum Level of Arousal Theory

1. The optimum level of arousal theory states that drives do not necessarily motivate an organism to seek the lowest level or arousal. Instead they provide motivation to seek an optimum level of arousal.
2. Robert Uerles and JD Dodson (1908), conducted an experiment to examine the effects of different arousal levels on learning. They varied arousal levels in mice by changing the intensity of electric shocks and by observing how well the animals performed in simple and complex mazes.
3. Yerkes-Dodson law states that performance on a learning task is related to arousal; the best performance results from intermediate levels of arousal. Performance is also related to the difficulty of the task.
4. Yerkes and Dodson found that the mice performed simple tasks better when the stimulation was more intense. For complex tasks, low to intermediate arousal was the best.

Cognitive Theories

1. A cognitive theory (the word comes from the Latin for knowing) emphasizes some sort of understanding or anticipation of events through perception, or thought, or judgment as in the estimation of probabilities, or in making a choice on the basis of relative value.
2. Any organism with memory is capable of recognizing some similarities between the present and the past, and hence is

able to form some sort of experience with regard to the consequences of its behavior.

3. According to a cognitive theory, motivated goal-seeking behavior comes to be regulated by these conditions, which are based on the past, modified by circumstances of the present and includes expectations about the future.
4. Cognitive dissonance theory: Festinger (1957) proposed a theory in which certain kinds of unbalanced cognitions are described as dissonant and the subject is under stress to remove this dissonance.

Expectancy Theory

1. Expectancy theory emphasizes the importance of rewards and goals as well as how person's expectations of consequences can influence his/her behavior. This theory stresses 'pull' rather than 'push.'
2. According to expectancy theory, the hunger drive is only part of the reason a hungry rat is motivated to find its way through a maze. It is also motivated because of previous learning experiences in which it has come to expect a bit of food at the end.
3. Motivation is composed of two major features, the valence or attractiveness of the goal and the expectancy or the likelihood that its behavior will lead to the goal.
4. The actions that hungry people take to satisfy their hunger depend very much on valence and expectancy. A simple way of explaining the expectancy theory is to say that:

   Motivation = Valence × Expectancy
5. Economic theories assume that the individuals can assign value or utility to possible incentives and that they make their decision according to the risk involved.

Psychoanalytic Theory of Modification

1. Freud believed that all behavior stemmed from two opposing groups of instincts, the life instincts (Eros) that enhance life and growth, and the death instincts (Thanatos) that pushes toward destruction.
2. The energy of the life instincts is libido, which involves mainly sex and related activities. The death instinct can be directed inward in the form of aggression towards others. Freud pointed to several forms of behavior:
   a. In dreams, we often express wishes and impulses of which we are unaware.
   b. Unconscious mannerisms and slips of speech may reveal hidden motives.
   c. Symptoms of illness (particularly symptoms of mental illness) often can be shown to serve the unconscious needs of the person.

Maslow's Hierarchy of Needs

1. The behavior of an individual at a particular moment is usually determined by his/her strongest need. These needs have a certain priority (Fig. 16.6).

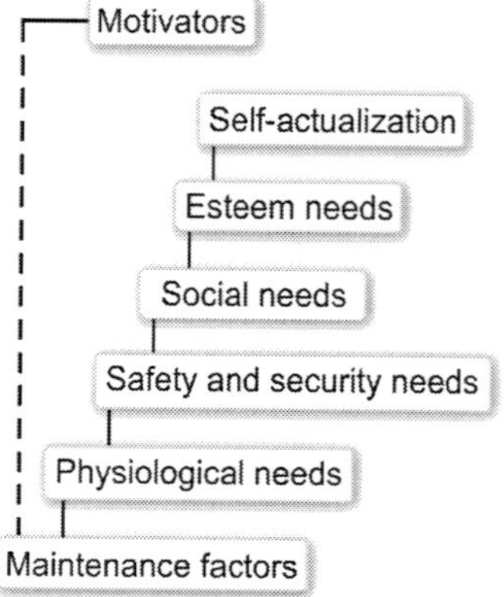

Figure 16.6: Relationship between Herzberg's and Maslow models

2. The lower level needs (e.g. physiological needs) have the highest strength until they are reasonably met. When the lower level needs are met, man goes to satisfy the higher needs.
3. The hierarchy needs organized step by step to the satisfaction of other needs such as physiological needs, safety and security needs, social needs, esteem needs and self-actualization needs. A satisfied need is no longer a motivator of behavior.

Herzberg's Two Factor Theory

1. According to Herzberg's (refer Fig. 16.6), there are ten factors called maintenance factors and six factors called motivational factors or satisfactory.
2. The absence of maintenance factors cause dissatisfaction in the employees, but their presence may not produce motivation in the employees.
3. The presence of motivational factors is necessary to produce motivation and job satisfaction in the individual, but their absence may not produce strong dissatisfaction.
4. The maintenance factors are policy and management, supervision, good interpersonal relationship with supervisor, good index of peer relations (IPR) with peers and subordinates, fair salary, job security, personal life, good working conditions and status.
5. The motivational factors are achievement, recognition, work itself, advancement and responsibility.
6. The Herzberg's model has given several insights. One of the insights is job enrichment. The idea behind job enrichment is to keep maintenance factors constant or higher, while increasing motivational factors by attaching more responsibility satisfying working conditions and power to the job.

McClelland's Needs Theory

1. McClelland identified three types of basic motivating needs. They are need for power, need for affiliation and need for achievement.
2. Power motive is the need to manipulate others or the drive for superiority over others. Such individuals are generally seeking positions for leadership.
3. The affiliation motive is concerned with maintaining pleasant social relationships, sense of intimacy and understanding, and enjoy in consoling and helping others who are in trouble.
4. Achievement motivated people can be the backbone of most organizations, because they progress faster. They are highly task-oriented and work to their optimum capacity.

Carrot and Stick Approach of Motivation

1. Carrot and stick approach of motivation comes from the old story that the best way to make a donkey move is to put a carrot out in front of him or beat him with a stick from behind.
2. The carrot is the reward for moving and the stick is the punishment for not moving.
3. In motivating people for better production in an organization some carrots (rewards) are used such as money, promotion and other incentives.
4. Some sticks (punishments) are used to push the people for desired behavior or to restrain from undesired behavior.

■ FRUSTRATION

When the pursuit of a goal is thwarted or blocked in any situation the result is frustration. That is, frustration is the consequence of the blockage of motives or when competing motives work at the same time and the individual is not in a position to make appropriate choice.

Definition

Frustration is defined as the blocking of a desire or need. It also refers to failure to satisfy a basic need because of conditions, either in the individual or external obstacles.

Meaning

1. Frustration is a condition of extreme tension; it is commonly interpreted as a strong emotional tension, caused by the blocking of impulses.
2. The individual is said to be frustrated because he/she does not to know how to rid of tension. These tensions make the frustrated person highly discomfort able.
3. Frustration involves an insurmountable obstacle and the inability to overcome it and a sense of defeat as well as feeling of stress and strain.

Sources (Fig. 16.7)

Environmental Forces

The frustration may be caused by environmental situations or conditions, which cannot control. Such environmental conditions include a contagious disease, the death of a friend or a beloved relative, usual rains and storms or floods.

Personal Inadequacies

Frustration may be in the form of poor ability or skill in the individual. On the other hand, the person's level of aspiration may be high; this may come in the way of reaching the goals. It may also be due to any physical handicap in the individual.

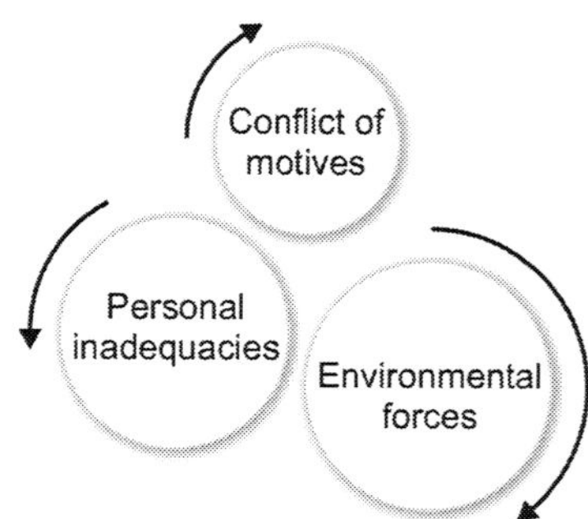

Figure 16.7: Sources of frustration

Conflict of Motives

Sometimes frustration results because of interference of one motive with other motives. For example, in our society sexual motivation is often in conflict with the society's standards of approved sexual behavior.

■ CONFLICT

Definition

Conflict is a state when two or more incompatible motivations or behavioral impulses compete for expression. In other words, the individual is faced with more than two incompatible demands, opportunities, goals or needs.

Mental conflict is a inner state characterized by tension as a result of the presence, at the same time, of mutually exclusive or opposing tendencies, impulses or desires.

Types (Fig. 16.8)

Approach-approach Conflict

Approach-approach conflict is a type of conflict faced by a person with two appealing/attractive goals or choices and he/she is forced to choose one of them. For example, a young computer engineer is offered jobs in two popular multinational companies. The young man is in a dilemma choosing between the two.

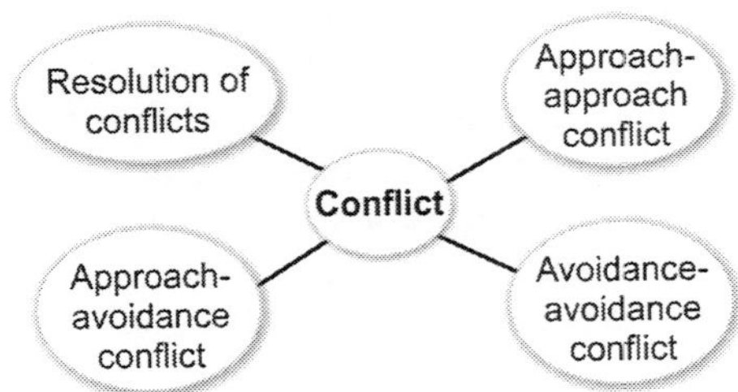

Figure 16.8: Types of conflict

Avoidance-avoidance Conflict

In avoidance-avoidance conflict, an individual has to make a choice between two unattractive goals. Here, the individual is repelled by two undesirable alternatives at the same time. For example, a person has a long history of painful backache for which he/she is advised surgery. Here the person is faced with the prospect of living with painful backache or undergoing dreadful surgery. This conflict is aptly described in the proverb caught between the devil and deep blue sea.

Approach-avoidance Conflict

The goal has both attractive and unpleasant aspects. The choice has pleasant and unpleasant consequences. A prospective young professional bride has an offer to marry an non-resident Indian in America. Here going to America is appealing and at the same time leaving the parents in India is distressing.

Resolution of Conflicts

Conflict often produces stress; stress includes a number of unpleasant responses. Every individual is equipped with capacity to overcome obstacles in order to avoid conflict, which is a source of frustration.

■ MOTIVATIONAL QUALITIES OF NURSE LEADER

1. Effective communication of ideas, confidence, commitment, energy, insight into the needs of others and an ability to take the action necessary to achieve goals important to others.
2. Knowledge and skill comes from preparation in the responsibilities of healthcare delivery and organizational duty. This leader has the ability to evaluate the likelihood of success in accomplishing goals and is able to support or suggest changes.
3. Confidence comes from an internal sense of security that one is competent to make a statement or take action and that there is a reasonable chance of success in accomplishing something of value. The motivational leader is secure enough to have a lower need to control and as a result is able to encourage autonomy, participation and the empowerment of staff in decision-making.
4. Commitment is the internalization of an idea and a resulting drive to accomplish specific goals. The mere setting of goals does not indicate leadership that motivates. It is the ability of the leader to translate the importance of the goal (or purpose) to others and to elicit actions from others that support reaching a goal.
5. Energy is also needed to empower and fire the imagination of others, and constantly invent, and move ahead toward future events as well as current needs. Different styles of energy can be motivational. The 'high-energy leader,' who is effective in one situation may be viewed as 'pushy and aggressive' in another situation.
6. Insight into the needs of others is the acute awareness of the reason behind events and an ability to anticipate results of actions. When a leader can put goals into a form that has real or personal value to each person, then motivation will exists.
7. Additional key qualities of a motivational leader are abilities to listen, reserve judgment, give direct and positive feedback,

recognize individual value through respect for others and use humor.

Professional practice and shared governance depend on the clinical leader to produce an environment that fosters autonomy in decision-making, and provides the skills, resources and information needed for others to make this transition (Fig. 16.9).

SEVEN RULES OF MOTIVATION

1. **Set a major goal, but follows a path:** The path has mini goals that go in many directions. When you learn to succeed at mini goals, you will be motivated to challenge grand goals.
2. **Finish what you start:** A half-finished project is of no use to anyone. Quitting is a habit. Develop the habit of finishing self-motivated projects.
3. **Socialize with others of similar interest:** Mutual support is motivating. We will develop the attitudes of our five best friends. If they are losers, we will be a loser. If they are winners, we will be a winner. To be a cowboy we must associate with cowboys.
4. **Learn how to learn:** Dependency on others for knowledge supports the habit of procrastination. Man has the ability to learn without instructors. In fact, when we learn the art of self-education we will find, if not create, opportunity to find success beyond our wildest dreams.

Effective communication
Additional key qualities
Knowledge and skill
Motivational qualities
Insight into the needs of others
Confidence
Energy
Commitment

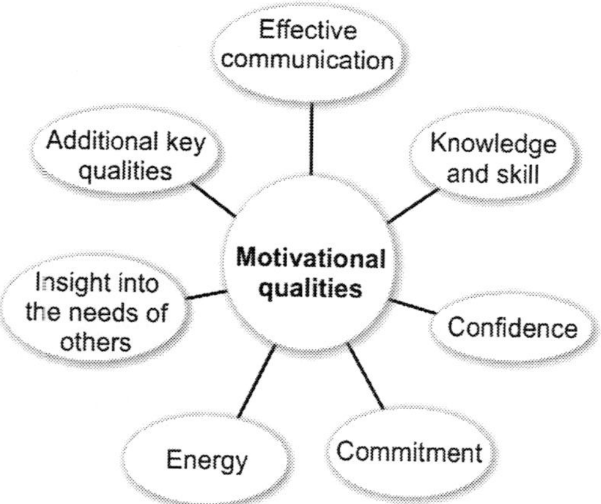

Figure 16.9: Motivational qualities of Nurse Manager

5. **Harmonize natural talents with interest that motivates:** Natural talent creates motivation, motivation creates persistence and persistence gets the job done.
6. **Increase knowledge of subjects that inspires:** The more we know about a subject, the more we want to learn about it. A self-propelled upward spiral develops.
7. **Take risk:** Failure and bouncing back are elements of motivation. Failure is a learning tool. No one has ever succeeded at anything worthwhile without a string of failures.

A TO Z STEPS IN MOTIVATION

1. **A:** Achieve your dreams. Avoid negative people, things and places. Eleanor Roosevelt once said, "The future belongs to those who believe in the beauty of their dreams".
2. **B:** Believe in yourself and in what you can accomplish.
3. **C:** Consider things from every angle and aspect. Motivation comes from determination. To be able to understand life, you should feel the sun from both sides.
4. **D:** Do not give up and do not give in. Thomas Edison failed once, twice, more than three times before he came up with his invention and perfected the incandescent light bulb. Make motivation your steering wheel.
5. **E:** Enjoy work as if you do not need money, dance as if nobody's watching, love as if you never cried and learn as if you will live forever. Motivational momentum takes place, when people are happy.
6. **F:** Family and friends are life's greatest 'F' treasures. Do not lose sight of them.

7. **G:** Give more than what is enough. Where does motivation and self-improvement take place—At work? At home? At school? Always give 110%.
8. **H:** Hang on to your dreams. They may dangle in there for a moment, but these little stars will be your driving force. Define your target and hit it, until you hit it.
9. **I:** Ignore those who try to destroy you. Do not let other people get the best of you. Stay away from toxic people; the kind of friends who hates to hear about your success. Stay away from negativity.
10. **J:** Just be yourself. The key to success is to be you and the key to failure is to try to please everyone.
11. **K:** Keep trying no matter how hard life may seem. When a person is motivated, eventually he/she sees a harsh life finally clearing out, paving the way to self-improvement.
12. **L:** Learn to love yourself. Now, is not that easy?
13. **M:** Make things happen. Motivation is when your dreams are put into work.
14. **N:** Never lie, cheats or steals. Always play a fair game.
15. **O:** Open your eyes. People should learn the horse attitude and horse sense. They see things in two ways—how they want things to be and how they should be?
16. **P:** Practice makes perfect. Practice is about motivation. It lets us learn repertoire and ways on how can we recover from our mistakes.
17. **Q:** Quitters never win and winners never quit. So, choose your fate—are you going to be a quitter or a winner?
18. **R:** Ready yourself. Motivation is also about preparation. We must hear the little voice within us telling us to get started before others will get on their feet and try to push us around. Remember, it was not raining when Noah built the ark.
19. **S:** Stop procrastinating. Do not put off until tomorrow what you can do today, we never know what tomorrow will bring.
20. **T:** Take control of your life. Discipline and self-control lives synonymously with motivation. Both are key factors in self-improvement.
21. **U:** Understand others. You know how to talk; you should also learn how to listen. Learn to understand first and to be understood the second. We have two ears and one mouth use them proportionately.
22. **V:** Visualize it. Motivation without vision is similar a boat on a dry land. You need to have a crystal clear path.
23. **W:** Want it more than anything. Dreaming means believing and to believe is something that is rooted out from the roots of motivation and self-improvement.
24. **X:** X Factor is what will make you different from the others. When you are motivated, you tend to put on 'extras' on your life such as extra time for family, extra help at work, extra care for friends and so on.
25. **Y:** You are unique. No one in this world looks, acts or talks exactly similar to you. Value your life and existence, because you only get to spend it once.
26. **Z:** Zero in on your dreams and go for it!

■ APPLICATION OF MOTIVATIONAL THEORY IN NURSING EDUCATION

Motivation theory proposes reasons for behavior. One classic approach is Abraham Maslow's *Toward a Psychology of Being* in 1946. Maslow explains in his later textbook *Motivation and Personality* in 1954 that individuals move through a hierarchy of motivating needs from physiological to safety, social, esteem and finally self-actualization. He suggests that individuals meet each category of needs in that order. Nursing students can identify situations where these needs are met in their practice of nursing.

Role Play Application of Theory

1. Teach the students the hierarchy of needs. Ask students to identify an experience to match each level of need. One example is to address the experience of safety in walking across a large hospital parking lot late at night.
2. Tell the students to list needs of patients in the same way. An example is the physiological need to address bleeding or pain from an injury.
3. Present a scenario of hospital duties that includes a nurse acting to address a need. One example is meeting the need for safety in the intake and medical history process.
4. Identify the roles played in the scenario, such as patient, parent and nurse. Assign the roles to students. Ask the role players to act out the scenario. In the discussion of the role play review the hierarchy of needs. Discuss these needs in the areas of physiological safety, social, esteem and finally self-actualization.
5. Instruct the other students to assess the nurse's behaviors that met the identified need. Give examples, such as meeting a safety need by asking about allergies to medicines.
6. Discuss what needs the nurse may have experienced, such as a need for esteem by being seen as competent.

▪ CONCLUSION

Motivation influences many aspects of our life and helps explain different causes of behavior. It aids survival, accounts for variations in any individual's behavior and guides our actions. Motivation operates in a cycle. Homeostasis involves maintaining various bodily processes within a narrow range of acceptability. Deviations from that norm lead to automatic corrective actions.

Motivation is the drive forces, which begins, sustain and directs human activities. Motivation is the way of human behavior. Motivation is made up of a need, drive, response and goal. All human being is motivated by something. Very little human behavior is completely random or instinctive. Most human behavior is goal directed. People do things for some reason to get certain results. Motivation drives the human beings to reach their goals and organization goals through every challenge and constraint they face in their workplace, considering it as an advantage to go ahead in the direction they have put for themselves. The need of achievement always results in a desire to do extra effort to have something done better and have the desire for success.

▪ REVIEW QUESTIONS

Long Essays

1. Define motivation. Explain the meaning and nature of motivation.
2. Explain physiological, general and social motives in detail.
3. Describe various theories of motivation.

Short Essays

4. Explain motivational process in detail.
5. Describe the components of motivation.
6. Define frustration. Explain the sources of frustration.
7. Define conflict. Describe the different types of conflicts.
8. Enumerate the motivational qualities of nurse.
9. Explain the need and importance of motivation in nursing.

Short Answers

10. Unconscious motives.
11. Instinctive behavior.
12. Hierarchy of motives.
13. Drive reduction theory.
14. Cognitive theories of motivation.
15. Maslow's hierarchy need.
16. Resolution of conflicts.
17. Seven rules of motivation.

CHAPTER

17 Emotion

■ INTRODUCTION

Emotions occupy an important place in our life. Life has become enjoyable because of the emotions such as love, affection, personal happiness and the preferences. But all emotions do not have pleasantly toned effect, which are just mentioned. Emotions such as fear, anger and jealousy bring about a good deal of disturbance. Our emotions have a great impact on others when we express them in ways that can be perceived by others. When we perceive the emotional responses of other people, we respond in appropriate ways, perhaps with an emotional expression of our own.

■ MEANING

1. An emotion is a strong feeling. It is a conscious stirred up state of our organism.
2. Emotions experienced as certain feelings, pleasant or unpleasant, accompanied by marked physiological changes that involves both visceral and peripheral areas.
3. The subjective experience of an emotion is the cognitive component. Here, the conscious experience could be pleasant or unpleasant.
4. The bodily arousal is the physical component; this is reflected by the activation of the autonomic nervous system, which regulates the activity of glands, smooth muscles and blood vessels.
5. Emotion is the mode of experience that accompanies the working of an instinctive impulse.

■ DEFINITION

1. Emotion is a distinct psychological state, which involves subjective experience, physical arousal and behavioral response. In other words, it has a cognitive component, physical component and a behavioral component.
2. Emotion is an affective experience that accompany generalized inner adjustment, mental and physiological stirred-up states in the individual, and that shows itself in his/her overt behavior.
3. Emotion is a complex affective experience that involves diffusion, physiological changes and can be expressed overtly in characteristic behavior pattern.

■ PHYSIOLOGY OF EMOTION

Physiological reactions and changes that are associated with emotions have their roots in our body chemistry. They are controlled by the endocrine glands, the autonomous nervous system (ANS) and brain.

Emotion and Autonomic Nervous System

1. The ANS plays a significant role in controlling and regulating the emotional behaviors.
2. The ANS consists of sympathetic and parasympathetic system.
3. The sympathetic system activation leads to dilated pupils, dryness of mouth, goose pimples of the skin, sweaty palms, dilation of the lung passages, increased heart rate, increased blood supply to the muscles, increased activity of the adrenal glands and inhibited digestion.
4. The parasympathetic system activation leads to constriction of the pupils, salivation, dryness of palm, absence of goose pimples, constriction of lung passages, decreased heart rate, increased blood supply to internal organs, decreased adrenal gland activity and stimulation of digestion.

Emotion and the Brain

1. The brain controls the autonomic responses that accompany emotions. The seat of emotion in the areas of brain is the hypothalamus, amygdale and the adjacent structures in the limbic system.
2. Emotions appear to be triggered by activity in the centers of the brain medicated by neurotransmitters. Dopamine has a major role in pleasant emotions.
3. Reticular formation: This mass of cells discharges impulses diffusely and some of them ascend to the cerebral cortex, where they have an alerting function. When the reticular formation is activated, the relaxed or passive organism becomes aroused or alert.
4. Hypothalamus: The limbic system consist series of interrelated brain structures, which include the hypothalamus and the sepal area both of which are important in emotions. Impulses from the hypothalamus also activate the viscera and muscles, as when the adrenal gland is stimulated to secrete adrenaline.
5. The hypothalamus, in every way, tries to coordinate the activities of the internal organs associated with the emotional behavior. Impulses that come from the hypothalamus increase both smooth muscle (involuntary) and skeletal muscle (voluntary) activities.
6. The connection between the emotional behavior and stimulation of the various parts of the brain has brought the electric stimulation of the brain as a method for treating violent behavior in human being, particularly epileptics whose brain malfunction causes unusual aggressive behavior.

■ CHANGES IN EMOTION

External Changes

1. Emotions are complex experiences; they are psychological as well as physiological or physical. As psychical experiences, the individual feels them as pleasant or unpleasant states of mind.
2. Emotion is a conscious and intellectual perception of a situation, intense and important enough to provoke one emotionally.
3. The body or organism gets stirred up, changes occur in our breathing, circulation of blood, heart rate and other physiological functions.
4. There are many external changes in the body—changes in our voice, gestures, postures, facial expressions, etc.
5. The changes in facial expressions serve as indices to the nature of emotions. The face of a person experiencing joy is radiated with a smile. The angry person's red face betrays anger.

6. There is a feeling tone accompanying these physical and physiological changes. All these result in some overt responses or behaviors such as laughing, crying, shouting, hitting, crouching and crying.
7. Bodily postures and gestures too can be used as clues to identify emotions. In sorrow, a person tends to slump his/her face downward and in joy, he/she holds head high and chest out.

Internal Changes

1. If there is a greater intensity on action of heart, it results in palpitation.
2. Blood pressure (BP) increases during emotional excitement.
3. There is a shift of blood from the viscera to the surface of the body causing flushing of face, e.g. anger.
4. There are many changes in the gastrointestinal (GI) tract. For example, churning movements slow down or stop in the stomach, and the flow of saliva and other gastric juices necessary for digestion is reduced by 85–90%.
5. There is a greater secretion of glycogen into the blood, sweat glands become more active.

Physiological Changes During Emotions

Psychologists believe that emotions can be measured quantitatively by observing different physiological responses (Fig. 17.1) of the individual, which are indicators of emotions. They also believe that they themselves are with different emotional states. The major physiological changes that occur during emotions are as detailed below.

Respiratory changes: The most apparent and obvious change during emotions. During emotions, respiration increases; it also occurs when the person is happy or excited. But the production and secretion of saliva decreases as the process of respiration increases.

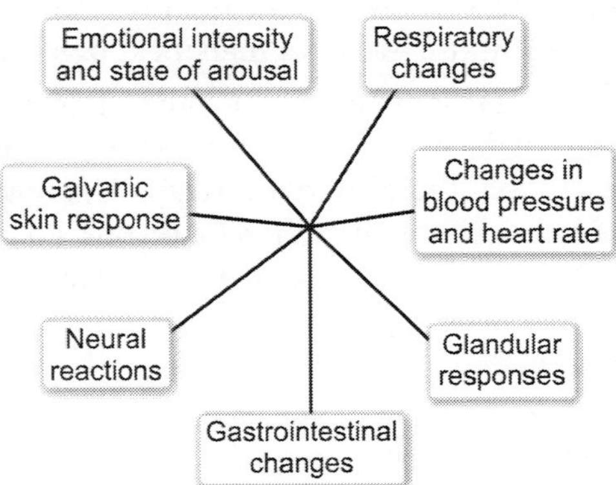

Figure 17.1: Physiological changes during emotion

Changes in BP and heart rate: Variations in BP occur during emotions; it usually increases during an emotional state. Heartbeat also increases during emotions. Increased BP and heightened heart rate for prolonged periods may lead to coronary heart disease.

Glandular responses: During strong emotional states such as anger or fear, excessive amounts of hormones adrenaline and noradrenaline are secreted into the bloodstream. Due to this secretion, liver secretes excessive amounts of glucose directly into the bloodstream that causes the blood to clot rapidly in case of injury or damage. Blood pressure and sugar level rises, pulse become fast, air passage of the lungs enlarges and causes more air into the lungs, pupils enlarge, sweat appears all over the body, particularly on hands and temperature of the skin rises. Noradrenaline helps to constrict the blood vessels, thus making it available to other parts of the body in case of injury. Pituitary and thyroid glands are also responsive to emotional states. All the glandular responses help to cope physically with the emotional as well as emergency situations.

Gastrointestinal changes: Stomach and intestines are also very responsive to emotional states. They either start working at a very high rate or stop entirely. During strong emotional arousal, its working speed decreases and flow of blood is more toward the brain and the skeletal muscles, rather than these organs.

Neural reactions: Besides affecting visceral organs of the body, emotions also bring changes in the neural/nerve activity. Autonomic division of the peripheral nervous system (PNS) is more effective in this regard in which sympathetic and parasympathetic nervous systems work successively.

Galvanic skin response: When perspiration appears during emotions, two important changes occur in skin's electrical stimulation; rapid generation of electromotive energy and the electrical resistance of skin changes. These changes can be measured through a measurement of galvanic skin response (GSR) formally called psychogalvanic response (PGR).

Emotional intensity and state of arousal: Most of the times, we are aware of our emotional states such as angry, excited or afraid; in all these states, the physiological conditions are the same, e.g. heartbeat increases, face blushes or becomes pale. Thus, people are unable, at times, to differentiate between different emotions and the associated arousals.

Other common bodily changes during emotions: As follows:

- Dryness of throat and mouth
- Muscle tension
- Weakness or fainting
- Trembling
- Sinking feeling in heart or stomach.

■ CHARACTERISTICS OF EMOTION

1. Emotions are universal; prevalent in every living organism at all stages of development from infancy to old age.
2. Emotions rise abruptly, but subside slowly; an emotion once aroused, tends to persists and leave behind emotional hangover.
3. Emotions are personal and thus differ from individual to individual.
4. An emotion can give birth to a number of other similar emotions.
5. The emotional experiences are associated with one or the other instincts or biological drives.

■ KINDS OF EMOTION

Kinds of emotions (Fig. 17.2) are different, which are as detailed below.

Pleasure

1. Pleasure is a reaction to the satisfaction of a motive or the attainment of a goal, i.e. satisfaction of motive states results in the emotion of pleasure.
2. We derive a great deal of pleasure from daydreams in which we think about attaining certain goals.
3. The emotion of pleasure manifest in smiling, laughing, hugging and kissing or in contentment, is evoked by situations, which give physical comfort to the infant or a young child.

Fear

1. In general, fear is triggered by situations that are perceived as physically threatening, damaging to one's sense of well-being.
2. Fear is produced in children by sudden happenings, when the child is not

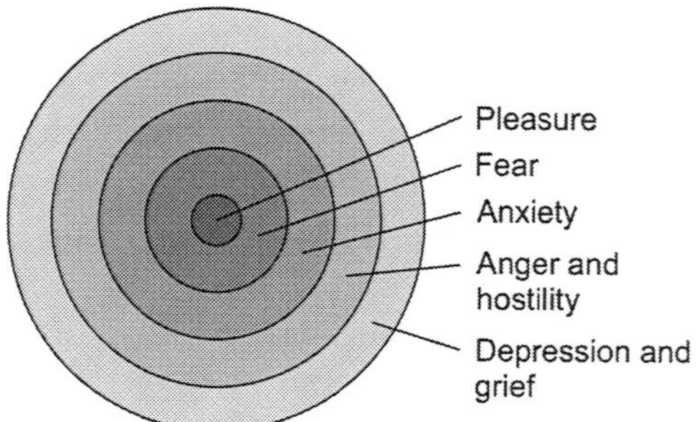

Figure 17.2: Kinds of emotion

prepared for what is coming. In infancy, strange and intense stimuli such as noise produce fear.

3. The adolescent boy or girl is afraid of social humiliation and ridicule. In adulthood, we are afraid of situation, which threatens our needs to obtain recognitions, prestige and economic security.
4. Several factors are important in determining what the specific sources of fear will be for an individual.

Anxiety

1. Anxiety is a vague fear experienced without knowing just what the matter is. One cause of anxiety can be unconscious memory of a fear stimulus.
2. When one learns a response to a particular situation, it means he/she learned a response to all situations that are of similar origin.
3. A child who learns to fear a strict father may later feel uneasy or anxious in the presence of other men.

Anger and Hostility

1. Anger and hostility are reactions to the frustration of motives, insults and threats.
2. Frustrating a motive by imposing restraints on behavior is likely to provoke anger in a person of any age—for infants, simple restraints, which frustrates exploratory motive is a common cause of anger.
3. Social frustrations are also common cause of adults' anger. We seldom observe outright displays of it. Most frequent are the feelings of anger are called 'annoyance'.
4. Ways of expressing anger change with age; among preschool children, anger is likely to take the form of temper, tantrums and fighting.
5. An adult feels angry when his/her prestige is at stake, when desires are being thwarted, when the plans are being spoiled.

Depression and Grief

1. When depressed, people often feel inadequate and worthless because of their failure to reach important goals. The depressed person losses the joy of living.
2. For most of us, depression does not last long, because the situation in the environment changes and we are able to reach at least some of our goals. But for some people, perhaps because of an innate predisposition, depression can be prolonged and serve enough to make suicide.
3. Grief or sorrow and depressions are closely related, but there are differences between them. We usually call the emotion grief, when it is triggered by a specific loss such as the death of a family member or friend.

■ CLASSIFICATION OF EMOTION (ROBERT PLUTCHIK)

Humans express a wide variety of emotions. Robert Plutchik, who was a professor emeritus at the Albert Einstein College of Medicine, researched emotions and designed a color wheel that depicts the intensity level of emotions. Eight primary emotions, in three strengths, for a total of 24 emotions, form this wheel. These are joy, trust, fear, surprise, sadness, disgust, anger and anticipation. Eight other secondary emotions are love, submission, awe, disapproval, remorse, contempt, aggressiveness and optimism. These emotions are as detailed below.

Serenity and its increasingly intense companions: Joy and ecstasy demonstrate increasingly positive feelings. Serenity is calmness, joy shows happiness or gaiety and ecstasy flows forth as pure delight or bliss.

Acceptance, trust and admiration: Show increasing feelings of respect. Acceptance means approval, trust means a firm belief in someone or something and admiration signifies esteem.

Apprehension, fear and terror: Signify emotional discomfort. Apprehension means a sense of uneasiness, fear represents aversion and terror means phobia.

Distraction, surprise and amazement: These are related to the unexpected. Distraction shows a lack of focus, surprise means unexpected usually in reference to a gift or event and amazement is astonishment or sudden wonder.

Pensiveness, sadness and grief: Represent intensified feelings of sorrow. Pensiveness shows sad thoughtfulness, sadness means unhappiness and grief generally relates to sorrow over death.

Boredom, disgust and loathing: These show aversion. Boredom represents a lack of interest, disgust is repugnance and loathing means extreme hatred.

Annoyance, anger and rage: Demonstrate levels of ire. Annoyance shows mild irritation, anger may be spoken or nonverbal, but demonstrates hostility and rage vents as intense fury.

Interest, anticipation and vigilance: These show increasing concern. Interest is beginning attention, anticipation marks a pleasurable expectation and vigilance signifies watchfulness.

Love and submission: Plutchik introduced the secondary emotions with love, although most people would consider it as a primary emotion. Love demonstrates strong affection and submission is a feeling of service.

Awe and disapproval: Awe represents wonder combined with slight fear and disapproval means censure.

Remorse and contempt: Remorse means deep sorrow or disappointment and contempt is disdain.

Aggressiveness and optimism: Aggressiveness signifies the powerful outward expression of strong emotion such as that shown by bullies, whereas optimism shows a positive belief in the best possible outcomes.

EMOTION AND HEALTH

1. Emotions play an important role in human life. People wish to influence another person's actions by raising the appropriate emotions. Emotions give energy to carry out the activity.
2. Modern discovers in medicine have shown to us that uncontrolled emotionality plays a vital role in the causation of many physical disorders.
3. Persistent emotional disturbances caused by anger, fear and worries have been found to be one of the causative factors of psychosomatic disorders.
4. The continuous worries, fears and anxieties cause perpetual tensions. As a result, one's mental health is found to be affected.
5. A relatively new field of investigation known as psychosomatic disease has thrown some light upon it. It has shown that how emotional strain can cause bodily harm.
6. Illness such as asthma, chronic headache, certain skin diseases, nervous pains, etc. are believed to have a psychosomatic origin. Their symptoms may be physiological, but origins are psychological.
7. Other illnesses in which emotions play a vital role are bronchial asthma, high BP, insomnia, chronic constipation and others.
8. Good and pleasant emotions contribute to good health. But intense and unpleasant emotions disturb person sometimes to a great extent if they persist. They may cause certain illnesses or may worsen the conditions of one already ill.

9. The responsibility of a nurse is not only to practice their nursing skills and provide physical comfort; it is also to reduce the intensity of emotional disturbances as much as it is possible for her.

■ THEORIES OF EMOTION

Theories of emotion can be categorized in terms of the context within which the explanation is developed. The standard contexts are evolutionary, social and internal. Evolutionary theories attempt to provide a historical analysis of the emotions, usually with a special interest in explaining why humans today have the emotions that they do. Social theories explain emotions as the products of cultures and societies. The internal approach attempts to provide a description of the emotion process itself. This article is organized around these three categories and will discuss the basic ideas that are associated with each. Some specific theories as well as the main features of emotion will also be explained.

James-Lange Theory

1. William James, an American psychologist and Lange, a Danish physiologist have independently brought forward a theory of emotion that explains the relationship between the components of emotions in just the opposite direction of the one given above.
2. According to this theory, an emotional experience has primarily a physiological basis. The psychical part is the resultant phenomenon.
3. Studies of patients with spinal cord damage have supported the James-Lange theory. These patients have no feedback from their muscles or viscera before the injury and many of them reported that their feelings of emotion changed considerably after the injury.
4. The James-Lange theory of emotions is subject to certain criticisms. The bodily changes in themselves are not seen to be the essential basis of emotions in experimental situations. Such changes brought about by drugs do not cause an experience of emotions.
5. Recently, some scientists have proposed the 'facial feedback hypothesis,' which suggests that feedback from the facial muscles and the viscera contribute to the experience of emotion.

Cannon-Bard Theory

1. Walter B Cannon objected to the James-Lange theory for several reasons. Cannon argued that people whose viscera were surgically separated from the central nervous system (CNS), still reported some kind of emotional experience (Fig. 17.3).
2. This theory emphasizes the role played by hypothalamus in emotional behavior. It says that both the feeling aspect and the bodily changes are set simultaneously by the hypothalamus.
3. Cannon's theory of emotions suggested that emotions originate in the activity of lower brain areas rather than in the viscera; these circuits then activate both the cortex and viscera. Activity in the brain is critically important for certain emotions.

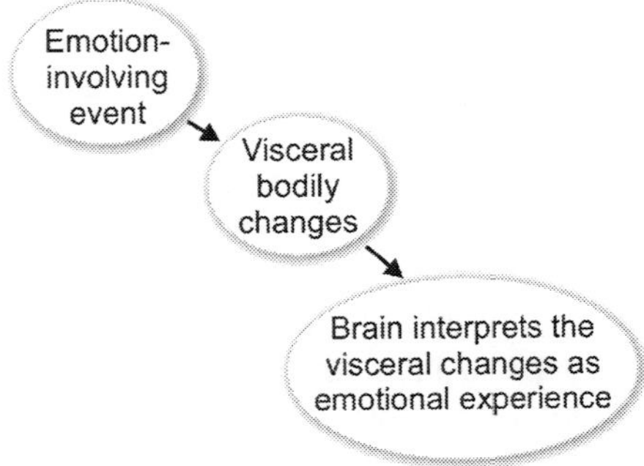

Figure 17.3: Cannon-Bard theory of emotion

Cognitive Theory

1. The American psychologists Stanley Schachter and Jerome E Singer, while adopting an eclectic approach to both the earlier theories of emotion, introduced a new theory named cognitive theory of emotion.
2. This theory suggested that whenever people are emotionally aroused, they decide, which emotion they are feeling by cognitively evaluating and appraising situational cues.
3. Network model of emotions is a recent view of the relationship between emotions and cognitions. This theory suggests that manifestations are linked in the brain to memories for the experience in which those emotions were aroused.

Cognitive Physiological Theory of Emotion

1. Schachter (1959) proposed that emotional states are a function of the interaction of cognitive factors and a state of physiological arousal.
2. Feedback to the brain from physiological activity gives rise to an undifferentiated state of affect. But the felt emotion is determined by the 'label' (cognition), the subject assigns to the aroused state. The assignment of a label is a cognitive process.
3. To interpret the feelings, the subject uses information from past experiences and his/her perception of what is going on around him/her.
4. Experienced and inexperienced users of alcohol and other drugs label their bodily sensations differently in terms of emotional tone. The initial users have to learn to label the physiological sensations as enjoyable. Hence, emotion is an internal physiological arousal in interaction with cognitive process.

Activation Theory

1. The term activation theory of emotion was actually coined in 1951 by Donald B Lindsley. In general, activation theory refers to the view that emotion represents a state of lightened arousal rather than a qualitative unique type of psychological, physiological or behavioral process.
2. Arousal is considered to lie on a wide continuum ranging from a very low level such as deep sleep, to such extremely agitated states as rage or extreme anger.
3. According to Lindsley (1951), emotion-provoking stimuli activate the reticular-activating system in the brainstem, which in turn sends impulses both upward toward the cortex and downward the musculature. For the occurrence of a significant emotional behavior, the reticular formation must be properly activated.

Somatic Theory of Emotions

1. Many psychologists held that consciousness was more directly associated with the muscles than with the brain. Jacobson trained his subjects to relax completely.
2. In this condition, their minds were blank. If the subject thought of moving his/her arm, the electrical potentials were showed up in their muscles. Similarly, tension in the region of the eyes accompanied visual images. These experiments clearly show that consciousness is intimately associated with muscular activity.

■ STRESS AND ADAPTATION

Stress is a term that is difficult to define; it is used loosely and means different things to different people. Some use it to describe an upset feeling or response; others use it to describe the source or stimulus for their feeling upset. Study in the field of stress and adaptation has been pursued by researcher in different disciplines, according to their individual conceptual views.

Definition

1. Hans Selye (1976) defined stress as the state manifested by a specific syndrome, which consists of all the non-specifically induced changes within a biological system.
2. George Engel (1960) defines stress as referring to all processes, whether originating in the external environment or within the person, which impose a demand or requirement upon the organism. The resolution or handling of which necessitates work or activity of the mental apparatus, before any other system is involved or activated.
3. Stress is a state produced by a change in the environment that is perceived as challenging, threatening or damaging to the individual's dynamic equilibrium. There is an actual or perceived imbalance in the individual's capability to meet the demands of the new situation.

Nature of Stress

1. Stress is mediated by two factors, the individual's ability to cope and the social support he/she receives.
2. The change or stimulus that evokes this state is the stressor. The nature of the stressor is variable.
3. Stress is any situation in which a nonspecific demand requires an individual to respond or take action. It involves physiological and psychological responses.
4. Stress can lead to negative or counterproductive feelings or threaten emotional well-being.

Sources of Stress (Fig. 17.4)

Physiological Stressors

- The primary physiological stressors are chemical agent, infectious agent, physical agent, faulty immune mechanisms, genetic disorders, nutritional imbalance and hypoxia
- All the stressors have both a general effect and a specific effect.

Psychosocial Stressors

- Accidents and the survivors
- The experience of others in our social networks
- Horrors of history
- Intrapsychic, unconscious conflicts and anxieties
- The fear of aggression, mutilation and destruction
- The events of history brought into the living room
- The changes of the narrower world in which we live
- Phase-specific psychosocial crisis
- Other normative life crisis—role entries and exits, inadequate socialization, underload and overload
- The inherent conflicts in all social relations
- The gap between culturally included goals and socially structured means.

Factors Influencing Stressors

The nature of the stressor involves the following factors such as intensity, scope, duration, number and nature of other stressors. Each factor influences the response to a stressor. A person may perceive the intensity or magnitude of a stressor as minimal,

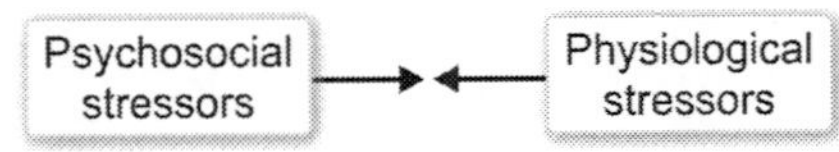

Figure 17.4: Sources of stress

moderate or severe. The greater the magnitude of stressor, the greater is the stress response. The response to any stressor depends on physiological functioning, personality and behavioral characteristics.

Models of Stress (Fig. 17.5)

Response-based Model

1. The response-based model is concerned with specifying the particular response or pattern of responses that may indicate a stressor.
2. Seyle's model or stress is a response-based model that defined stress as a non-specific response of the body to any demand made on it.
3. Stress is demonstrated by a specific physiological reaction, the general adaptation syndrome (GAS). Thus, the response of a person to stress is purely physiological and is never modified to allow cognitive influences.
4. The response-based model does not allow individual differences in response patterns. This lack of flexibility may produce some differences that must be identified in the assessment phase.

Adaptation Model

1. The adaptation model proposes that four factors determine whether a situation is stressful. The ability to cope with stress, the first factor, usually depends on the person's experience with similar stressor, support systems and overall perception of the stressor.
2. The second factor deals with the practices and norms of the person's peer group. If the peer group considers it normal to talk about a particular stressor, the client may respond by complaining about it or discussing it.
3. The third factor is the impact of the social environment in assisting an individual to adapt to a stressor.
4. The last factor involves the resources that can be used to deal with the stressor.
5. The adaptation model is based on the understanding that people experience anxiety and increased stress when they are unprepared to cope with stressful situations.
6. Using this model and appropriate interventions, nurses can help clients and families to promote health in all human dimensions.

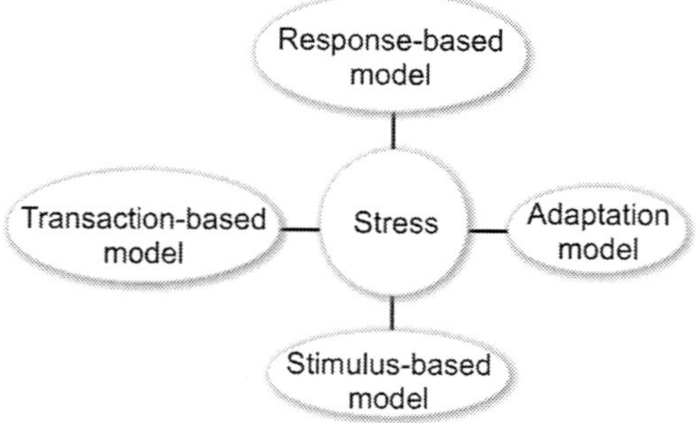

Figure 17.5: Models of stress

Stimulus-based Model

The stimulus-based model focuses on disturbing disruptive characteristics within the environment. The classic research that identified stress as a stimulus has resulted in the development of the social readjustment scale, which measures the effects of major life events on illness. Assumptions of the stimulus-based model:

1. The life-changing events are normal, and they require the same type and duration of adjustments.
2. People are passive recipients of stress and their perceptions of the event are irrelevant.
3. All people have a common threshold of stimulus and illness results at any point after the threshold.
4. As with the response-based model, the stimulus-based model does not allow for individual differences in perception and response to stressors.

Transaction-based Model

1. The transaction-based model views the person and environment in a dynamic, reciprocal and interactive relationship.
2. This model, developed by Lazarus and Folkman, views the stressor as an individual perceptual response rooted in psychological and cognitive process.
3. Stress originates from the relationship between the person and the environment. This model focuses on stress-related process such as cognitive appraisal and coping.

Response to Stress

The classical research by Selye has identified the two physiological responses to stress, the local adaptation syndrome (LAS) and the GAS. The LAS is a response of a body tissue, organ or part to the stress of trauma, illness or other physiological change. The GAS is a defense response of the whole body to stress.

Local Adaptation Syndrome

The body produces many localized responses to stress. These include blood clotting, wound healing, accommodation of the eye to light and response to pressure.

Characteristics of LAS

1. The body produces many localized responses to stress that include entire body systems.
2. The response is adaptive, meaning that a stressor is necessary to stimulate it.
3. The response is short term. It does not persist indefinitely.
4. The response is restorative, meaning that the LAS assist in restoring homeostasis to the body region or part.

Reflex pain response

The reflex pain response is a localized response of the CNS to pain. It is an adaptive response and protects tissue from further damage.

Inflammation response

1. The inflammatory response is stimulated by trauma or infection. This response localizes the inflammation, thus preventing its spread and promoting healing.
2. The inflammatory response may produce localized pain, swelling, heat, redness and changes in functioning.

General Adaptation Syndrome (Fig. 17.6)

The general adaptation syndrome is a physiological response of the whole body to stress. It involves several body systems, primarily the ANS and the endocrine system.

Alarm reaction

1. The alarm reaction involves the mobilization of the defense mechanisms of the body and mind to cope with the stress.
2. Hormones levels rise to increase blood volume and thereby prepare the person to act. Other hormones are released to increase blood glucose levels to make energy available for adaptation.
3. This extensive hormonal activity prepares the person for the fight-or-flight response.
4. During the alarm reaction, the person is faced with a specific stressor. The person's physiological response is extensive, involving major systems of the body and it may last from a minute to many hours.

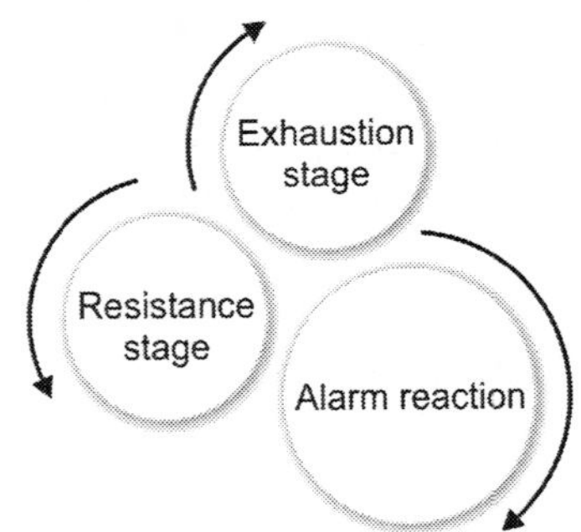

Figure 17.6: General adaptation syndrome

Resistance stage

1. In the resistance stage, the body stabilizes and hormones levels, heart rate, BP and cardiac output return to normal.
2. The person is attempting to adapt to the stressor. If the stress can be resolved, the body repairs damage that may have occurred.
3. If the stressor remains present, as in continued blood loss, debilitating disease or long-term severe mental illness and adaptation fails, the person enters the third phase of GAS, i.e. exhaustion.

Exhaustion stage

1. The exhaustion stage occurs when the body can no longer resist stress and when the energy necessary to maintain adaptation is depleted.
2. The body is unable to defend itself against the impact of the stressor, physiological regulation diminishes and if the stress continues, death may result.

Types of stimuli

Focal stimuli: These provoking stimuli command the attention of the person. Stimuli become focal because of size, intensity, position, novelty, quality, movement and internal predisposing factors such as set and attitude.

Contextual stimuli: This category includes those stimuli that surround the focal stimulus. These are all the other environmental stimuli present, i.e. physical surroundings, other people present and so on.

Residual stimuli: These are recalled remnants of past experiences that influence the meanings attached to other stimuli. It includes attitudes, values, beliefs and other factors that influence an individual's behavior in a given situation.

Adaptation to Stress

Adaptation is a constant, ongoing process that occurs along the time continuum, beginning with birth and ending with death. Also existing along this lifetime continuum is the dimensions of health and illnesses. Adaptation is a continuous process of seeking harmony in an environment. The desired end goals of adaptation for any system are growth and reproduction. A major nursing objective is to support and promote the efforts of the individual to achieve a healthy adaptation.

Concept of Adaptation

1. Adaptation is a term used to describe the work expended by the body in attempting to maintain homeostasis and to ward off the effect of the stressor.
2. The current usage of the term includes the multiplicity of genetical, physiological, psychical and social phenomena through which adjustment (homeostatic balance) is achieved in response to changes within the environment.
3. According to Helsen's concept of adaptation, constant and varied stimuli impinge on each individual at all times.
4. The basic premise of the adaptation level theory is that an individual's attitudes, values, ways of structuring experiences, judgments of physical, esthetic and symbolic objects, intellectual and emotional behavior, learning and interpersonal relationships, all these represent modes of adaptation to environmental and organism forces.

Modes of Adaptation

In the Roy's adaptation theory, humans are conceptualized as having four modes of adaptation as detailed below (Fig. 17.7).

Basic physiological needs: As human respond to environmental changes, they need to keep balance in exercise, nutrition, elimination, fluid and electrolytes, oxygen, circulation and regulation (temperature, sense, endocrine system).

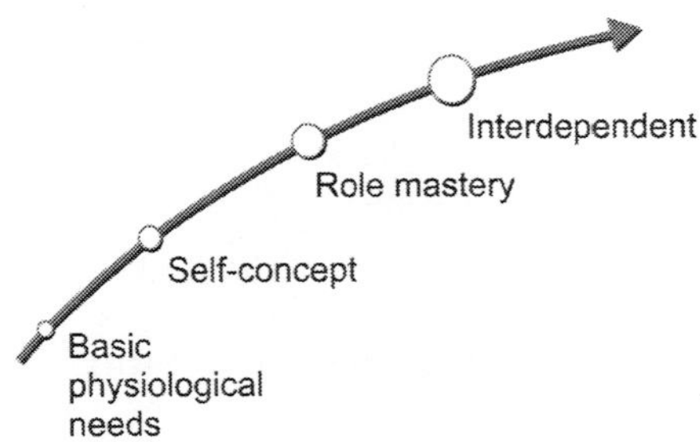

Figure 17.7: Modes of adaptation

Self-concept: It includes all the ideas, feelings, beliefs and attitudes that persons have about them. To maintain psychological adaptation, defense mechanisms may be used to protect the ego when the self-concept is threatened.

Role mastery: In this mode of adaptation, humans are viewed as regulating their performance of duties according to their varying positions in society.

Interdependent: Environmental changes may threaten conflict in a person's interactions with other persons.

Adaptation Concept in Nursing

In the conceptual framework of adaptation, nursing intervention becomes the means through which the nurse's knowledge and skill are interposed in supporting and promoting the patient's adaptive potential to the highest level of effectiveness.

Assessment

First level: Recognizing patient's level of wellness behavior in each adaptive mode.

Second level: Identifying positive and negative behaviors related to problem areas.

Planning

Selecting appropriate intervention from basic seven objectives:

1. Reducing or limiting stress.
2. Preventing additional stress.
3. Supporting adaptations.
4. Limiting and supporting adaptation.
5. Altering, limiting and supporting adaptations.
6. Interrupting, altering, limiting and supporting adaptations.
7. Supplementing, interrupting, altering, limiting and supporting adaptations.

Intervention

Saxton and Hyland pointed out seven objectives to nursing intervention related to stress and adaptation:

1. Reduce or limit the extent and intensity of the present stress.
2. Prevent additional stress.
3. Support the individual's adaptations to assist in sustaining and maintaining the defensive responses.
4. Limit and support the individual's adaptations to confine and restrict the compensatory responses.
5. Interrupt, alter, limit and support the individual's adaptations to modify, and adjust the symptoms or response.
6. Interrupt, alter, limit and support the individual's adaptations to discontinue or stop the responses that have become stresses.
7. Supplement, interrupt, alter, limit and support the individual's adaptations to complement or replace the responses that are failing to control stress.

Evaluation

Reassessing patient's level of wellness behavior in each adaptive mode to determine satisfactory resolution of problem area or need for reassessment and replanning.

Nursing Implications on Stress Reduction

Coping behavior should be remembered that the individual is in constant interaction with his/her environment, both internal and external. This implies that change is constant and that change is necessary for optimal psychosocial and physiological growth. The development of a nursing database that supplies the essential information for making decisions about patient care is a necessity.

Strategies of Stress Reduction

Modification of the situation: Techniques to reach these goals may include changing jobs if the workplace is the source of excessive stress. Through health appraisals, nurses may identify patient stressors. The stress control requires self-care and motivation, and therefore the patient must actively and willingly participate in appraising, identifying and managing his/her sources of stress.

Modification of the meaning of the problem: It may require taking a longer range view of situation or putting it into perspective. Compulsive behavior, deadlines and clock watching may need to be re-evaluated.

Control or management of the symptoms of stress: The individual needs to be able to anticipate the development of stress and to know how to typically react.

Stress Reduction Methods (Fig. 17.8)

Self-regulation of stress: Sutterley (1982) has described six categories or approaches to self-regulation of stress. Proper nutrition, adequate rest and regular exercise improve one's well-being and help develop resistance to stressors. Regular exercise assists in weight control, decrease a sense of fatigue and monotony, and increase the exercise tolerance for patients with angina pectoris and peripheral arterial disease.

Biofeedback: The purpose of biofeedback is to gain some degree of mental control over the ANS and possibly decrease BP, control heart rate and prevent migraine headaches, hyperactive stomachs, etc. Some form of electronic instrumentation is used to monitor a biological function such as measuring skin conductance with the galvanic skin responder.

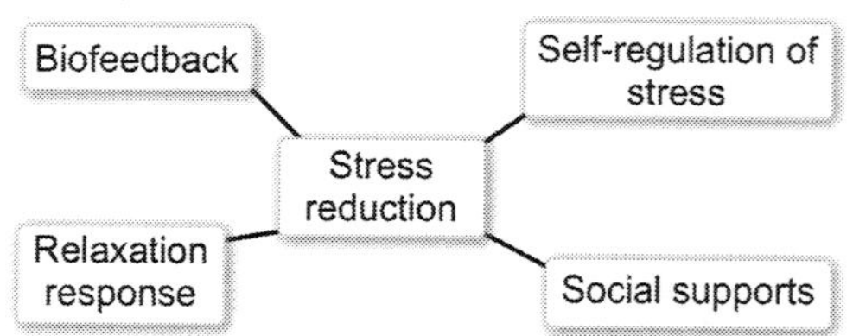

Figure 17.8: Stress reduction methods

Relaxation response: Benson (1975) has described what he calls the 'relaxation response,' which is a calming state opposite to the arousal state or stress. Four elements are necessary to produce the relaxation response, a quite environment, a comfortable position, a passive attitude and a mental device or object such as a word, sound or phrase occupy the mind and keep out thoughts.

Social supports: The importance of social support as a mediating resource in stress has already been identified. To reinforce the information, the function of social networks includes the maintenance of positive social identity, the provision of emotional support, the provision of material aid and tangible services, access to information and new social contacts and new social roles.

Role of Nurse in Emotional Control

A number of patients show emotional reactions such as anxiety, worry, fear, irritability, anger and resentment. Such negative feelings need to be replaced by hope, courage and cooperation. A nurse should listen sympathetically, develop cooperative relationship with the patient and help him/her reduce to tensions. Emotions are controlled as follows:

1. The causes, reactions and consequences of emotions are studied.

2. Emergency situations are avoided because they cause strong emotional reactions. Adequate planning is useful in preventing emergencies.
3. Mental conflicts and emotional tensions are avoided by adopting a sound philosophy of life.
4. Hobbies and sound social relationships are developed, so as to direct one's attention away from emotion-provoking situations.
5. Unreasonable and uncontrolled external expression of emotions is avoided, since it increases the intensity of emotions further.
6. A sense of humor is developed. It helps overlook irritations and petty annoyances.

■ CONCLUSION

In hospitals and clinics, there are clients of different ways of behavior. Sometimes nurses face some situations whereby they will be stimulated to change their behavior. There are situations whereby nurses will be ordered to give patient medication at a certain time; some patient will be refusing to take it due to some reasons such as religious believes. Some nurses will come into the extent of being angry. Some nurses will use the defense mechanism called denial. They normally deny whatever is happening by doing as if nothing has happened. They normally control their anger by talking to the patient with low and slowly explaining them the importance of the medication. Nurses face different emotions each and every day. Patients show unhappiness, confusion, anger and sadness. So, nurses must be able to manage their own emotions, so that they can be able to remain calm during unstable conditions. Nurses have to suppress any negative feelings toward patients in order to demonstrate a non-judgmental manner with patients.

Basically, emotions are socially very important, because through it, people can work together or bind to each other and they are what make life worth living or sometimes ending. So, I consider it important for each and everyone to know and understand more about emotions. For nurses is a must for them to acquire knowledge and more understanding about emotions, since they are dealing with people of different characters, who can just arouse their feelings in any other way. Hence, by understanding it, they may know how to cope with situation they encounter in their working places. Least, but not last, emotions are similar to wild horses, so people have to consider it before they take a step forward.

■ REVIEW QUESTIONS

Long Essays

1. Define emotion. Explain the physiological reaction and changes in emotion.
2. Describe internal and external changes in emotion.
3. Discuss various theories of emotion.

Short Essays

4. Discuss the types of emotion.
5. Describe the characteristics of emotion.
6. Enumerate health and emotion.
7. Cannon-Bard theory of emotion.
8. James-Lange theory of emotion.
9. Define stress. Explain the sources and factors that influence stress.
10. Enumerate the models and response of stress.
11. Describe adaptation of stress.
12. Describe the adaptation concept in nursing.
13. Nurse's role in emotional control.

Short Answers

14. Fear.
15. Anxiety.
16. Activation theory.
17. Adaptation model.
18. Alarm reactions.
19. Mode of adaptation.
20. List out the nursing implications of stress reduction.
21. Biofeedback.
22. Self-regulation of stress.

CHAPTER

18 Attitude

■ INTRODUCTION

Attitudes are not innate or unlearned as those of physiological motives or some emotional reactions. They are acquired by people. Some of them are built by people by their effort. Others are absorbed by us passively and spontaneously from the social environment into which a person is born and in which he/she grow. Many of the people's attitudes are the result of reflection and purposeful thinking or the outcome of training and suggestion from others, especially their parents and teachers. Attitude is the evaluation of an object, person, behavior or event based on beliefs, guiding behavior of an individual. Psychologists have defined an attitude in any diverse ways. Kimball Young defines an attitude as a predisposition to respond in a persistent and characteristic manner in reference to some situation, idea, value, material objects or class of objects, or person or group of persons. This can be positive, negative or neutral views of an attitude object. For example, person, behavior or an event.

■ DEFINITION

1. An attitude denotes an adjustment of the individual toward some selected person, group or organization. —*Kuppusamy*
2. An attitude is the entire package of particular beliefs, feelings and response tendencies of the individual toward the appropriate object. —*Kerch and others*
3. Attitude is a mental structure of framework that includes motivational, perceptual, emotional and cognitive reactions. The positive or negative reaction of a person to his/her environment, other persons and objects is based on his/her attitude.
4. Attitude is a permanent disposition of a person toward an object, subject or thought that tends him/her to react in accordance with his/her interests.
5. Attitudes are the manifestation of a person's concepts, thoughts or imaginations, which direct person's behavior toward a specific direction.

■ COMPONENTS OF ATTITUDE (Fig. 18.1)

Cognitive Component

The opinion or belief is segment of an attitude. It is made up of thoughts and beliefs the people hold about the object of the attitude. It is therefore, what one has learned about something. It is what a person believes to be true about it. For example, vegetarian food is healthy.

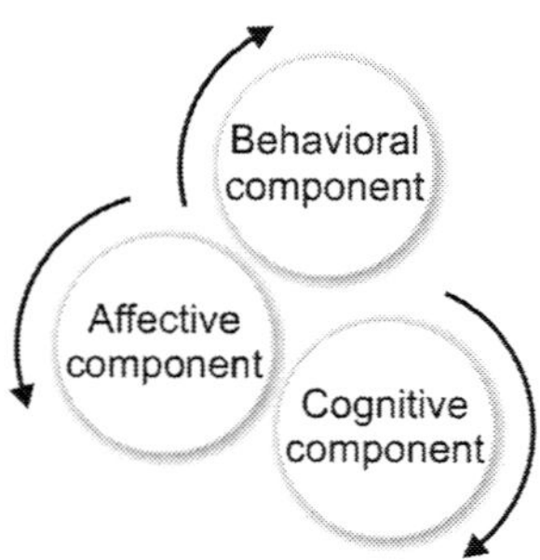

Figure 18.1: Components of attitude

Affective Component

Affective component is the emotion or feeling segment of an attitude. The affective component is the matter of liking or disliking something. This consists of the emotional feelings stimulated by the object of the attitude. For example, "I prefer vegetarian food".

Behavioral Component

Behavioral component is an intention to behave in a certain way toward someone or something. The action component of attitude refers to a readiness to respond. Thus, expressed attitudes usually have a consistent relationship to behavior. For example, "I always eat vegetarian food".

■ NATURE OF ATTITUDE

Attitudes are universal; they are either positive or negative and are found toward social as well as non-social aspects of the environment. These attitude are not innate, they are acquired. It implies subject-object relationship. Attitude of respect toward our elders is a positive attitude, whereas an attitude of hatred toward a certain community is a negative attitude. It is a way we perceive, think and feel more or less permanently in relation to something. It is a sort of mental readiness or a tendency to react to certain situations, in a more or less consistent manner. We have acquired certain set ways of reacting to religious rituals, to political democracy, to social equality, to our parents and teachers, to various racial, communal and religious groups, to people exercising authority over us, to our colleagues who work with us, to our own profession and its prestige, and to other professions, which are as follows:

1. Attitude is evaluation expressed by terms such as liking-disliking, pro-anti, favoring-not favoring and positive-negative. They are the feeling tone aroused by any attitude object.
2. Attitudes are thought to guide behavior. For example, if one is unfavorable toward smoking, he/she shows negative attitude toward smokers.
3. The expressions that one makes publicly to others are not always the same as the expressions one makes privately to oneself.
4. They are feeling tones aroused by any attitude object. Attitudes can be formed about many things. The objects of attitude can be certain entities (a lecture, a restaurant), people (parents, siblings, Prime Minister, oneself) or abstract concepts (abortion, civil rights, foreign aid).
5. The attitude may be similar toward some of the objects and different toward others. Thus, attitude varies with everyone.
6. Individuals are not fully aware of their attitudes and these accounts in part for possible inconsistency of attitudes with one another.
7. The attitude attempts to understand the motives they serve for the individual.
8. It provides a ready basis for interpreting the world and processing new information.
9. It is a way of gaining and maintaining social interaction.
10. Attitude is a hypothetical construct that represents an individual's likes or dislikes for an item.

11. Attitudes that are accompanied by strong feeling tones are called sentiments. These can be positive or negative. One may have sentiments of love for respective country, a sentiment of respect for elders or a sentiment of hatred for dishonesty and lying.

■ MOTIVATIONAL FUNCTIONS OF ATTITUDE

Katz (1960) has suggested four motivational functions of attitudes; they are knowledge, social adjustment, value expression and ego defenses:

1. **Knowledge function:** People seek a degree of practicability, consistency and stability in their perception of the world.
2. **Social adjustment function:** It refers to the favorable responses and the individual achieves from others by displaying socially acceptable attitudes.
3. **Value expression function:** Through this, the individual achieves self-expression with regard to cherished values.
4. **Ego-defensive function:** This allows the individual to be protected from acknowledging personal deficiencies.

■ DEVELOPMENT OF ATTITUDE (Fig. 18.2)

Attitudes of person are the permanent ways of one's behaving. These are the acquired characteristics of a person, which are reflected in his/her work and behavior. Many of people's attitudes are the result of reflection and purposeful thinking or the outcome of training and suggestion from others, especially their parents and teachers. Children whose parents show respect and courtesy to other acquire attitudes of respect and courtesy to most human being without being specially told about it. They simply take suggestions from their parents unconsciously.

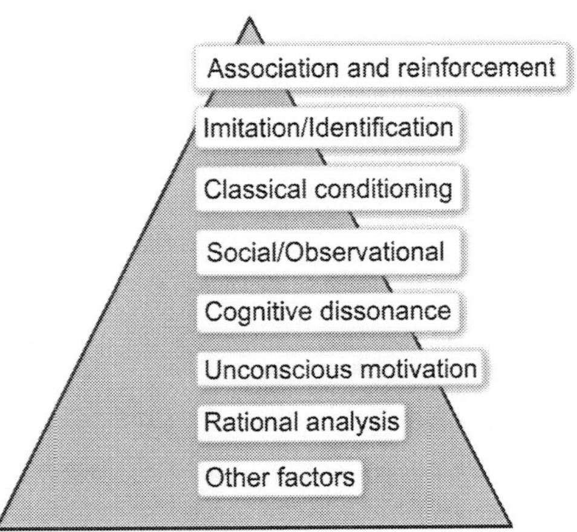

Figure 18.2: Development of attitude

Motives, emotional conditions, schooling, cultural norms, the type of parent-child relationships that is obtained in childhood, the way they have been taught to perceive things and propaganda—all these factors affect the growth of people attitudes.

Attitude is also influenced by the type and quantity of the factual knowledge that is acquired about situation, things and person. Many times, people may develop hostile attitudes toward a person because what we have been told about him/her does evoke hostility or aggression. Many of the people's attitudes are the result of wrong or false knowledge that is available to them. The best example is people's prejudices and biases. People may have acquired this knowledge from newspaper, journals, books, movies or the political speeches. The cognitive components of attitudes are assumed to be learned in the same ways as are any facts, knowledge of beliefs. The basic processes of association, reinforcement and imitation determine this acquisition.

Association and Reinforcement

The child is exposed to certain things about the world. He/She is reinforced for expressing some cognitions or attitudes or for actual acting; on the basis of this, they learn them.

Imitation/Identification

Imitation/Identification is important in the learning process. A child spends a great deal of time with their parents and after a while begins to believe as they do simply by copying them, even when they do not deliberately try to influence him/her.

Classical Conditioning

Classical conditioning involves involuntary response and is acquired through the pairing of two stimuli. Two events that repeatedly occur close together in time become fused and before long the person responds in the same way to both events. For example, pleasant and unpleasant experiences with members of a particular group could lead to positive or negative attitudes toward the group.

Social/Observational

Social (observational) learning is based on modeling. We observe others. If they are getting reinforced for certain behaviors or expression of certain attitudes, it makes it more likely that we too will behave in this manner or express the same attitude.

Cognitive Dissonance

When two contradictory feelings, beliefs or behaviors exist, it creates a state of tension and the person tries to reduce tension by changing their feelings, beliefs or behaviors.

Unconscious Motivation

Some attitudes are held because they serve some unconscious function for an individual. For example, a person who is threatened by his/her homosexual feelings may employ the defense mechanism of reaction formation and become a crusader against homosexuals.

Rational Analysis

Rational analysis involves the careful weighing of evidence against a particular attitude. The nurse giving health education to slums will influence their attitude for personal hygiene when informing about rationale of unhygienic conditions.

Other Factors

Even after a child develops attitudes, he/she continues to be exposed primarily to information that supports it. At this stage, various socioeconomic factors determine what he/she hears. His/Her neighborhood, newspaper, school, friends, etc. tend to be more homogeneous than the rest of the world.

■ CHANGING ATTITUDES

An individual's attitude is formed during the childhood stages as a result of socialization and later on when he/she meets and interacts with the peer group in later childhood, adolescence and early childhood. When an individual sees a smoker is confronted with communication from the communicator that cigarette smoking causes lung cancer. Now, the stress is produced by the discrepancy between the individual's attitude and the attitude expressed in the communication. This stress has been called conflict, incongruity, imbalance or just inconsistency. Therefore, there is pressure on the individual to resolve the discrepancy. If the individual changes his/her attitude in the direction advocated by the communication, the discrepancy is reduced. Hence the stress is resolved. Thus, attitude change can be either:

1. **Congruent change:** For example, negative attitude will increase too negatively or positive attitude will increase too positively, i.e. change in the same direction.
2. **Incongruent change:** For example, change in attitude from positive to

negative or from negative to positive. In other words, the change will be in the same direction.

Change of Attitude

Once the attitudes and beliefs have been formed, they have a tendency to persist or continue. Therefore, it is difficult to change the attitudes that have been established. There are many reasons of our inability that cannot be changed easily. One of the reasons is that a person do not want to change on account of the social support he/she has acquired. For them in order to change attitudes and beliefs, they should:

- Change perceptions by new experiences and factual knowledge
- Control emotions and motivational factors in early childhood, when most of the daily attitudes are formed
- Tap the various formative agencies.

■ CHARACTERISTICS OF ATTITUDES

- Attitudes are related to the needs and problems of the person
- Unconscious mind plays an important role in the formation of attitudes
- A series of emotional experiences is attached to attitudes
- Attitudes direct the activities or actions of person
- The reaction of a person toward an object, issue or environment can be predicted by knowing a person's attitudes
- Attitudes are related to some thoughts, images and external objects.

■ EFFECTS OF ATTITUDES ON BEHAVIOR

Attitudes manifest the nature of person and they direct the behavior of person. Hence, favorable or positive attitudes (kindness, service and assistance) are the indicators of good behavior, while unfavorable or negative attitudes (hatred, noncooperation, selfishness, etc.) express the bad behavior of a person. It is easy to provide nursing to the patients having favorable attitude toward hospital, while the behavior of patients with negative attitudes toward hospital, may create obstacles in their nursing treatment. Similarly, nurses and doctors should adopt a professional attitude toward the patients.

■ THEORIES OF ATTITUDE CHANGE (Fig. 18.3)

Balance Theory

1. Balance theory given by Heider (1946, 1958) emphasized the positive and negative balances of attitudes toward one or more persons, which might not agree with one another.
2. There is always movement toward a balance state, a situation in which the relations fit together harmoniously and then there is no stress.
3. The basic concept of the balance is that a tendency exists for individuals to restore balance to attitude, which are not of the same sign.
4. Heider's P-O-X model explains situations in which there are two person, a perceiver 'P' and another 'O', each of whom might have an attitude toward a given object 'X'.
5. If 'P' likes 'O', the assumption is that O's attitude toward 'X' should be the same as P's. For example, two staff nurses might share a common positive attitude

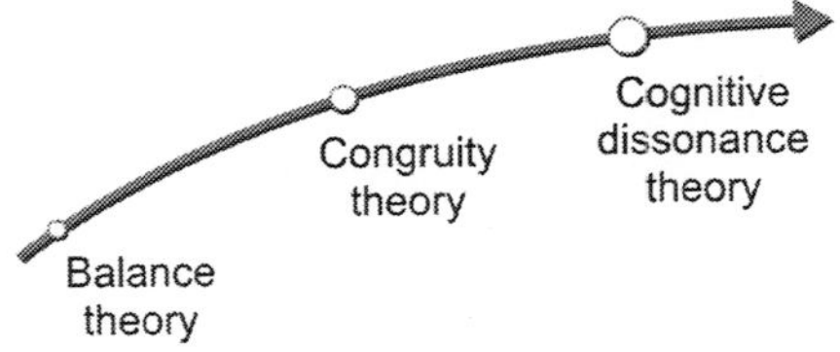

Figure 18.3: Theories of attitude change

toward ward sister. If they differed on that issue, then an imbalance state would exist. In that case, they might try to persuade each other or also avoid the topic until the duty was over in order to retain at least apparent balance.

6. These theory statements are shown by plus (+) or minus (-) signs. It predicts that when all signs are positive, a state of balance exists. If there is one negative sign or three negative signs, the outcome is negative leading to an imbalance state (just as the multiplication of two minuses yields a plus). Therefore balance occurs when there are either two positive signs or two negative signs.

Congruity Theory

1. Osgood and Tannenbaum (1955) postulates that imbalance between attitudes is resolved by summing the amount of their positive or negative quality. There is a pair of attitudes on which one has a positive sign and one has a negative sign.
2. The greater the amount of the positive or negative quality of an attitude, the less likely it is to change when paired with something of an opposite sign. The valence goes from +3 to -3 on the usual attitude scale.
3. Suppose a person dislikes a public figure at the highest scale value of +3 and then learn that he/she favors a policy, which that person may dislike at the relatively moderate level of -1.
4. The prediction is that the person is more likely to alter the attitude toward the policy, in a more favorable, a positive direction, rather than the attitude toward the political figure in an unfavorable direction.
5. However, the actual results may be a less negative or neutral attitude, rather than a positive one. Abelson's and Rosenberg (1958) gave three rules of cognitive interaction, they are:
   a. A likes B and B likes C implies that A likes C also.
   b. A likes B and B dislikes C implies that A dislikes C.
   c. A dislikes B and B dislikes C implies that A likes C.

Cognitive Dissonance Theory

1. Festinger (1957) states that when related cognitions, feelings or behaviors are inconsistent or contradictory, it creates an unpleasant state of tension that motivates people to reduce their dissonance by changing their cognitions, feeling or behavior.
2. For instance, a person who starts out with a negative attitude toward marijuana and finds himself/herself enjoying the experience.
3. The dissonance they experience is thus likely to motivate to change their attitude toward marijuana or to stop using marijuana.

■ MEASUREMENT OF ATTITUDES

Self-report Methods

1. It includes attitude scales, questionnaires, interviews and projective tests. For example, when a person is asked to express his/her preferences, likes and dislikes to an interviewer or to write the evolution of something on a questionnaire.
2. Attitudes are measured by attitude scales, which deal with an issue or set of related issues. These depict the direction of an attitude, the degree or extent in that direction and the intensity of feeling that goes with the attitude.
3. Sometimes these components may be a part of questionnaire, studies and interviews in which people are asked. First, how (pro or con) they feel about something and then how strongly they feel. Finally these rates are highly related.

4. Attitude scales typically consist of a number of statements with which a person may agree or disagree with several scale points, usually ranging from highly agree or highly disagree. In this way, both the direction and the degree are indicated by the response to each statement or item.
5. Typically, these items relate to some common social thing, person, issue and person's overall attitude.
6. Attitude scales commonly used are Thurstone scale, Likert scale, paired comparison method and rank order method.

Thurstone Scale

1. Louis L Thurstone and EJ Chave (1929) in their classic study of attitudes toward the Church developed an interval scale by using the method of equal-appearing intervals.
2. Since the scale represents an evenly graduated series of attitudes as in the foot rule the method is named so.
3. Every statement in Thurstone scale has a numerical value, already determined.
4. The subject has to place a tick mark against each item with which he/she agrees. The attitude score is the mean of the scale value.

Likert Scale

1. For the Likert scale (summated rating), various opinion statements are collected, edited and then given to a group of subjects to rate the statements on a five-point scale, strongly disagree, agree, undecided, disagree and strongly disagree.
2. The subject expresses the degree (1–5) of their personal agreement or disagreement with each of the statements.
3. The respondent's attitude score in the sum of her/his rating of all the statements. For this reason, the Likert scale is also known as the scale of summated ratings.

Bogardus Social Distance Scale

1. Bogardus ES developed an attitude scale in 1933, called social distance scale, which become a classic instrument to measure attitudes toward ethnic group.
2. He was the first person to design a technique for the specific purposes of measuring and comparing attitudes toward different nationalities, particularly measuring tolerance of outgroup.
3. The subject is asked to indicate the extent of his/her willingness to accept members of different social groups into various social institutions.

Observations of Behavior

1. It is a method of studying the behavior, consists of the perception of an individual's attitude under conditions by the other individuals and analysis of his/her perceived attitude by them.
2. By this method, one can infer the mental processes of other persons through the observation of their behavior.
3. For example, observing the actual overt behavior of students in natural situation.

Involuntary Behavioral Measures

1. These study body's physiological responses to attitude.
2. Galvanic skin response (GSR) measures the electrical resistance of the skin.
3. Electromyography (EMG) measures major facial muscle movements.

▪ ATTITUDE AND NURSE

While giving nursing services in the hospital, the nurse has to deal with patients having all kinds of attitudes; simultaneously he/she also has to adjust with the personal and professional attitudes. A nurse should try to understand the patient's attitudes. Some of them enter hospital ready and willing to cooperate;

others enter hospital afraid or resentful, or even definitely antagonistic to the ideas of receiving treatment and to the rigidity of ward routine. Kempf and Averill have listed the following attitudes for a successful and efficient nurse:

1. Ambition to do the task.
2. Conformity with the rules and regulations of the profession for which nurse is preparing.
3. Willingness to work and to work with effectiveness.
4. Cheerfulness and optimism.
5. Interest in the problems and difficulties of other people.
6. Cooperativeness, industriousness, respect for the opinion and judgment of others.
7. Interest in increasing the fund of knowledge underlying effective nursing care.
8. Determination to grow professionally.
9. Maintenance of poise and self-control in all professional situations.
10. Maintaining a consistent pride in their profession.
11. Arising to the unexpected without undue panic.
12. Determination to make the patient comfortable by giving attention to small details that mean so much to the patient's well-being.

■ CONCLUSION

Attitudes are not inborn, but acquired. A person develops his/her behavior pattern in accordance with knowledge, experiences and emotions. Such behavior becomes a relatively permanent basis of his/her actions. Parents, teachers, religious leaders, literature and media, etc. have an extensive impact on the development of attitudes. Healthy attitudes such as kindness, generosity, selfless service, etc. must be encouraged. The nurse needs to develop and cultivate professional attitude, which will contribute to him/her being successful in the work. The nurse should try to find out the cause of unfavorable attitudes and should change them to favorable ones, because favorable attitudes help in treatment and recovery.

■ REVIEW QUESTIONS

Long Essays

1. Define attitude. Explain the various components of attitude.
2. Describe the characteristics of attitude in detail.

Short Essays

3. Explain motivational functions of attitude.
4. Describe development of attitude.
5. Enumerate changing attitude.
6. Discuss the effects attitude on behavior.
7. Explain self-reporting methods of attitude measurement.
8. Enumerate nurse's role in attitude.

Short Answers

9. Association and reinforcement.
10. Balance theory.
11. Cognitive dissonance theory.
12. Thurstone scale.
13. Likert scale.

■ BIBLIOGRAPHY

1. Arnel B Salgado. Psychology for Nurses: Emotions, 1st edition. Malaysia: McGraw-Hill Companies; 2009.
2. Bhatia HR. Elements of Educational Psychology. New Delhi: Orient Longman Ltd; 2000.
3. Bingham WVD. Aptitude and Attitude Testing. New Delhi: Harper and Brothers; 1937.
4. Boring EG. Foundations of Psychology. New York: John Wiley and Sons Inc.
5. Burnard P. Counseling: A Guide to Practice in Nursing. Oxford: Butterworth-Heinnemann; 1994.
6. Carrothers RM, Gregory SW Jr, Gallagher TJ. Measuring emotional intelligence of medical school applicants. Acad Med. 2000;75(5):456-63.

7. Caruso DR, Mayer JD, Salovey P. Relation of ability measure of emotional intelligence to personality. J Pers Assess; 2002;79(2):306-20.
8. Cruze, Wendell W. Psychology in Nursing. New York: McGraw-Hill.
9. Dennis Coon. Introduction to Psychology: Emotional Intelligence, 9th edition. United State of America; 2003.
10. Dennis Coon. Psychology: A Modular Approach to Mind and Behavior, 10th edition. United State of America: Wadsworth Thomson Learning; 2004.
11. Diana I Cordova, Mark RL. Intrinsic Motivation and the Process of Learning: Beneficial Effects of Contextualization, Personalization, and Choice; 1995.
12. Edward P Sarafino. Health Psychology: Biopsychosocial Interaction, 4th edition. San Francisco: John Wiley & Sons; 2001.
13. Garderner, Lambert. Attitudes and Motivation in Second Language Learning. Rowley; MA: Newbury House. 1972.
14. Henry L, Roediger, Elizabeth, et al. Psychology, 3rd edition. Canada: Little Brown & Company; 1996.
15. In: Jones, Marshall R (Eds). Nebraska Symposium on Motivation. Vols. 4, 8, 10. Lincoln: University of Nebraska Press; 1956-1962.
16. In: Lauridsen K, Whyte CB (Eds). An Integrated Counseling and Learning Assistance Center. New Directions Sourcebook; Jossey-Bass.
17. Janis, Irving L. Psychological Stress: Psychoanalytic and Behavioral Studies of Surgical Patients. New York: Wiley; 1958.
18. Jones EE. Ingratiation, A Social Psychological Analysis. New York: Appleton; 1964.
19. Jung CG. The Integration of the Personality. New York: Farrar & Rinehart; 1939.
20. Lester M Sodorow, Rickabaugh CA. Psychology, 4th edition. United State of America: McGraw-Hill; 1998.
21. Mangal SK. Statistics in Psychology and Education. New Delhi: Prentice Hall of Indian; 2002.
22. Morgan, King. Introduction to Psychology. New Delhi: McGraw-Hill; 1993.
23. Philip GZ, Richard JG. Psychology and Life, 14th edition. New York: Harper Collins College Publishers; 1996.
24. Raty H, Snellman L. Does gender make any difference? Commonsense conceptions of intelligence. Social Behavior and Personality. 1992;20(1):23-34.
25. Rita LA, Richard CA, et al. Introduction to Psychology, 12th edition. United State of America.
26. Robert A Bason. Psychology. New Delhi: Prentice Hall of India Pvt Ltd; 2001.
27. Rogers C, Freiberg HJ. Regarding Learning and its Facilitation. Freedom to Learn. Columbus: Merrill. pp. 157-16.
28. Samuel EW, Ellen GW, Denise Boyd. Mastering the World of Psychology, 12th edition. United State of America: Pearson Education; 2006.
29. Seligman, Martin EP. Learned Optimism. New York: Alfred A Knopf Inc: p. 101.
30. Stout GF. A Manual of Psychology. London: University Tutorial Press; 1938.
31. Susan Harter. A New Self-Report Scale of Intrinsic versus Extrinsic Orientation in the Classroom. Motivational and Informational Components; 1981.
32. Thomas JP. Guide to Managerial Persuasion and Influence. Upper Saddle River NJ: Pearson Prentice Hall; 2004.
33. Troland, Leonard T. The Fundamentals of Human Motivation. New York: Van Nostrand; 1928.
34. Vernon PE. The Structure of Human Ability. London: Methuen; 1950.
35. Walker, Edward L, Heyns, et al. An Anatomy for Conformity. Englewood Cliffs, NJ: Prentice-Hall.
36. Watson JB. Psychology From the Standpoint of a Behaviorist. Philadelphia: JB Lippon Otta Co; 1919.
37. Weiten W, Lloyd M, Dunn D, et al. Psychology Applied to Modern Life: Adjustment in the 21st Century, 6th edition. Canada: Engaged Learning; 1999.
38. White RW. Motivation reconsidered: the concept of competence. Psychol Rev. 1959;66:297-333.
39. Whyte, Cassandra B. An Additional Look at Orientation Programs Nationally. National Orientation Directors Association Journal. 2007;15(1):71-7.
40. Whyte, Cassandra B. Effective Counseling Methods for High-risk College Freshmen. Measurement and Evaluation in Counseling. 1979;6(4):198-200.

CHAPTER 19

Personality

■ INTRODUCTION

Etymologically, the word personality has been derived from the Latin word 'persona.' Persona means mask used by actors on the stage. Personality in the modern usage of the terms means the real individual. Personality covers the whole nature of an individual and hence it is very difficult to define it. The personality system is a complex product of biological endowment, cultural shaping, cognitive style and spiritual groups. When psychologist talk of personality, they mean a dynamic concept describing the growth and development of person, as a whole, which is composed of habits, interests, attitudes, will, character, etc. Watson (1930), the Father of behaviorism, taking clues from his behavioral studies, tried to conclude that personality is the sum of activities that can be discovered by actual observations over a long enough period of time to give reliable information.

■ DEFINITION

1. Personality is the dynamic organization within the individual of those psychophysical systems that determine his unique adjustments to the environment. —*Gordon Allport*
2. Personality is defined as the most characteristic integration of an individual's structure, modes of behavior, interests, attitudes, capacities, abilities and aptitudes. —*Munn MN*
3. The more or less stable and enduring organization of a person's character, temperament, intellect and physique that determines his unique adjustment to the environment. —*Eysenck*
4. Personality is that, which permits a prediction of what a person will do in a given situation. —*Cattell*
5. Personality is a person's unique pattern of traits. —*Guilford*
6. Personality is the most adequate conceptualization of a person's behavior in all its detail. —*McClelland*
7. Personality is a study concerned with the interaction of the biological organism with the social interaction. —*Gardener Murphy*
8. Personality is the sum total of all the biological innate dispositions, impulses and tendencies acquired by experience. —*Morton Prince*
9. Each individual's characteristically recurring patterns of behavior are known as personality. —*Kolb*
10. Personality refers to the aggregate of the physical and mental qualities of the individuals as these interact and function in characteristic fashion with his environment. —*Taylor*

11. Personality consists of the distinctive patterns of behavior including thoughts and emotions that characterize each individual's adaptation to the situations of his/her life. —*Walter Mischel*
12. Personality is the sum of activities that can be discovered by actual observations over a long enough period of time to give reliable information. —*Watson*
13. Personality refers to deeply ingrained patterns of behavior, which include the way one relates to, perceives and thinks about the environment and oneself.
—*American Psychiatric Association (APA)*
14. Personality is defined as enduring patterns of perceiving, relating to, and thinking about environment and oneself.
—*Diagnostic and Statistical Manual of Mental Disorders-IV (DSM-IV) (APA)*
15. Personality refers to the organized, consistent and general pattern of behavior of a person which helps us to understand his/her behavior as individual.
—*Indira Gandhi National Open University (IGNOU)*
16. Personality is a united multiplex, which means a unit composed of elements. He further stated that personality is continuous in an individual's life, a perpetual and a consistent whole, which represent his entire life pattern. —*William Stern*

▪ CONCEPTS OF PERSONALITY

1. Personality is a combination of all the behavioral, emotional, temperamental and mental attributes that shape the unique character of a person.
2. Personality includes both physical, mental characteristics of the person, which determine his/her general and specific qualities. The distinct identity of the person is only determined by the personality.
3. The impact of personality can always be seen on the behavior, thoughts, conducts, actions and activities of the person.
4. Personality is also described as the unique pattern of traits, which characterize the individual. Traits are characteristics of an individual such as good natured, calm, anxious, shy and irritable.
5. Personality includes the behavior patterns, a person shows across the situation or the psychological characteristics of the person that lead to those behavior patterns.
6. Personality includes the cognitive, affective and psychomotor behavior, and covers all the conscious, subconscious and unconscious also.
7. Personality is not static, but dynamic in nature. Personality of an individual keeps adjusting itself to the environment on a continuous basis. A fine balance is maintained between the inner and environmental forces.
8. Personality is the individual characteristic and relatively during organization or integration of ways of behaving (or trait, motives, interests, abilities, attitudes), and modes of adjustment to others and to his/her total environment.

▪ COMPONENTS OF PERSONALITY (Fig. 19.1)

Physical Appearance

Physical appearance refers to the physique of an individual. Some people give much emphasis on looks and judge mental alertness from personal appearances. It cannot be denied that to some extent, success and failure is determined by personal appearance, which includes not only weight, height, complexion but also voice, dress and other characteristics of personal nature.

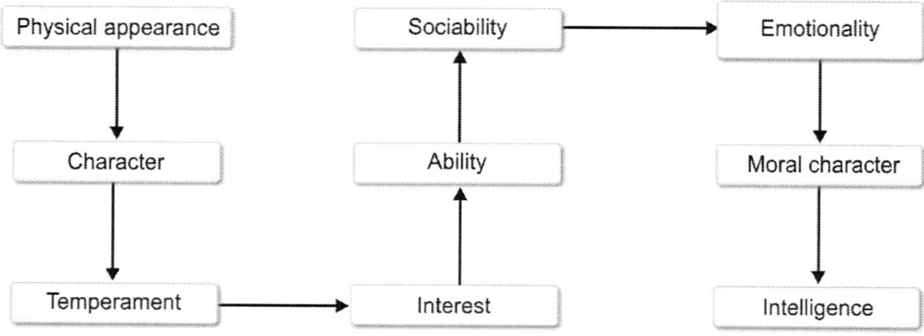

Figure 19.1: Components of personality

Character

Character refers to the ethical or moral aspect of a personality, which one possesses. The character of an individual is judged by the level of consistency exhibited in his/her behavior.

Temperament

Temperament refers to the deep-rooted emotional trends present in an individual. It is a result of secretion of endocrine glands as well as habit formation. Temperament plays an important role in one's ability to adjust to his/her environment.

Interest

Interest refers to a felt need. It is connected to three aspects, the need to know, feel and perform.

Ability

Ability refers to a special natural power to do something well, physical or mental.

Sociability

Sociability refers to an ability of the individual to socialize himself/herself in a social environment and how others perceive his/her presence in the group. This trait is present in varying degree in different people. The young child is inclined to be extremely selfish and self-centered, but gradually he/she learns to share the things and experiences with others. He/She plays with other children and shares his/her toys with them. This give-and-take cooperation in childhood lays the foundation of social solidarity at the adult level.

Emotionality

Emotionality refers to the ability of an individual to show mature emotional behavior in suitable situations. Emotionality has a powerful role to play in personality. The emotional stability and maturity is required for healthy personality.

Moral Character

Moral character trait refers to social approval as to whether we have a balanced personality pursuing well-defined goals that benefit to the individual society.

Intelligence

Intelligence is the capacity of an individual to learn and solve problems, and adjust to relatively new and changing conditions. These are individual differences, but it is desired from well-balanced personality in which intelligence is supplemented by healthy social being.

■ VARIABLES OF PERSONALITY

There are three basic factors or variables, which have to be considered in describing or analyzing of the personality:

1. The internal aspects of the individual or organism is the basic drives, covert feelings, the physiological systems, glands and his/her inherently determined physical features.
2. The social and material stimuli or situations exterior to the individual. These modify and direct his/her impulses and needs. They include the influence of family and other groups to which one belongs, the influence of customs, traditions and culture.
3. The reaction of behavior or conduct, which results from the interaction of the individual and the stimuli.

From these three basic variables, it will be clear that personality is a dynamic thing. It grows in a social setup, through social experiences. These variables do not stand apart from each other; they are related to each other, they are interconnected and as well as a result of this integration give rise to a characteristic behavior pattern or quality called personality.

■ FACTORS INFLUENCING PERSONALITY

Physiological Factors (Fig. 19.2)

Physiological factors include the physique of the individual size, strength, looks and constitution. They also include the physical deficiencies and nature of glandular functioning. The physiological conditions of the body, influenced by drugs, disease, diet, toxins and bacterial infections, may also shape our behavior and personality. The changes are detailed below.

Physical Appearance

Physical appearance is the first thing that attracts our attention, when we meet a person and our judgment of him/her is inevitably colored by it. An attractive physical appearance helps to create self-confidence, poise, self-reliance and other similar personality traits in the individual. A well-built person generally enjoys a forceful and impressive personality. He/She may develop a tendency to bully or to dominate or to protect. The smaller person may feel belitted in the presence of large and tall people. He may try to compensate for this by being hard worker.

Physical Attractiveness

Physical attractiveness, strength and general health may determine certain reactions and traits. But it must be remembered that these things, in themselves, are not the major factors that determine one's personality.

Physical Handicaps

Physical handicaps such as orthopedic defects, a bad squint in the eye, snub nose or deafness may cause shyness, reserve and unsociableness in persons.

Endocrine Glands

The endocrine glands produce hormones, which have the power to raise or depress the activity of the various organs. They influence emotional behavior and hence color our personality. They bring about changes in physical appearance, motor functioning, intelligence and emotional stability. The parathyroid gland regulates calcium metabolism. Excitability of nervous system is directly dependent on the amount of calcium in the blood. Deficient working of this gland leads to the development of an irritable, quick-reactive, distracted, nervous and a tense

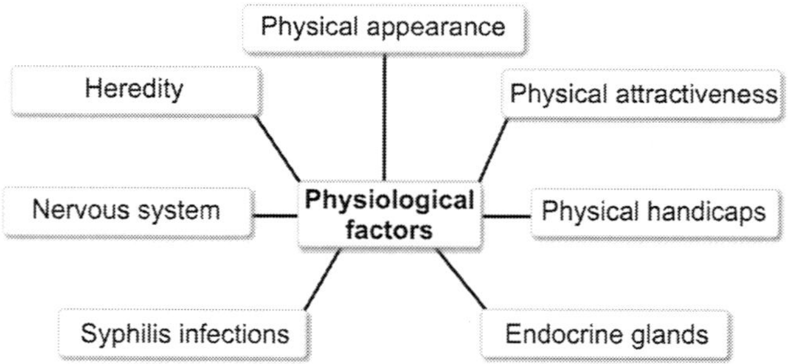

Figure 19.2: Physiological factors influencing personality

person. Similarly other glands namely pituitary, the adrenal and the gonads have their tremendous impact on various personality traits.

Syphilis Infections

Syphilis infections of the brain or general paralysis may change a truthful, meticulous person into one who is dishonest and unreliable. Encephalitis lethargic or sleeping sickness may cause serious behavior problems in a child who has been a joy to parents and teachers.

Nervous System

Entire behavior is effectively managed and controlled by the coordination and functioning of the nervous system. The sense impressions, which are received through sense organs, do not bear any significance unless they are given meaning by the nervous system.

Heredity

At conception, when the egg cell of the female is fertilized by the sperm cells of the male, each new human being receives a genetic inheritance that provides potentialities for development and behavioral traits throughout a life time. The principle raw materials of personality such as physique, intelligence and temperament are the result of heredity.

Environmental/Social Factors (Fig. 19.3)

The social aspects of an individual's environment affect personality significantly. Cruze says, "an individual's personality is influenced more by the reactions of other people towards him/her and the reactions to other people than by any other factor in the environment". Of these social factors, the most important are the relationship at home and with the family, the influence of school and playground, social codes and roles, which the individual has to play in the family environment and community.

Family

The reaction of the family environment towards an individual and the role of parents are very important in molding of personality. Parents serve as a model for the child to

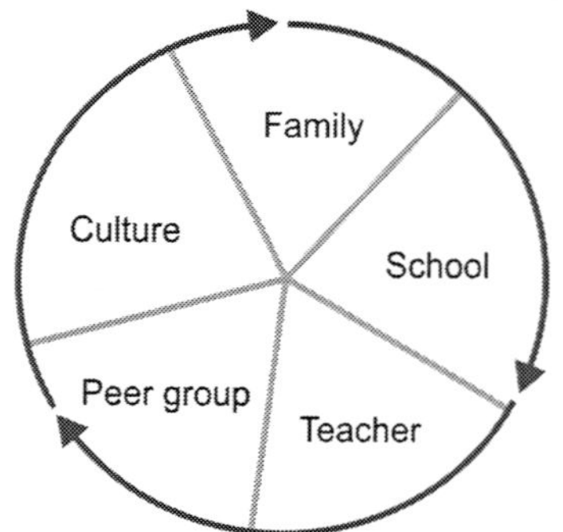

Figure 19.3: Environmental/Social factors

imitate and their influence is much considerable on the child. Parents influence the development of a child's personality in a wide variety of ways. Children learn the moral values, code of contact, social norms and methods of interacting with others from parents.

School

The children spend much of their time in the schools and hence it can play a very significant part in the formation of the personality of the child. A nurturing school atmosphere provides for all-round development of the child.

Teacher

A teacher is the most important person in the school who can help in modifying the children's personalities. He/She is the most powerful source of stimulation for the child.

Peer Group

Peer group refers to other children of the same age who study or play with the child. Peer group is much more influential than sibling or parents. The peer group serves as an important reference group in shaping personality traits and characteristics of the growing child. As peer group grows up, peers become progressively more influential in molding the child's self-concept.

Culture

Culture influences personality because every culture has a set of ethical and moral values, beliefs and norms, which considerably shapes behavior. Cross-cultural studies have pointed out the importance of cultural environment in shaping one's personality.

Psychological Factors

Psychological factors include a person's motives, acquired interests, attitudes, will power and character, intellectual capacities such as intelligence, reasoning, attention, perception and imagination. These factors determine our reaction in various situations and thus, affect our personality growth and direction.

■ TYPES OF PERSONALITY

Hippocrates Classification (400 BC)

Hippocrates was a great physician and known as Father of medicine, classified human beings into four characteristic groups according to their temperaments (Table 19.1).

Kretschmer's Classification

Kretschmer classified all human being into certain biological types according to their physical structure (Table 19.2).

Table 19.1: Hippocrates classification of personality

Type of fluids in the body	Personality type	Temperamental characteristics
Blood	Sanguine	Optimistic, happy, hopeful, accommodating and lighthearted
Phlegm	Phlegmatic	Cold, calm, slow and indifferent
Black bile	Melancholic	Sad, depressed, pessimistic, dejected, deplorable and self-involved
Yellow bile	Choleric	Irritable, passionate, strong, active, imaginative

Table 19.2: Kretschmer's classification of personality

Physical structure	Personality type	Characteristics
Fatty body	Pyknic	Sociable, jolly, easy going and good natured
Balanced body	Athletic	Energetic, optimistic and adjustable
Lean and thin	Leptosomatic	Unsociable, reserved, shy, sensitive and pessimistic

Sheldon's Classification

Human beings were classified by their physical body structures and attached certain temperamental characteristics to them (Table 19.3).

Jung's Classification

Carl G Jung proposed to classify the personality based on complex network of ideas bound together by a common emotions or a set of feelings (Table 19.4).

Table 19.3: Sheldon's classification of personality

Name	Description	Characteristics
Endomorphic	Person having highly developed viscera, but weak somatic structure—fat, soft, round (as pyknic type)	Easy going, sociable, affectionate and fond of eating
Mesomorphic	Balanced development of viscera and somatic structure—muscular, strong (as athletic type)	Craving for muscular activity, self-assertive, loves risk and adventure, energetic, assertive and bold tempered
Ectomorphic	Weak somatic structure as well as undeveloped viscera—thin, long fragile (as Kretschmer's leptosomatic)	Pessimistic, unsociable, reserved, brainy, artistic and introvert

Table 19.4: Jung's classification of personality

Emotions/ Feelings	Extrovert	Introvert
Interest	Extroverts are interested in the world around them	Introverts are interested in themselves, their own feeling, emotions and are unable to adjust easily to social situation
Social interaction	Involves in social participation, they are sociable, not easily upset by difficulties	Socially they are aloof and withdrawn
Adjustment	They are successful in adjusting to the realities of their environment, socially active and more interested in leaving a good impression on others	They prefer to work alone and avoid social contacts; they are inclined to worry and get easily embarrassed
Influencing factor	Their behavior is influenced more by physical stimulation than by their inner thoughts and ideas	Introverts are the persons who seek the manifestation of their life through inner activities by going inward or dragging up things within themselves
Area of occupation	Politicians, social workers, lawyers, insurance agents, salesmen, etc. fall in this category	Philosophers, scientists, writers, etc.

Hans Eysenck's Classification (1967)

The distinct types in Eysenck's theory of personality are introversion, extraversion, neuroticism and psychoticism (Table 19.5).

Gordon Allport's Classification (1937)

Gordon Allport counted 18,000 trait-like terms designated as distinctive and personal forms of behavior and divided into three parts (Table 19.6).

■ THEORIES OF PERSONALITY

There are six paradigms that have been chosen to represent personality theories (Hergenhahn, 1944). Each paradigm is named after its central theme. All paradigms provide useful information about personality and contribute to understand personality (Fig. 19.4), as detailed below:

1. **Psychoanalytical paradigm:** For example, personality theories of Sigmund Freud and Carl Jung. This paradigm focuses on the analysis of the psyche.
2. **Sociocultural paradigm:** For example, personality theories of Alfred Adler,

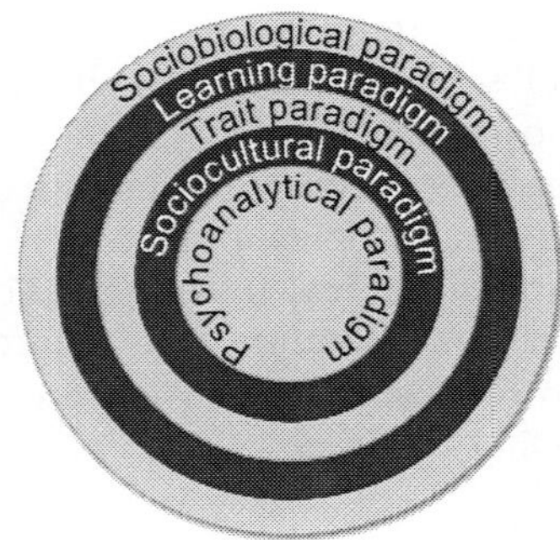

Figure 19.4: Theories of personality

Table 19.5: Hans Eysenck's classification of personality

Sl No.	Types of personality	Characteristics
1.	Type A personality	Competitive drive, restlessness, hostility, sense of urgency, impatience, hard driving, live under constant pressure Seeks recognition and advancement, multiple activities with deadliness to meet and cope up more constructively with stressors might be useful
2.	Type B personality	Calmer, more philosophical, easy going, noncompetitive, little dull, longer life, struggle to control situation, but when they fail to do so, they stop coping

Table 19.6: Gordon Allport's classification of personality

Sl No.	Traits	Characteristics
1.	Cardinal traits	Cardinal traits are the traits, which are so dominant that nearly all of the individual's actions can be traced back to them Each term describes a trait so broad and so deep in its impact that it overshadows the influence of other traits in the same individual He believed that most people have no true cardinal traits
2.	Central traits	Central traits are traits, which are major characteristics of a person such as trust, worthiness, honesty or conscientiousness
3.	Secondary traits	Secondary traits are less important characteristics that are not central to our understanding of an individual's personality such as particular attitudes, performance and style of behavior

Karen Horney and Erik Erikson. This paradigm emphasizes the importance of sociocultural factors influencing personality.

3. **Trait paradigm:** For example, personality theories of Gorton Allport and Raymond B Cattell. This paradigm emphasizes the importance of various traits that a person possesses.
4. **Learning paradigm:** For example, personality theories of BF Skinner, John Dollard and Neal Miller, Albert Bandura and Walter Barash. This paradigm emphasizes the importance of learning in personality development.
5. **Sociobiological paradigm:** For example, Albert Bandura and Richard Walters gave altogether a new approach to personality.

Psychoanalytical Theory (Freud)

Freud (1939), Father of psychoanalytical theory, is believed to be the first to identify the development by stages. He believed that the first 5 years of a child's life to be the most important, as he believed that an individual's basic character had been formed by the age of five (Table 19.7).

Structure of Personality

1. **Id:** It contains all our biologically based drives—the urge to eat, drink and eliminate especially to be sexually stimulated. The id operates according to the pleasure principle. It aims to achieve immediate gratification. Id-driven behaviors are impulsive and may be irrational.
2. **Ego:** This is based on rational self or reality principle. It develops between ages of 4 and 6 months. It acts as a mediator to maintain harmony among the external world. It experiences the reality of the external world, adapts to it and responds to it.
3. **Superego:** This is based on perfection principle. It develops between 3 and 6 years, internalizes the values and morals set forth by primary caregivers. The superego is important in the socialization of individual, as it assist ego in the control of id impulses. When superego becomes rigid and punitive, problems with low self-confidence and low self-esteem arise.

Dynamics of Personality

1. Consciousness: Refers to the perception, thoughts and feelings existing in a person's immediate awareness. The conscious includes all memories that remain within an individual's awareness. It is thought to be under the control of ego, rational and logical structure of personality.
2. Preconsciousness: It includes all memories that may have been forgotten or not in present awareness, but that with attention can be recalled into consciousness. Preconscious content on the other hand, is not immediately accessible to awareness.
3. Unconsciousness: It includes all memories that one is unable to bring to conscious awareness. Unconscious material consists of unpleasant or non-essential

Table 19.7: Freud's personality theory conceptualization

Sl No.	Theories	Description
1.	Structure of personality	Id, ego and superego
2.	Dynamics of personality	Conscious, preconscious, semiconscious and unconscious
3.	Topography	Psychic energy, Cathexis, anticathexis
4.	Stages of personality development	Oral stage, anal stage, phallic stage, latency stage and genital stage

memories that have been repressed and can be retrieved only through therapy, hypnosis and with certain substances that alter the awareness and have the capacity to restructure repressed memories.

Stages of Personality Development/ Psychosexual Development

Sigmund Freud (1856–1939) described formation of personality through five stages of psychosexual development:

1. **Oral stage** (infancy) (1–18 month): During this stage, infant's mouth is the focal point of pleasure; children suck, bite and chew anything that fits into their mouth. Infant obtains gratification by taking in, begins to develop self-concepts from the response of others. Infant interests in oral gratification from sucking, eating, mouthing and biting.
2. **Anal stage** (early childhood) (18 month to 3 year): Gratification from expelling and withholding feces; coming to terms with society's controls relating to toilet training. In early part of his/her period, the child freely gratifies the love of self with the pleasurable sensation involved in evacuating the bladder and bowels naturally and without restriction. Freud believed that if great success is placed on the child in relation to remaining clean during this period, he/she may grow up compulsively clean. Other adult attitudes thought to be rigid toilet training include stubbornness, hoarding, collecting excessive concern with bowel function and sadistic or masochistic tendencies.
3. **Phallic stage** (later childhood) (3–6 year): Interest in the genitals; coming to terms with oedipal conflict, leading to identification with same sex parent. The focus of pleasurable sensation has shifted from the mouth and the excretory organs to the genitalia. Freud proposed that the development of the Oedipus complex occurred.
4. **Latency stage** (6–12 year): Sexual concerns are largely unimportant; during the elementary school years, the focus changes from egocentrism to more interest in group activities, learning and socialization with peers. Sexuality is not absent during this period, but remains obscure and imperceptible to others. The preference is homosexual; children of this age show a distinct preference for same sex relationships, even rejecting members of opposite sex.
5. **Genital stage** (12–18 year): Re-emergence of sexual interests and establishment of mature sexual relationships. During puberty and adolescence, final stage of personality development is characterized by a reactivation of libidinal energy and focusing of this energy on the genital area. The adolescent is simultaneously drawn towards his/her parents and driven away from them. This ambivalence is manifested by much conflict between behaving in a dependent, immature, child-like way and in an independent, mature, adult manner.

Topography of the Mind

1. **Psychic energy:** It is the force or impetus required for mental functioning. The psychic energy originates in the id and instinctually fulfills basic physiological needs called libido. As the child matures, it is diverted from id to form ego and then from ego to form superego.
2. **Cathexis:** It is the process by which the id invests energy into an object in an attempt to achieve gratification.
3. **Anticathexis:** It is the use of psychic energy by the ego and the superego to control id impulses.

Psychosocial Theory (Erikson)

Erik H Erikson, born in 1902, built psychosocial theories on the basis of Freud's theories by identifying eight development stages that encompasses the entire life span, referred as eight ages of man.

Trust vs Mistrust (Birth to 18 Month)

The major development task during this stage is to develop a basic trust with the mothering figure and be able to generalize it to others. The trust depends not on absolute quantities of food or demonstrations of love, but rather on the quality of maternal relationship, when needs met and trust develops. Distrust can develop if the infant's world is filled with insecurity due to unmet needs, caused by lack of caring on the part of parents and significant others.

Autonomy vs Shame (18 Month to 3 Year) (Early Childhood)

The major developmental task during this stage is to gain some self-control and independence within the environment. Achievement of the task results in a sense of self-control and ability to delay gratification. Autonomy is achieved when parents encourage and provide opportunities for independent activities. Nonachievement results in the lack of self-confidence and lack of pride in the ability to perform, a sense of being controlled by others and a rage against the self.

Initiative vs Guilt (4–5 Year) (Middle Childhood)

The major development task during this stage is developing a sense of purpose and ability to initiate and direct own activities. Achievement of the task results in ability to exercise restraint and self-control of inappropriate social behavior; enjoys learning and personal achievement. Achieve initiative when creativity is encouraged and performance is recognized and positively reinforced. If this initiative and curiosity are discouraged, the child may be prevented from setting future goals by a sense of guilt and shame for holding such ambitions.

Industry vs Inferiority (6–11 Year) (Late Childhood)

The major developmental task during this stage is to achieve a sense of self-confidence by learning, competing, performing successfully and receiving recognition from significant others, peers and acquaintances. Achievement of the task results in a sense of satisfaction and pleasure in the interaction and involvement with others; masters reliable in work habits and develops attitudes of trustworthiness; feels pride in achievement. This industry is achieved when encouraged for activities and responsibilities given in home, school and community. Nonachievement results in difficulty in interpersonal relationships owing to feeling of personal inadequacy; neither cooperate and compromise with others in group's activities for problem solver or complete task successfully.

Identity vs Role Confusion (12–20 Year) (Adolescence)

The major developmental task during this stage is to integrate the tasks mastered in the previous stages into a secure sense of self. Childhood comes to an end during this stage and youth begins. Puberty brings on a physiological revolution with each adolescents must learn to cope. Achievement of this task results in a sense of confidence, emotional stability and a view of self as unique individual. Identity is achieved when adolescents are allowed to experience independence by making decisions that influence their values. Nonachievement results in sense of self-consciousness, doubt and confusion about one's role in life.

Intimacy vs Isolation (20 –30 Year) (Young Adolescence)

The major development task during this stage is to form as intense, lasting relationship or a commitment to another person. Intimacy achieved by the task results in the capacity for mutual love and respect between two people, and the ability of an individual to pledge a total commitment to another, personal sacrifices are made for another; capacity for giving of oneself to another. This is learned when one has been the recipient of this type of giving within the family unit. Nonachievement results in withdrawal, social isolation, aloneness unable to form lasting intimate relationships, often seeking intimacy through numerous superficial sexual contacts.

Generativity vs Stagnation (30–65 Year) (Adulthood)

The major development task during this stage is to achieve the life goals established for oneself, while also considering the welfare of future generations. Achievement of the task results in a sense of gratification from personal and professional achievements, and from meaningful contributions. Nonachievement results in lack of concern for the welfare of others and total preoccupation with the self, becomes withdrawn, isolated and highly self-indulgent with no capacity for giving of self to others.

Ego Integrity vs Despair (65 Year to Death) (Old Age)

The major developmental task during this stage is to review one's life and derive meaning from both positive and negative events, while achieving a positive sense of self-worth. Achievement of task results in a sense of self-worth and self-acceptance, as one reviews life goals; derives a sense of dignity from his/her life experiences and does not fear death. Nonachievement results in a sense of self-contempt and disgust with how life has progressed; feels worthless and hopeless to change; feels anger, depression, loneliness and fears death.

Learning Theories of Personality

Social Learning Theory (Bandura and Walters)

1. Albert Bandura and Richard Walters in 1963 gave altogether a new approach to personality in the shape of a social learning theory.
2. The theory emphasizes that what one represents through his/her personality is very much acquired through a process of continuous structuring and restructuring of his/her experience through social learning.
3. Observational learning from social situations may involve both real and symbolic models. Children, for example, may learn social etiquette by watching their parents and elders as well as by direct instructions.

Learning Theory of Personality (Dollard and Miller)

1. John Dollard and Neal Miller (1950), in the Institute of Human Relations at Yale University, provided their own theory of personality. In this theory, they tried to substitute Freud's concept of a pleasure principle with the principle of reinforcement, concept of ego with the concept of learned drive and skills, concept of conflict with competing reinforces, etc.
2. It emphasizes that what we consider as a personality is learned. The child at birth is equipped with two types of basic factors; reflexes and innate hierarchies of

response and a set of primary drives, which are internal stimuli of great strength and are linked with known psychological processes.
3. Dollard and Miller's theory of personality stressed the acquisition of personality in the same way as learning of most of the responses and behavior through the process of motivation and reward.

Self-theory (Carl Rogers)

1. Carl Ransom Rogers, an American psychologist, in 1947 brought out a new theory of personality named self-theory, quite distinct from the earlier theories of personality.
2. He stressed the importance of an individual's self for determining the process of his/her growth and development, and unique adjustment to the environment. There are two basic systems underlying his personality theory—the organism and the self.
3. Rogers considers them as a system operating in one's phenomenological field (a world of subjective experience, the personal and separate reality of each individual). The organism is an individual's entire frame of reference. This represents the totality of experience—both conscious and unconscious available with him/her.
4. In second system, the self is the accepted, awareness part of experience. The self as a system of one's phenomenal field can perhaps best be understood in terms of one's concepts of 'I,' 'me' or 'myself.' Human being has inherited a tendency to develop their self in the process of interpersonal and social experiences, which they have in the environment.
5. Rogers does not propose a set of specific stages in the development of personality as proposed by Freud in his history, rather his advocate's continuity of growth in terms of the continuous evolution of the concept of self.
6. Once a concept of self is formed, the individual strives to maintain it. In order to do this, he/she regulates his/her behavior. What is consistent at conscious level, while what threatens the image of self may be totally ignored or buried deep in his conscious.
7. The most unfortunate results in the environment of one's personality lie in the cases where an individual develops some false self-images. This false image is often so strong that obvious reality can be stoutly denied.

Trait Approach Theory

Trait Approach (GB Allport)

GB Allport (1897–1967) was the first personality theorist who adopted 'Trait Approach' in providing a theory of personality. According to him, an individual develops a unique set of organized tendencies or traits; generally, these traits are organized around a few cardinal (primary) trait. Allport's theory asserts that no two individuals are alike. Allport regarded traits as responsible for these individual differences; trait is a predisposition to act in the same way in a wide range of situations. Allport deeply committed to study of individual traits. He started calling them as personal dispositions. Common traits were simply called traits. Allport proposed three types of personal dispositions (Table 19.8).

Trait Theory (Raymond Cattell's)

The most recent advanced theory of personality based on trait approach has been developed by Raymond B Cattell, a British-born American researcher. He defined trait as a structure of the personality inferred from behavior in different situations and describes four types of traits (Table 19.9).

Table 19.8: Allport's types of personal dispositions

Sl No.	Types	Description
1.	Cardinal disposition	A cardinal disposition is so dominant that all actions of the person are guided by it Very few people possess cardinal dispositions
2.	Central disposition	These are not so dominant as cardinal dispositions, but they influence the person's behavior in a very prominent way, therefore, they are called the building blocks of personality
3.	Secondary disposition	These are not very consistent and are thus less relevant in reflecting the personality of the individual

Table 19.9: Cattell's types of traits

Sl No.	Types	Description
1.	Common traits	The traits found widely distributed in general population such as honesty, aggression and cooperation
2.	Unique traits	Unique to a person as temperamental traits and emotional reaction
3.	Surface traits	Able to recognize by one's manifestations of behavior such as curiosity, dependability and tactfulness
4.	Source traits	Underlying structures of sources that determine one's behavior such as dominance, submission, emotionality, etc.

According to Cattell, personality is that which permits us to predict what a person will do in a given situation. In line with his mathematical analysis of personality, prediction of behavior can be made by means of a specification equation,

$R = f(S, P)$

where,

R is the person

f is a function

S is the stimulus at a given moment of time

P is the existing personality structure.

This equation conveys Cattell's strong belief that human behavior is determined and can be predicted.

Trait-type Theory of Personality (Hans Eysenck)

Trait-type theory of personality approach tries to synthesis the type and trait approaches. Eysenck gave it more specification by grouping traits into definite types. The essence of personality can be arranged hierarchically. In this scheme, certain supertraits and types such as extroversion exert a powerful influence over behavior. According to Eysenck, focus has been on a small member of personality types, defined by two major dimensions, i.e. introversion-extraversion, stability-instability (neuroticism) (Table 19.10).

Based on his categorization of personality types, Eysenck constructed an inventory called Eysenck personality questionnaire (EPQ). It covers items from each of the personality types identified by them throughout his writing. Eysenck consistently emphasized the role of genetic factors and neurophysiologic factors, role of the cerebral cortex, autonomous nervous system, limbic system and reticular activating system in explaining individual differences in behavior.

Table 19.10: Trait-type theory of personality

Sl No.	Types	Stable	Unstable
1.	Introvert	Calm	Moody
		Anxious	Anxious
		Controlled	Rigid
		Peaceful	Pessimistic
		Careful	Reserved
2.	Extrovert	Leader	Restless
		Easy going	Aggressive
		Talkative	Impulsive
		Outgoing	Optimistic
		Sociable	Active

■ PSYCHOMETRIC ASSESSMENT OF PERSONALITY

Personality testing is done for various reasons. A personnel psychologist may want to identify people for a salesman's job. A clinical psychologist often uses personality tests to evaluate psychological disorders. We have to describe it and know what type of personality or the personality traits possessed by us or others. It needs the knowledge and skill for the assessment or measurement of personality.

Subjective Methods of Personality Assessment

Subjective methods of personality assessment are the approach where methods employed provide an opportunity to the individuals to speak about themselves. The methods followed under this approach are called subjective methods.

Autobiography

The subject (individual) is asked to write his/her autobiography either on a structured pattern or an unstructured pattern. Generally, only those subjects should be asked of guidance. Such autobiographical material provides data on the personal qualities of an individual, for instance, goals, aspirations, hopes, wishes, disappointments, frustrations, etc.

Case History Method

The case history method takes into consideration the time factor and the changes in personality of an individual during this time. Following steps should be followed in the case history method:

- Identification data
- Family background
- Health history
- Educational achievement
- Emotional and social behavior
- Interpretation of the data
- Evaluation treatment.

The above information helps in making predictions about the personality of an individual; this method has a limited application for educational institutions, but it is more useful in clinics for the treatment of patients.

Case Study Method

Case study method is concerned with the intensive study of an individual with the aim of having a holistic view of that individual. The causes of the problems of an individual are found on the basis of the collected information and remedial treatment is suggested for better adjustment in the society, school or home environment. Following steps should be taken into consideration, while following the case study methods:

- Selection of the subject/case
- Reason for the selection of case/subject
- Tools for recording data such as cumulative records, tests, medical reports, etc.
- General information about the subject
- Health records
- Family background
- Educational data
- Social relations

- Hobbies, interests, attitudes, etc.
- Interpretation of data.

Remedial treatment to the case/subject under study: The following points should be taken into consideration for selecting a case for case study:

1. Preferably problem children, i.e. those who are truants, delinquents, low-achievers, shy, quiet and retiring, etc. should be selected for the case study. The teacher is free to select any student for case study depending upon the situation.
2. Selection of the case by the teacher should be made from his/her class.
3. Time and facilities should be taken into consideration for the case study in question.

Questionnaires

A questionnaire is a valuable tool for collecting information directly given by a person. Such information may consist of personal knowledge, likes and dislikes (values and preferences), attitudes and beliefs, experiences (biography) and present status of things or event. This information can be both qualitative (verbal, description, comments or views) and quantitative (numbers or scores as in the case of rating scale, or opinion scores elicited by attitude scales).

Any assembly of questions cannot be called questionnaire. It must reflect an objective, design and framework. It is a way of obtaining data about persons by asking them rather than watching them behave or by sampling a portion of their behavior. A good questionnaire embodies a beginning, middle and an end. There is an introductory section comparing a note on the purpose of the questionnaire, an appeal and a direction for responding to the various questions and a basic data part of which is to be filled in accurately by the respondents.

Interviews

An interview is face to face talking with a purpose. It is a systematic method by which one person enters more or less imaginatively into the inner life of another who is generally a comparative stranger to him/her. An interview can be formal or informal. For good interview, there is a need for establishing a rapport between the interviewee and the interviewer.

Objective Methods of Personality Assessment (Fig. 19.5)

Objective data are collected by experts using specific tools or devices based upon certain methodologies. These methods, which are used to collect objective data regarding varied personality aspects of an individual, are called objective methods of assessing the personality of an individual. These methods are also known as observational methods, as these are based upon the observation of experts rather than the answers given by individuals in the case of the subjective methods. The observation methods are rating scales, verbal behavior, situation tests and sociometric methods.

Observation Method

The observation method can be used to observe intellectual functioning, emotional development, interest, hobbies and to study habits, etc.

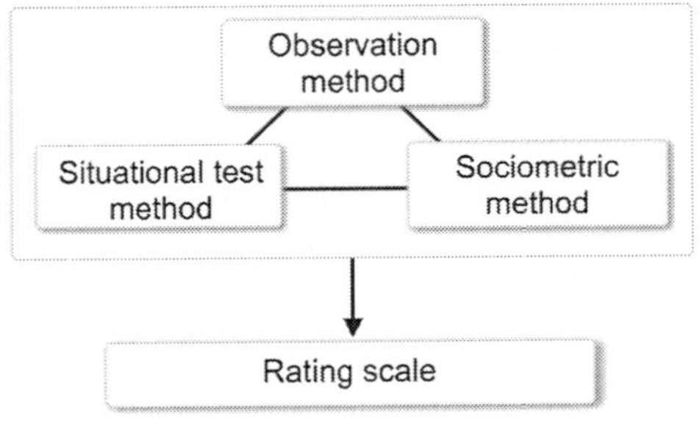

Figure 19.5: Objective methods of personality assessment

Psychological process involved: Four psychological processes are involved in collecting data in the observation method—attention, sensation, perception and conception:

1. **Attention:** It implies a mental set or a state of alertness, which an individual assumes in order to perceive selected events and conditions of things.
2. **Sensation:** It means the awareness of the internal and external environment through one's senses. It is the immediate results of a stimulus to the sense organs.
3. **Perception:** It is the art of liking what is sensed with some past experience to give meaning to sensation.
4. **Conception:** It is that quality of the mental activity associated with observing by which one removes blocks to perception through the creation of imaginative concepts. It is an intellectual representation of some aspects of reality, which is derived from the perception of a phenomenon.

Steps of observation method: Following are the four elements of the observational method:

1. Deciding the major phenomenon to be observed:
   a. Defining the major phenomenon to be observed.
   b. Modalities for the observation of the phenomenon—structured, semistructured or unstructured.
   c. Person conducting the observation.
   d. System involved in recording various features of the phenomenon—videotape, tape recorder or any other type of devices.
2. Recording.
3. Organizing.
4. Interpreting the observations.

Precautions: As follows:

1. Training of the observer is a must.
2. Subjective of the observer should be involved to the minimum possible extent.
3. The observer should have knowledge of personality aspects.
4. A member of observations should be taken for the purpose of making the observation more reliable.

Phenomena amenable of observations: It includes the following:

1. **Characteristics and conditions of individuals:** People's attributes and states such as physical appearance, physiological symptoms that can be observed directly through the senses or with the aid of observational apparatus such as radiography.
2. **Verbal communication behaviors:** Observing the content and structure of people's conversations, e.g. nurses giving information to parents, nurses conversation with grieving relatives.
3. **Non-verbal communication behaviors:** This includes facial expressions, touch, posture, gestures and other body movements.
4. **Activities:** Patient's eating habits and trends, and aggressive actions among children in the hospital playroom.
5. **Skill attainment and performance:** Behavior assessment through skill development by patients and nurses.
6. **Environmental characteristics:** Noise levels in different areas of a hospital, cleanliness in homes in a community, safety hazards of children's classroom, shelters of homeless, etc.

Situational Test Method

In situation tests, certain artificial situations resembling real life situations are created before the students. The reaction of the students are recorded and interpreted. The interpretations on the recorded responses under certain situations reveal the personality of the individual. These tests provide opportunities to observe the behavior in life situations. Traits such as leadership, initiative, cooperation, persistence, risk-taking capacity, honesty, flexibility, imagination, etc. can be assessed.

Reliability and validity of these tests have not been ascertained.

Group discussion: It is a general part of the selection procedure for admission. Group discussion is a situational test. A group is given a problem on a certain theme. No one is assigned the duty of a group leader. Everyone in the group is free to express ideas on the problem. In this situation, qualities such as initiative, imagination, accommodation, suggestibility, flexibility, etc. can be assessed.

Created situations to assess honesty: A teacher may create the following situations in the class to assess the honesty traits of his/her students:

1. The teacher holds a class test.
2. He/She evaluates the written performance, but does not show marks on the answer books.
3. He/She distributes the answer book to the student expressing the inability to mark the answer books due to certain reasons. The teacher asks his/her students to handover the answer books for the next day.
4. The answer books are collected again.
5. Those students are located whose awards are found higher due to additions. Thus, some students may reveal their dishonesty traits or honesty trait.

Imaginary situations: This can be created and responses of students to these imaginary situations may reveal personality aspects of the individuals. For example, suppose one of us comes across an individual who inquire about a certain place and the approach road to reach that place.

Situational test by May and Hartshorne: They mentioned a number of situational tests in their book studies in deceit. One example related to honesty from this book is mentioned. The teacher had a box containing coins. Then the coins from the box were distributed to some of the students in a class. The coin left in the box was counted and then the box was placed in a corner. Students were asked to place back the coins given to them. The coins were again counted. Some students kept the coins with themselves.

Sociometric Method

The sociometric method involves studying relationship among the members of a group, which helps in assessing the personality traits of the members of that group. Moreno devised this method. Social preferences with specific references to a specific criterion are recorded. For example, social preferences of students are recorded on the following questions:

1. With whom would you like to sit in the class?
2. With whom would you like to go on the educational tour?

The sociometric data, so obtained, can be expressed graphically. Such graphical expression is called sociogram. A sociogram reveals information regarding subgroups, cliques, stars, isolated, neglected and rejected. Appropriate steps can be taken on the basis of the sociometric data to improve the personality of the individuals.

Rating Scale

A rating scale is an instrument designed to facilitate appraisals of a number of traits or characteristics by reference to a common quantitative scale of values. The rating scale is used to know from others where an individual stands in terms of some personality traits. Three points are taken into consideration in this method:

1. The specific traits or trait to be rated are specified.
2. The scale range is also decided, i.e. 3-point scale, 5-point scale, 7-point scale or 11-point scale.
3. Those persons are decided who are required to use the scale to quantify the trait regarding a specific person whose

personality is to be measured, for example, One may decide that these specific persons will submit their observations on the scale for a particular trait(s) regarding a person.

Precautions while using a rating scale: The rating scale method can be made more effective if the following precautions are taken:

1. The raters should be impartial.
2. A number of raters should give their rating and these should be taken into consideration for framing the final assessment on the traits.
3. Generally, the halo effect is rating of the raters for different traits. It should be checked. It is a tendency for transfer to occur, so that a rater may rate the same individual high or low for many different traits. One impression may color the rest.
4. Avoid being too lenient or too strict in standard.
5. Avoid the tendency to either remain at the neutral points or the extreme points in the rating scale.

Purposes of rating scale: According to Freemen (1965), the purposes of rating scales are as follows:

1. Rating scales are chiefly useful for finding out what impression an individual has made of people with whom he/she has come in contact, with respect to some specified traits or attitudes.
2. It is a device that rates social values, occupational efficiency, group status and the similar in certain specified areas.
3. It reflects the impression the subject has made upon the people who do the rating.
4. For the evaluation of an individual, rating scales are submitted to teachers, counselors, employers, colleagues, parents and others who have had sufficient contact with the person in question.
5. Rating scales may be devised for a variety of traits such as tact, generosity, leadership, cooperativeness, resourcefulness, punctuality, industriousness, honesty, personal attractiveness, etc.

Points for the construction and use of rating scale: As follows:

1. Each trait should be clearly defined.
2. The degree of the trait should be defined. Each trait should be rated on a scale, most frequently of five or seven intervals.
3. The mean or the median of the rating by different judges should be taken for having a reliable rating.
4. Guidance counselors, employers and personnel officers find them helpful, if the judges are carefully selected and if the rating are properly made.
5. Overt traits are more reliably rated than convert traits. For example, overt traits such as emotional expression, social acceptability, manifest fear and anxiety, aggressive or impulsive acts are related with greater reliability than the covert traits such as a person's inner life and feeling about one's self.
6. Degree of certainty of rating should be stated, for example, very strong, strong and moderate.
7. Extroverted persons are more reliably judged than introverted ones.

Types of rating scales: As follows:

1. Scoring rating scale.
2. Ranking rating scale.

Projective Tests

Projective tests technique has been developed by Swiss psychologist, son of an art teacher Hermann Rorschach. Projective methods involve an unstructured stimulus or situation. In this process, the individual projects the unconscious desires, fears, motives, drives, needs, etc. Subjective and objective methods do not clearly study the unconscious mind of an individual. Projective methods deal with the conscious as well as the unconscious mind. The unconscious mind is 9/10th of the mind and the inner urges, wishes, emotions, etc. are not visible to the outsiders and the individual himself/herself.

According to Lindsey, projective test is an instrument that is considered sensitive to covert or unconscious aspect of behavior. It permits or encourages a wide variety of subject's responses. It is highly multidimensional' it invokes rich and profuse response data with a minimum of subject's awareness, concerning the purpose of the test.

Characteristics of Projective Test

According to Rastogi (1983), following are the characteristic features of a projective test:

1. Brief instructions are given to the subjects who are necessary for him/her to respond.
2. The test material is kept ambiguous, which projects his/her characteristic ideas, attitudes, strivings, fears, conflicts, aggressiveness, hostility, etc.
3. The purpose of the test is hidden from the subject.
4. The projective tests reflect the influence of psychoanalytical school.
5. The test reveals emotional and social characteristics, maladjustments, attitudes and motives. Certain intellectual aspects of individual behavior are also revealed.

Projective Methods of Personality Assessment (Fig. 19.6)

Rorschach ink-blot test (Table 19.11)

Description

Ink-blot test was developed by H Rorschach, which had 10 cards with vague ink-blot on them. Five of the cards were chromatic stimuli, while rests of the five were achromatic stimuli; subjects were asked to tell what they see on those cards. Each response had elaborate scoring system and well-developed interpretation. Rorschach IB test revealed structural aspects of personality such as individual stability, value system ego-strength, etc.

Procedure

1. The card is presented one at a time in a specific order. When the subject takes his/her seat, the examiner gives him/her first card with necessary instruction. He/She is asked to say what the person sees in it, what it looks like, etc.
2. The subject is allowed as much time as he/she wants of a given card and it is permitted to give as many responses to it as he/she wishes. The person is also allowed to turn the card around and look at it from any angle to find things in it.
3. Besides keeping a record of the response of the subject concerning these ink-blots on different pieces of paper, the examiner notes the time taken for each

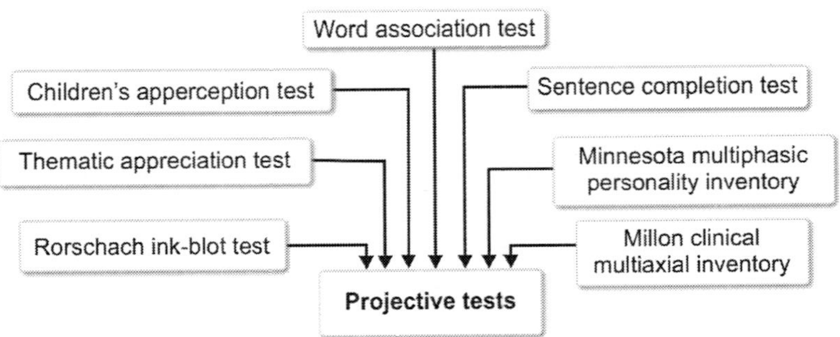

Figure 19.6: Projective methods of personality assessment

Table 19.11: Responses and interpretation of Rorschach ink-blot test

Sl No.	Response	Interpretation
1.	Associated with the whole ink-blot (location)	The subject has the ability to solve his/her problems in a comprehensive manner; he/she possess high mental ability
2.	Linked with large details (location)	The subject has a practical approach towards problems of life
3.	Linked with small details (location)	The subject expresses emotional conflicts
4.	It involves too many colors (determining quality)	The subjects are impulsive
5.	Predominance of human figure movement (determining quality)	The subject has vivid imagination
6.	It frequently involves animal figures (determining quality)	The subject has stereotyped thinking and perhaps he/she is of low intelligence

response, position in which cards are being held, emotional expression and other incidental behavior of the subject during the test period, etc.

4. After all, the cards have been presented; the second phase of inquiry follows. It is intended to seek clarification or addition to original responses.

Verbal projective test: It present subjects with an ambiguous verbal stimuli rather than a pictorial one. There are two types of verbal methods as detailed below:

1. **Association technique:** An example of an association technique is word-association method, which represents subjects with a series of words to which the individual respond with the first thing comes to mind. The word list often combines both neutral and emotionally tinged words, which are included for the purpose of detecting impaired thoughts, processes or internal conflicts, anxiety or any problems in relationships.
2. **Sentence completion test:** This test includes a list of incomplete sentences generally open at the end and is asked to complete them in any desired manner. This approach is frequently used as a method of measuring attitudes or some aspect of personality.

Expressive methods: These techniques encourage self-expression through the construction of some product out of raw materials. The major expressive methods are play techniques, drawing and painting, and role playing. It is believed that people express their feelings, needs, motives and emotions by working with or manipulating various materials.

Scoring of responses: Responses to the test are scored in terms of location, determinants, content and popularity or originality taken for responses, which are as follows (Table 19.11):

1. **Location:** The response of the subject in context of the whole ink blot or a part of it is recorded. The subject may observe the whole ink for giving a response or a part of it. The subject may give large or small details.
2. **Determining quality:** Scoring is done with specific responses of the subject on the form or shape, shades, movements (human movement, inanimate movement or animal movement) perceived by the subject.
3. **Contents:** The subject may respond on the ink-bolt on the basis of human figures and details, parts of human figure, animal figure, details of animal figure, inanimate objects, plants, maps, clouds,

blood, nature (light), sexual objects and other symbols. The responses are recorded keeping in view of the above contents of the ink-blot.

4. **Popularity or originality:** Some responses are given frequently by normal subjects. These are called popular responses. Some responses may be extremely different, which can be considered as original responses.

Analysis

The recorded responses are analyzed in the light of location, determining quality, contents and popularity or originality.

Interpretation

Interpretation is done on the basis of the analyzed data. Interpretation of the responses is a different job. Generally, subjectivity comes in the way and reduces the validity of the test as such. There is need for further experimentation on the test to make it valid. A few examples of responses are subjected to Rorschach ink-blot test and the corresponding interpretation.

Thematic appreciation test

The test consisting of perception of a certain picture in a thematic manner (revealing imaginative themes) is called thematic appreciation test (TAT). This test was developed by Murray and Morgan in 1935.

Description

The standard test contains 30 pictures of which 10 pictures for men alone, 10 for women alone and 10 mixed ones for both men and women. All the pictures are more or less vague. Each picture shows a dramatic or emotional scene that might have a number of explanations.

Administration of the test

1. The picture is shown to the subject one by one and he/she is asked to develop a story about each picture. The subject is asked to explain the picture and to give an imaginary reconstruction of what went before and what followed. Although a good deal of emotion is portrayed in each picture, yet it is not clear just what the excitement is all about.
2. Thus, a man may be shown pointing excitedly towards something, but there is no clue as to what he/she is pointing at. The subject therefore, reads into the pictures some fantasies or interpretations of his/her own.
3. In giving meaning to the pictures, a person is certain to reveal something about him/her.
4. The raw material for a pupil's story comes from one's own experiences and is colored by own personality needs. The stories are scored for evidence of basic, unsatisfied urges and for environmental pressures.
5. The nature of the outcome is also examined, since it is the product of needs and pressures. Environmental and psychological aspects can be analyzed.

TAT type pictures: As follows:

- Achievement motivation
- Need for affiliation
- Parent-child relationships
- Inner fantasies
- Level of aspiration
- Social and family relationships
- Functioning of sex urge
- Emotional conflicts
- Attitudes to work, minority groups or authority
- Outlook towards future
- Frustration
- Creativity
- Fear of success.

Modifications of TAT

1. The number of pictures can be reduced depending upon the nature of subjects and experience of the expert.
2. Some other pictures can be combined with the original ones.

3. The test can be determined to act as a group test. Pictures can be projected and the group of individuals can be required to write stories after necessary instructions. Stories are evaluated individually to assess the personality of concerned students.
4. Leopold Bellak modified TAT for using it for children of 3–11 years. This test is known as children's apperception test (CAT). The test consists of 10 pictures depicting situations of family relationships, toilet training, feeding habits, etc.

Children's apperception test

Children's apperception test was developed by Leopold Bellak. The TAT test is used among adults and adolescents, but not suitable for children between 3 and 10 years.

Description

The CAT consists of 10 cards. The cards have pictures of animals instead of human character, since it was thought that children could identify themselves with animal figures more readily than with persons. These animals are shown in various life situations. For both sexes, all the 10 cards are needed. Whatever story the child makes, he/she projected himself/herself. The pictures are designed to produce fantasies relating to the child's own experiences and reactions.

Administering the test

All the 10 cards are presented one by one and the subject is asked to make up stories on them. The child should have confidence and he/she should take story making a pleasant game to play with.

Interpretation

Interpretation of the stories is centered round the following variables:

1. **Hero:** The personality traits of the hero as revealed by the story.
2. **Theme of the story:** What particular theme has he/she selected for the story building?
3. **End of the story:** Happy ending or unhappy, wishful, realistic or unrealistic.
4. **Attitude towards parental figures:** Hatred, respectful, devoted, grateful, dependent, aggressive, fearful, etc.
5. **Family role:** With whom in the family the child identifies himself/herself.
6. **Other outside figures introduced:** Objects of the elements introduced in the story, but not shown in the picture.
7. **Omitted or ignored figures:** Which figures are omitted or ignored should be not, as they may depict the wish of the subject that the figures were not there.
8. **Nature of the anxieties:** Harassment, loss of love, afraid of being left alone, etc. should also be noted.
9. **Punishment for crime:** The relationship between a crime committed in the story and severity of punishment given for it.
10. **Defense and confidence:** The types of defenses, flight, aggression, passivity, regression, etc. the child takes nature of compliance or dependence, involvement in pleasure and achievement of sex desire, etc.

Word association test

A word is presented to a subject and he/she is asked to answer as quickly as possible with the first word that comes in his/her mind. The interpretation depends upon two factors, responses and the reaction time. In this technique, there are a number of selected words. The subject is told that:

1. The examiner will utter a series of words, one at a time.
2. After each word, the subject is to reply as quickly as possible with the first word that comes to his/her mind.
3. There is no right or wrong responses.

The examiner then records the reply to each word spoken by him/her, the reaction time and any unusual speech or behavior manifestations accompanying a given response. The contents of the response along with other recorded things give clues for evaluating the human personality and thus help a psychologist in his/her work.

Sentence completion test

The tests include a list of incomplete sentences, generally open at the end, which require completion by the subject in one or more words. The subject is asked to go through the list and answer as quickly as possible (without giving a second thought to the answer). For example, we can have the following sentences:

1. I am worried over ....
2. My hope is ....
3. I feel proud when ....
4. My hero is ....

The sentence competition tests are regarded as superior to word association because the subject may respond with more than one word. Also it is possible to have a greater flexibility and variety of responses, and more area of personality and experiences may be tapped.

In addition to the projective techniques mentioned above, there are some others, which may prove useful in many situation. These are play technique; drawing and painting tests, etc. both of these techniques are very useful in the case of small children. In the former, the examiner observes spontaneous behavior of children, while playing or constructing something with the help of given material and in the later, the natural freehand drawing and painting of children are the matter of study. Both of these techniques provide a good opportunity for the careful analysis of a child's personality.

Minnesota multiphasic personality inventory

One of the most commonly used personality test in the Minnesota multiphasic personality inventory (MMPI). It was developed during 1930's. This test asks for answers of true or false, i.e. 567 statements (one for men and another for women) about different personality traits such as attitudes, emotional reactions, physical and psychological symptoms, and past experiences. The answers are quantitatively measured and personality assessment is done based on the normal scores. NH Murthy of National Institute of Mental Health and Neurosciences (NIMHANS), Bangalore has reduced it to 100 items called multiphasic questionnaire.

Millon clinical multiaxial inventory

Items on this test correspond more closely than those on the MMPI to the categories of psychological disorders currently used by psychologists. This makes the test especially useful to clinical psychologist, who must find or identify individual's problems before recommending specific forms of therapy for them.

■ IMPORTANCE OF PERSONALITY IN NURSING

An understanding of personality will help the nurse to predict his/her behavior as well as the behavior of others. Major decisions in life depend upon this knowledge. For example, selection of a career, spouse, etc. his/her relationship with friends and relatives depend upon the expectations of their behavior from an understanding of their personalities.

The nurse should not only acquire skills and knowledge but also develop a pleasing and strong personality, if he/she should be successful. Patients, doctors, co-workers and other important members of the society want certain behavior patterns and certain qualities from them. In particular, patients appreciate a nurse who brings physical comfort to them with the skills, and who is prepared to understand their emotional reactions and difficulties, which have been caused by illness.

Besides possessing such professional qualities as integrity, dignity, mental alertness, self-confidence, caring attitude, empathy, approachability, respect for the patient, ability to build trust and accepting the patient as he/she is; the nurse ought to have such personal qualities as sympathetic understanding, friendliness of spirit, gracious manner, kindliness, adaptability, genuineness, optimism, sincerity and self-awareness.

Besides these qualities mentioned above, good health, fresh and neat appearance, a strong purpose and will power, high standard of values, healthy work habits, sense of humor, teaching as well as managerial abilities, ability to control one's emotions, healthy and friendly interpersonal relationship are important traits that the professional nurse should cultivate. The nurse deals with different age groups. A good, sensitive nurse should be aware of their personality. A sick person is very emotional, sensitive, dependent and demanding. A warm, sincere outlook can help them out.

Nurse and Personality

1. The nurse needs to know the basic structure of personality for providing effective care in the community and hospital setup.
2. The nurse interacts with different individual every day, so evaluation of character and personality is essential in planning the care.
3. The nurse should have basic understanding about the uses of defense mechanisms. It is important in making determinations about maladaptive behaviors, in planning care clients should assist in creative change, if desired or in helping clients accept themselves as unique individuals.
4. The nurse should not only acquire skills and correct knowledge but also he/she should have develop a pleasing and strong personality, if wants to be a successful nurse.
5. Possessing professional qualities are the essential characteristics of a nurse such as integrity, dignity, mental alertness, poise, self-confidence and dependency. She ought to have such personal qualities as sympathetic, understanding, friendliness of spirit, gracious manners, kindness and adaptability.
6. The nurse interacts with patients, doctors, co-workers and other important members of society, who need certain behavior patterns, so the nurse should develop and practice well-adjustable personality.
7. The patient appreciates a nurse who brings physical comfort to them with his/her skills, and is prepared to understand their emotional reaction and difficulties, which have been caused by illness.
8. Personality is the total quality of an individual's behavior, as it is shown in the habits of thinking, attitudes, interests, members of acting and personal philosophy, which facilitates quality patient care.
9. Personality is dynamic, growing thing, which is different in each person. Individuals are different from each other even at birth, in physical appearance, motility or temperament, the needs to understand the individual differences, while planning the care or education.
10. Many individuals with mental health problems are still struggling to achieve tasks from a number of developmental stages. Nurses can plan care to assist these individual in fulfilling these tasks and moving to a higher developmental level.
11. Assisting teaching and advising the parents, teachers and family's responsibility in developing and achieving developmental task in personality.
12. It incorporates sociocultural concepts into the development of personality.

PERSONALITY DISORDERS

Deviate from the characteristic trait, which goes beyond normal.

Meaning

Personality disorders are recognized in early adolescence.

Definition

An abnormal personality is one in which there are deeply ingrained maladaptive patterns of behavior recognizable by the time of adolescence or earlier and continuing through most of adult life (ICD-9).

Classification (DSM-IV)

- Cluster A: Schizoid, paranoid, schizotypal
- Cluster B: Histrionic, antisocial and borderline, narcissistic
- Cluster C: Avoidant, dependent, obsessive compulsive, aggressive and passive.

Etiology

- Hereditary: Chromosomal abnormality or genetic predisposition
- Biological factors: Brain dysfunction and changes in neurotransmitters
- Developmental factors: Emotional, physical and sexual abuse
- Sociocultural factors: Involuntary isolation, long-term psychiatric diseases
- Precipitating stressors: Instability in the family or divorce
- Psychological stressors: High anxiety.

Treatment

Group psychotherapy: Widely used in antisocial personality.

Individual psychotherapy: Effective in antisocial, dependent and inhibited personality disorder.

Behavior therapy: It is useful in anger control and social skills training of some valve.

Cognitive behavior therapy: Effective in antisocial personality disorder.

CONCLUSION

Personality is something that enables a person to stand out him/her distinct from others. It is the total quality of an individual's behavior. It includes his/her physical, mental, emotional and temperamental make up and how it shows itself in behavior. Personality is a dynamic thing; it grows in a social setup. It is different in each person. The growth is affected by one's physique, glandular functioning, physical appearance, physiological conditions of the body brought about by drugs, disease and toxins. The growth is also influenced by one's environmental and social factors, as the relationships in the home, school, social codes and roles which one has to play; cinema, agencies of social communication and radio. Maternal factors influence the growth of a person's motives, acquired interests, attitudes, will or character and intellectual capacities. Personality can be assessed or evaluated by means of interview, observation of behavior, rating scales, questionnaire and case study method. A successful nurse needs to develop a pleasing and strong personality; qualities such as dignity, mental alertness, self-confidence, dependability, sympathetic understanding, a strong desire to help, a high standard of values and the ability to develop healthy interpersonal relationships, are generally associated with the personality of a successful nurse.

REVIEW QUESTIONS

Long Essays

1. Define personality. Explain concepts and components of personality.

2. Describe physical, environmental and psychological factors of personality.
3 Discuss the psychometric assessment of personality. Describe the types of personality disorders.

Short Essays

4. Describe the variables of personality.
5. Discuss various types of personality.
6. Enumerate the theories of personality.
7. Explain psychoanalytical theory.
8. Enumerate psychosocial theory of Erik Erikson.
9. Describe the learning theories of personality.
10. Explain different types of projective test in detail.
11. Importance of studying personality in nursing.

Short Answers

12. Sheldon's classification of personality.
13. Jung's classification personality.
14. Structure of personality.
15. Dynamic personality.
16. Unconsciousness.
17. Psychic energy.
18. Cathexis.
19. Phallic stage.
20. Industry vs role confusion.
21. Case study method.
22. Sociometric method.
23. Rating scale.
24. Verbal projective test.

■ BIBLIOGRAPHY

1. Eysenck HJ. Dimensions of Personality. London: Kegan Paul; 1947.
2. Eysenk HJ. The Structure of Human Personality, 3rd edition. New York: Methuen and Co; 1971.
3. Hall CS, Lindzey, Garner. Theories of Personality, 2nd edition. Wiley and Sons Inc.; 1970.
4. Kuppusamy B. Advanced Educational Psychology. Delhi: University Publication.
5. Mangal SK. Advanced Educational Psychology, 2nd edition. New Delhi: Prentice hall; 2002.
6. Siagner R. Psychology of Personality. New York: McGraw-Hill.
7. Travers, Robert MW. Educational Psychology. New York: Macmillan; 1973
8. Williams, Jessie. Psychology for student Nurses. New York: Methuen and Co Ltd.
9. Young Kimball. Personality and Problems of Adjustment. London: Kegan Paul, Trench, Trubner and Co Ltd; 1947.

Section V

Developmental/Educational/Social Psychology

CHAPTER

20 Developmental Psychology

■ INTRODUCTION

Developmental psychology is the scientific study of changes that occur in human beings over the course of their life. Originally concerned with infants and children, the field has expanded to include adolescence, adult development, aging and the entire life span. This field examines change across a broad range of topics including motor skills and other psychophysiological processes cognitive development involving areas such as problem solving, moral understanding and conceptual understanding language acquisition social, personality and emotional development, and self-concept and identity formation.

Developmental psychology examines issues such as the extent of development through gradual accumulation of knowledge versus stage-like development and the extent to which children are born with innate mental structures, versus learning through experience. Many researchers are interested in the interaction between personal characteristics, the individual's behavior and environmental factors including social context and their impact on development; others take a more narrowly focused approach.

■ DEFINITION

Developmental psychologists study the human growth and development that occurs throughout the entire life span. This includes not only physical development but also cognitive, social, intellectual, perceptual, personality and emotional growth. The study of human development is important not only to psychology but also to biology, anthropology, sociology, education and history. Developmental psychologists help us better understand how people change and grow, and then apply this knowledge to helping us live up to our full potential.

■ NEED OF DEVELOPMENTAL PSYCHOLOGY

The specific tasks performed by developmental psychologists may vary somewhat based on the specialty area in which they work. Some developmental psychologists focus on working with a specific population such as developmentally delayed children. Others specialize in studying a particular age range such as adolescence or old age. Some of the tasks that a developmental psychologist might do include:

- Evaluating children to determine, if they have a developmental disability
- Investigating how language skills are acquired
- Studying how moral reasoning develops in children
- Exploring ways to help elderly individuals remain independent.

Developmental psychologists can work in a wide range of settings. Some work in educational settings at colleges and universities, often conducting research on developmental topics, while also teaching courses. Others may work in government agencies to help assess, evaluate and treat individuals suffering from developmental disabilities. Other possible areas of employment include assisted living homes for the elderly, teen rehabilitation clinics, centers for the homeless, psychiatric clinics and hospitals.

ISSUES IN DEVELOPMENTAL PSYCHOLOGY (Fig. 20.1)

There are a number of important issues that have been debated throughout the history of developmental psychology. The major questions include the following:

1. Is development due more to genetics or environment?
2. Does development occur slowly and smoothly or do changes happen in stages?
3. Do early childhood experiences have the greatest impact on development or later events equally important?

Nature vs Nurture

The debate over the relative contributions of inheritance and the environment is one of the oldest issues in both philosophy and psychology. Philosophers such as Plato and Descartes supported the idea that some ideas are inborn. On the other hand, thinkers such as John Locke argued for the concept of tabula rasa a belief that the mind is a blank slate at birth, with experience determining our knowledge. Today, most psychologists believe that it is an interaction between these two forces that causes development. Some aspects of development are distinctly biological such as puberty. However, the onset of puberty can be affected by environmental factors such as diet and nutrition.

Early Experience vs Late Experience

A second important consideration in developmental psychology involves the relative importance of early experiences versus those that occur later in life. Are we more affected by events that occur in early childhood or do later events play an equally important role? Psychoanalytic theorists tend to focus upon events that occur in early childhood. According to Freud, much of a child's personality is completely established by the age of 5 years. If this is indeed the case, those who have experienced deprived or abusive childhoods might never adjust or develop normally. In contrast to this view, researchers have found

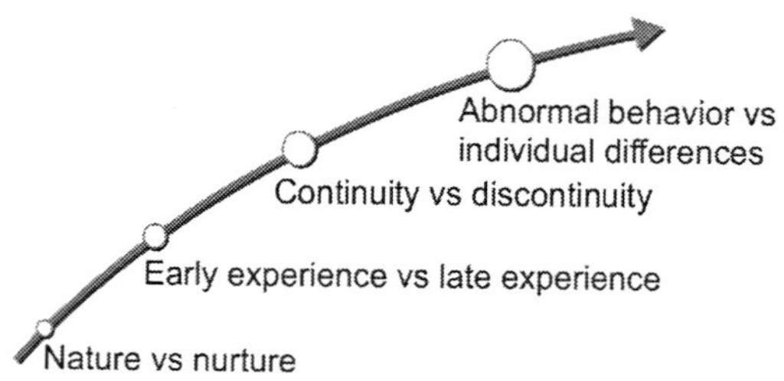

Figure 20.1: Issues in developmental psychology

that the influence of childhood events does not necessarily have a dominating effect over behavior throughout the life. Many people with less than perfect childhoods go on to develop normally into well-adjusted adults.

Continuity vs Discontinuity

A third major issue in developmental psychology is that of continuity. Does change occur smoothly overtime or through a series of predetermined steps? Some theories of development argue that changes are simply a matter of quantity; children display more of certain skills as they grow older. Other theories outline a series of sequential stages in which skills emerge at certain points of development. Most theories of development fall under three broad categories, which are as follows.

Psychoanalytic Theories

Theories influenced by the work of Sigmund Freud, who believed in the importance of the unconscious mind and childhood experiences. Freud's contribution to developmental theory was his proposal that development occurs through a series of psychosexual stages.

Theorist Erik Erikson expanded upon Freud's ideas by proposing a stage theory of psychosocial development. Erikson's theory focused on conflicts that arise at different stages of development and unlike Freud's theory, Erikson described development throughout the life span.

Learning Theories

Focus on how the environment impacts behavior. Important learning processes include classical conditioning, operant conditioning and social learning. In each case, behavior is shaped by the interaction between the individual and the environment.

Cognitive Theories

Focus on the development of mental processes, skills and abilities. Examples of cognitive theories include Piaget's theory of cognitive development.

Abnormal Behavior vs Individual Differences

One of the biggest concerns of many parents is whether or not their child is developing normally. Development milestones offer guidelines for the ages at which certain skills and abilities typically emerge, but can create concern when a child falls slightly behind the norm. While developmental theories have historically focused upon deficits in behavior, focus on individual differences in development is becoming more common. Psychoanalytic theories are traditionally focused upon abnormal behavior, so developmental theories in this area tend to describe deficits in behavior. Learning theories rely more on the environment's unique impact on an individual, so individual differences are an important component of these theories. Today, psychologists look at both norms and individual differences when describing child development.

▪ INFANCY

Infancy is traditionally designed as the period from 1 month to 1 year of age. This year is one of rapid growth and development, with the infant tripling birth weight, and increasing length by 50%. During this period the baby's senses sharpen and the process of attachment.

Stages of Infancy

Rapid Growth and Development

1. Infancy is the period of rapid growth and development, inner as well as outer organs developed rapidly at this stage.

2. There is a rapid growth in terms of height, weight and size.
3. There is rapid development of emotions and almost all the emotions are developed in the child during this stage.
4. This stage is marked by intensive motor activity and restlessness.

Dependence

1. Infant depends up on their mother, father and family members for the satisfaction on their basic needs.
2. The infant is helpless to move and function without the help of others. Even for the emotional satisfaction, infant depends upon others.
3. They expects that everybody around, should love them with entire affection and attention.
4. Infants want to love and to be loved, and in this exchange they totally depend on the mercy of others.
5. In this way the child at this stage is dependent, but as the child moves into the later years of their infantile behavior, they slowly proceed toward independence.

Self-assertion

1. The child is helpless one and depends upon others for the satisfaction of their needs, they are quite self-assertive.
2. Infants try to dominate superior and elder their wishes must be fulfilled.
3. They think, they are always right and all around them should obey them.
4. They are the prince although without crown and try to assert themself all the time in all situations.

Period of 'Make Believe and Fantasy'

1. Infant live in the world of their own creation, i.e. a period of rich, but baseless imagination.
2. As on this stage, infant has limited potentialities and aspires more than, what they can actually get in the actual life.
3. They compensate themself in fantasy and makes believe.

Selfish and Unsocial

1. In infancy, the child is almost completely egocentric and selfish.
2. They do not want to share their toys or give any of their possessions to anyone else.
3. They want to have all the things even love, admiration and affection reserved for them.
4. They do not care for the social and its moral codes, principles and places; themself interests at the premium.

Emotionally Unstable

1. Infancy is the period of violent emotional experiences.
2. The emotions at this stage are marked by intensity, frequency and instability.
3. There are spontaneous and the infant is hardly able to exercise control over them.
4. Infants are not able to hind their feelings and in this way, the emotion of the infant is generally in the overt form.

Mental Development During Infancy

Developing Curiosity and Questioning Attitude

1. At this age, the child is very much curious about knowing so many things around them. The world and the environment are new for them.
2. Infant is in the habit of questioning such as "What is this?" Answers do not interest them as much as asking questions.

3. Infant speed of questioning is so rapid that they do not wait for the previous answers.

Intellectually Not Developed

1. The child at this initial stage is very immature in intelligence.
2. They lacks in the reasoning and abstract understanding.
3. They can think only in concrete terms and is not developed in abstract reasoning and thinking.
4. Their powers of observation, perception and concentration, etc. are also not developed.

Rate Memory

1. The child though not developed much intellectually has a very good memory, but this type of memorization is without reasoning.
2. It is purely based on role of memory; they can cram and reproduce the matter easily.

Creativity

1. The period of infancy is also characterized by the tendency of creative impulse in the child.
2. Infants develop a creative attitude and often engage themself in making or collecting so many things.
3. They tries to take satisfaction in realizing that they can make, construct and perform the activities as their elders do.

Time Concept Not Developed

For the child at this stage, the divisions of time such as yesterday, today, tomorrow, month, year, etc. are meaningless as they not yet developed the concept of time.

Sexual Development

1. Although, the sex organs at this stage are not developed, yet the sex tendency is in a continuous stage of development.
2. The findings of psychoanalysis such as Freud and others have clearly shown that the sexual life of the infant is rich as that of an adolescent.
3. An infant passes through the three stages of sexual development—stages of self-love, homosexual and heterosexual.
4. At the initial stage, the child derives pleasure from their own body by sucking his/her thumb or touching the sex organs.
5. Later on the child seeks the satisfaction of his/her sex impulse outside and develops sentiments of love, for the mother and father depending upon his/her sex.
6. Finally, the child develops heterosexual tendency and the male gets itself attached to the mother, and the female child to the father.

Physical Growth

Weight

1. As a rule, most infant double their weight at 4–6 months, they triple it by 1st year.
2. During the first 6 months, infants typically average a weight gain of 2 lb per month.
3. During second 6 months, weight gain is approximately 1 lb per month.
4. The average 1-year-old male baby weigh 10 kg (22 lb), the average female baby weigh 9.5 kg (2 lb).

Height

1. The infant increases in height during the 1st year by 50% or grow from the average birth length of 20 inch to about 30 inch (50.8–76.2 cm).

2. Weight for height is best assessment, if it is plotted on a standard growth chart.

Head Circumference

1. Head circumference increase rapidly during the infant period, reflecting rapid brain growth.
2. By the end of the 1st year, the brain has already reached two third of its adult size.

Body Proportion

1. Body proportion changes during the 1st year from that of a newborn to a more typical infant appearance.
2. The mandible becomes more prominent as bone grows.
3. The circumference of the chest is generally less than that of the head at birth by about 2 cm. It is even with the head circumference in some infants as early as 6 months and in most by 12 months.
4. The abdomen remains protuberant until the child has been walking well.

Body Systems

1. In the cardiovascular system, heart rate slows from 120–160 beats per minute (bpm) to 100–120 bpm by the end of the 1st year.
2. Respiratory rate of the infant slows from 30–60 breaths per minute to 20–30 breaths per minute by the end of the 1st year.
3. At birth, the gastrointestinal tract (GIT) is immature in its ability to digest food and mechanically move it along. These functions mature gradually during the infant year.
4. The immune system becomes functional by at least 2 months of age; the infant is able to produce both immunoglobulins (Ig), IgG and IgM antibodies, by 1 year of age.
5. Ability to adjust to cold is mature by age 6 months.
6. Kidneys, liver and endocrine glands remain immature, and not as efficient at eliminating body wastes as in the adult.

Teeth

1. The first baby tooth usually erupts at age of 6 months, followed by a new one monthly.
2. Teething pattern can vary greatly among children.

Motor Development

Gross Motor Development

1. **Ventral suspension position:** The infant's appearance when held in midair on a horizontal plane, supported by the hand under the abdomen. The 3-month-old child lifts and maintains the head well above the plane of the rest of the body in ventral suspension.
2. **A landfall reflex:** It develops at 3 months. When the infant held in ventral suspension, the infant's head, legs and supine extends. When the head is depressed, the hips, knees and elbows flex. This reflex continues to be present in most infants.
3. **Neck-righting reflex:** It begins at 4-month-old children. The infant turns the head to the side, shoulders, trunk and pelvis turn in that direction. This reflex causes the baby to lose his/her balance and roll sideways when lifting the head up.
4. **Sitting position:** A 5-month-old child can be seen to straighten his/her back when held or propped in a sitting position. By 6 months, children sit momentarily without support.
5. **Standing position:** The 9-month-old child can stand holding onto the coffee

table if he/she is placed in that position. At 12 months, a child stands alone at least momentarily.

Fine Motor Development

1. **Thumb position:** It an ability to bring the thumb and fingers together. It occurs at 4th month.
2. **Pincer grasp:** It is a major milestone, which occurs at 9th month. It is a perforce for use of one hand over the other.
3. At 12th month, the infant can play pat a cake and peek-a-boo, holds a crayon to make a mark on paper and helps in dressing such as putting arm through sleeve.

Developmental Milestones

Language Development

1. A child begins to make small, cooing sounds by the end of the 1st month.
2. By 4th month, an infant is very talkative, cooing, babbling and gurgling, when spoken to he/she definitely laughs out loud.
3. The infant can imitate vowel sounds well, for example, oh-oh, ah-ah and oo-oo at 7 months.
4. By 9th month, the infant usually speaks a first word dd-da or ba-ba.
5. At 12th month, the infant can generally say two words besides ma-ma and dd-da; they use those two words with meaning.

Play During Infancy (Solitary Play)

1. Safety is chief determinant in choosing toys (aspirating small objects is one cause of accidental death).
2. The 1-month-old infant spend a great deal of time in watching the parent's face, appearing to enjoy this activity so much that the face may become their favorite 'toy'.
3. A 3-month-old infant can handle small blocks or small rattles.
4. A 6-month-old infant can sit steadily enough to be ready for bathtub toys such as rubber ducks or plastic boats.
5. Many 9-month-old infant begin to enjoy toys that go inside one another.
6. The 12-month-old infant enjoying putting things in and taking things out of container, they like little boxes that fit inside one another or dropping objects such as blocks into cardboard box.

Sensory Development

Vision

1. A 1-month-old infant regards an object in the midline of vision.
2. Eye movement coordinated most of the time, follows a light to midline. Visual acuity is from 20/100 to 20/50 at 1 month.
3. Follows a light to the periphery and has binocular coordination (vertical and horizontal vision) at 3 months.
4. Recognizes familiar object and people at 5 months.
5. A 7-month-old infant pat their image in a mirror. Their depth perception has matured to the extent that they can perform such tasks as transferring toys from hand to hand.
6. By 10 months, the infant looks under a towel or around a corner for a concealed object (beginning of the object performance).

Hearing

1. Hearing is demonstrated by the 1-month-old infant who quiets momentarily at a distinctive sound such as a bell or a squeaky rubber toy.
2. Most of the 3-month-old infants will turn their heads to attempt to locate a sound.

3. At 5 months of age, the infant demonstrate that he/she can localize a sound downward and to the side, by turning the head and looking down.
4. By 10 months, the infant can recognize his/her name and listen acutely when spoken to.
5. By 12 months, the infant can easily locate a sound in any direction and turn toward it.

Emotional Development

1. At 1 month, watches face intently, while being spoken to.
2. Smiles in response to person or object occur in 3 months.
3. Coos and gurgles when talked to; enjoy social interaction at 5 months.
4. At 6 months, infants are increasingly aware of the difference between people, who regularly care for them and strangers.
5. At 7 months, children show obvious fear of strangers. They may cry, when taken from their parent, attempt to cling to him/her and reach out to be taken back.
6. Fear of strangers appears to reach its height during the 8th month, so much so that this phenomenon is often termed '8th month anxiety' or 'stranger anxiety'.
7. By 12 months, most children have overcome their fear of strangers and are alert and responsive again when approached. They like to play interactive nursery rhymes and rhythm games, and dance with others.

Cognitive Development

1. **Primary circular reaction:** During this time, he/she explores objects by grasping them with the hands or by mouthing them. At this stage, the infant appears to be unaware of what actions he/she can cause or what actions occur independently. It occurs in 3rd month of life.
2. **Secondary circular reaction:** It occurs at 6 months of age. During this time, the infant is able to realize that his/her actions can initiate pleasurable sensations.
3. Piaget describes the cognitive process of infant as sensorimotor intelligence for until an individual is about 2 years old. He/She concentrates on regularizing his/her sensation and controlling his/her motor activity.

Social, emotional and behavior problems of infant

Teething

Most infants have little difficulty with teething. Generally gums are sore and tender before a new tooth breaks the surface. Because of this pain, a baby might be resistant to chewing for 1–2 days.

Thumb Sucking

The need is so intense that may infants begin to suck a thumb or finger at about 3 months of age and continue the habit through the first few years of life.

Headbanging

Some infants rhythmically bang their heads against the bars of crib for a period of time before falling asleep. Excessive headbanging done to the exclusion of normal development or activity, or headbanging past the preschool period, suggests a pathological basis. Such children need a referral for counseling and further evaluation.

Sleeping Problems

Sleep problems develop in early infancy because of colic or because an otherwise healthy infant takes longer than usual to adjust to sleeping through the night. Breastfeed babies tend to wake more often than those who are formula fed because breast milk is more easily digested. In late infancy, the problem of waking at night, the remaining awake for an hour or more becomes common.

Nurse's Role in Health Promotion of the Infant

Promoting Infant Safety

Accidents are a leading cause of death in children. Most accidents in infancy occur because parents either underestimate or overestimate the child's ability. Nursing intervention is to establish sound parent-child relationship and provide anticipatory guidance for the child's safety.

Preventing Aspirations

The accident that leads to the greatest number of infant deaths is aspiration. Round, cylindrical objects are more dangerous than square or flexible object in regard.

Preventing Fall

Falls are a second major cause of infant accidents. No infant, beginning with the newborn, should be left unattended on a raised surface. Normal wiggling can bring a baby to the edge of a bed, couch or table top, resulting in a fall. Teach parents to be prepared for their infant to roll over by 2 months of age.

Nutritional Health

The best food for the infant during the first 12 months of life is breast milk. Breast milk is the most complete diet for the first 6 months, but requires supplements of fluoride and iron by 6 months. Iron-fortified commercial formula is an acceptable alternative to breastfeeding. Solids can be introduced by about 6 months.

Activities of Daily Living

In the 1st year, caring for the infant feeding, bathing, dressing and so forth occupies what may seem in case of nearly all parent's waking hours. All these basic care-related activities provide important opportunities for caregivers and infants to get to know one another, and to become used to each other's personalities and patterns. Nurses play a key role in teaching parents about these activities, stressing their importance.

Vaccinations

The diphtheria, pertussis and tetanus (DPT) vaccination are given at 2, 4, 6 months, boosters given at 15 months and 5 years of age. Measles, mumps and rubella (MMR) live attenuated vaccine, generally given at 12 months of age because of the presence of natural immunity from mother; a second dose should be administered at 4–5 years of age. Polio, trivalent oral polio vaccine infant receives at 2, 4 and 6 months. *Haemophilus influenzae* type B should be given at 2, 4, 6 and 15 months of age. Chickenpox vaccine (Varivax) 1 dose should be given before 12 months.

■ TODDLER

The toddler period is usually considered from age 1 to 3 years, enormous changes takes place in the child and consequently in the family. During the toddler period, the child accomplishes a wide array of developmental tasks. Promoting toddler health and maintaining wellness involves knowledge of normal growth and development processes, an understanding of common significant milestones and the ability to anticipate deviations.

Physical Development

1. A child gains only about 5–6 lb (2.5 kg) and 5 inch (12 cm) a year during toddler.

2. Physical growth is slow during toddlerhood. This is because of the toddler's decline in appetite and erratic eating habits.
3. Head circumference equals chest circumferences at 6 months to 1 year of age. At 2 years, chest circumferences are greater than of the head.
4. Toddler tend to have a prominent abdomen a pouch belly because, although they are walking, their abdominal muscles are not yet strong enough to support abdominal contents as well as they will later.
5. They also have a forward curve of the spine at the sacral area (lordosis). As they walk longer, this will correct itself naturally.
6. The toddler waddles or walks with a wide stance, this stance seems to increase the lordotic curve, but it keeps the child on his/her feet.

Physiological Development

1. Brain growth continues slowly, corresponding to advancing intellectual skills and fine motor development.
2. Improved coordination and equilibrium parallels the most complete by 2 years. Myelination of the spinal cord is evidenced by refined walking, jumping and climbing.
3. Respirations slow slightly, but continue to be mainly abdominal.
4. The heart rate slows from 110 to 90 bpm; blood pressure increases to about 99/64 mm Hg.
5. In the respiratory system, the lumen of vessels increases progressively so that threat of lower respiratory infection is less.
6. Stomach capacity increases to the point that the child can eat three meals a day.
7. Stomach secretions become more acidic; therefore, gastrointestinal infections also become less common.
8. Urinary and anal sphincter control becomes possible with complete myelination of the spinal cord.
9. In the immune system, IgG and IgM antibody production become mature at 2 years of age, the passive immunity effects from intrauterine life are no longer operative.
10. The sense of hearing, smell, taste, touch and vision develop, and begin to connect, since toddler utilize all fine senses to explore the world, and exert autonomy and independence.
11. Bladder and bowel control is typically achieving during this time period, and children are able to retain urine up to 4 hours before needing to void.

Common Problems

Sibling rivalry: It is defined as intense feeling of jealousy between siblings; often is seen when an infant is born into a family with a toddler.

Temper tantrums: It is an outward explosive reaction to inward stressful or frustrating situations that are a normal part of toddler life.

Psychosexual Development

1. According to Freud, toddlers are in the anal stage of development. Freud first pointed out the tension resolving around toddler, bladder training and viewed toilet training as a possible way of resolving conflict and handling stress.
2. Freud believed, improperly managed toilet training could lead to lifelong psychological trauma with accompanying physical bowel/bladder responses.
3. Toddler is generally able to recognize gender differences by 2 years of age and begin to explore and recognize body parts during toilet training.

Psychosocial Development

1. The three major psychosocial tasks of toddlerhood are gaining self-control, developing autonomy and increasing independence.
2. A 15-month-old toddler are still enthusiastic about interacting with people, provided those people are willing to follow the toddlers where they want to go.
3. By 18 months, toddler imitates the things they see a parent doing such as study or sweep; so they seek out parents to observe and initiate reactions.
4. At 2 or more years, children become aware of gender differences and may point to other children and identify them as 'boys' or 'girls.'

Emotional Development

1. Toddler who does not develop a sense of autonomy may manifest feeling of shame or doubt.
2. Children who learned to trust themselves and others during the infant year are better prepared to do this than those who cannot trust themselves or others.

Cognitive Development

1. The toddler enters the fifth and sixth stages of sensorimotor thought.
2. During the toddler years, language ability develops rapidly.
3. In tertiary circular reaction stage, i.e. 12–18 months, the toddler is described as 'a little scientist' because of the child's interest in trying to discover new ways to handle objects or new results different actions can achieve.
4. At the end of the toddler period, children enter a second major period of cognitive development, the preoperational thought. During this period, children deal much more constructively with symbols then they did, while still in the sensorimotor period of cognition.
5. Cognitive toddler is able to recognize and distinguish between shapes of objects, as they are only beginning to classify objects, i.e. classify objects into categories of use.

Play Behavior

1. The toys toddler enjoys most are those they can play with themselves and that require action.
2. A 15-month-old child are still in a put in, take out stage, so they continue to enjoy stacks of boxes or balls that fit inside each other.
3. They enjoy throwing toys out of a playpen or from a highchair tray as long as someone will pick them up and return them again and again.
4. By age 2, toddler began to spend time, imitating adult action in their play, e.g. wrapping a doll and putting into bed, setting the table or driving the car.

Spiritual Development

1. Fowler defined faith as a relational phenomenon, an active relationship with another, a commitment, belief, love and/or hope, which may be directed toward family, religion, God or friends.
2. Attending religious programs similar to a nursery school that emphasize appropriate behavior and positive self-esteem rather than a lesson is important as well.
3. Children at this stage know that imitating or confirming to rituals results in approval of others who are important to the child.

Major Learning Events

Toilet Training

1. Physical maturation must be reached and attitude of parents play a vital role.

2. Psychological readiness of a child such as able to inform the parent of the need to urinate or defecate.
3. Process of training should begin usually with bowel and bladder.
4. Parental response is to choose a specific word for the act.

Need for Independence Without Overprotection

1. Parents should be consistent and set realistic limits.
2. Reinforce desired behavior.
3. Be constructive, geared to teach self-control.

Health Promotion for Toddlers

Childhood Nutrition

1. Provide adequate nutrient intake to meet continuing growth and development needs.
2. Provide a basis for support of psychosocial development in relation to food patterns, eating behavior and attitudes.
3. Provide sufficient calories for increasing physical activities and energy needs.

Injury Prevention

1. Children under 5 years of age account for over half of all accidental deaths during childhood.
2. More than half of accidental child deaths are related to automobiles and fire.
3. Aspirating small objects and putting foreign bodies in ear or nose.
4. Prevention through parent education and child protection is the goal.

Common Health Problems in Toddler

Burns

1. Second and third common causes of death by individuals less than 15 years of age for boys and girls respectively.
2. Causative agents are thermal, chemical, electrical and radiation.
3. The clinical features are edema formation, fluid loss, circulatory stasis, burn shock and decreased cardiac output.

Poisoning

1. Ingestion of toxic substances or an excessive amount of substances.
2. More than 90% of poisoning occurs in the home and highest incident occurs in children under age of 4 years.
3. Improper storage is the major contributing factor of poisoning.

Fracture

1. In children, bones are more easily injured; fracture can result without major injury to surrounding tissues.
2. Healing occurs rapidly in children, rapidity of healing is inversely related to the age of the child.
3. The clinical features of facture are generalized swelling, pain or tenderness, diminished function or use of part.

Aspiration of Foreign Objects

1. Obstruction of the airway by a foreign object can occur anywhere from larynx to bronchi.
2. It is most common in children 1–3 years of age; leading cause of fatal injury in children less than 1 year of age.

3. Foods causing asphyxiation, e.g. round candy peanuts, grapes and popcorn.
4. The clinical findings of complete obstruction are substernal retractions, inability to cough or speak, increased pulse rate, respiratory rate and cyanosis.
5. Turn the small child upside down, head lower than chest and deliver up to five quick, sharp back blows with the heel of the hand.
6. Abdominal thrust for children aged 1 year and older (Heimlich maneuver).

Child Maltreat

1. One of the most significant social problems affecting children.
2. Majority of abused children are under 4 years of age; about 70–80% of abuse is by parents or other caregivers.
3. It may be intentional physical abuse or neglect, emotional abuse or neglect and sexual abuse of children.
4. Therapeutic intervention includes treat injury and identify and protect child from further abuse.

Mental Retardation

1. The Diagnostic and Statistical Manual of Mental Disorders, 5th edition (DSM-IV) defines cognitive impairment on the basis of two criteria; significantly subaverage general intellectual functioning and an intelligence quotient (IQ) of 70 or below.
2. The common causes of cognitive impairment are chromosomal abnormalities, infection in utero, anoxia at birth, fetal alcohol syndrome and head trauma.
3. Assessment done by using standardized tests notably the Wechsler Intelligence Scale for Children (WISC) or the Stanford-Binet Intelligence Scale.

Cerebral Palsy

1. Non-specific term for a neuromuscular disability or difficulty in controlling voluntary muscles.
2. Major causes are anoxia of the brain, congenital or neonatal infection, trauma, or prematurity.
3. Clinical findings are delayed motor/speech development, reflex abnormalities and difficulty in sucking and swallowing.
4. Management includes multidisciplinary approach, mobility devices and surgery to correct spastic muscle imbalance, medication, speech, physiotherapy and occupational therapy.

Role of Nurse in Care of Toddlers

Immunization

Caregivers should be encouraged to complete the initial immunization series in a timely manner to protect their child from infectious diseases.

Nutrition

Calorie and nutrient requirements increase with age, so that caretaker should consider for child's appetite, choices and motor skills.

Elimination

The nurse should educate parents about the signs of readiness for toilet training, which include the ability to demonstrate cognitive awareness of elimination.

Hygiene

Toddlers are usually bathed either every day or every other day, depending on their activity and state of cleanliness. It is always important to check the temperature of the bath water with a thermometer, if possible.

Dental Health

An important aspect of the visit is assessment of oral health, education of caretaker regarding correct methods of dental hygiene and counseling on strategies to prevent caries.

Rest and Sleep

Most 2-year-old children require 12–14 hours of sleep each day with one or two naps a day. Nightmare is also common in toddlerhood since their dreams seem very real.

Safety and Injury Prevention

Prevention can be done through parent education and child protection.

■ CHILD (PRESCHOOLER)

The preschool years span 3-6. Although physical growth slows, this is a time characterized by reinforcement of the cognitive and social skill begun during the toddler years. The preschooler establishes control of body systems as indicated by the ability to toilet, dress and feed self and is also able to tolerate longer periods of separation from caregivers, and interact cooperatively with adult and other children.

Characteristics of Preschooler

1. **Period of rapid and intensive growth:** The preschooler is the period of rapid and intensive growth, whereas the stage of childhood is characterized as the period of slow, steady and uniform growth occurs.
2. **Independence:** In fact at this stage he/she feels more at home with the world and takes satisfaction by doing his/her work with his/her own efforts. By acquiring experiences and developing physically and socially he/she tries to adjust themself in the environment.
3. **Emotional stability and control:** The preschoolers exercise control over his/her emotions and express them in appropriate and socially approved ways. The emotional behavior is not guided by instinctive causes, but has an appropriate notion behind it.
4. **Developing social tendency:** They like to play in group and share their toys with others. Feeling of mutual cooperation, team spirit and group loyalties are developed among children of their age.
5. **Realistic attitude:** Child at this stage begins to accept and appreciate the hard realities in place of imaginative idealist. He/She begins to take close interest in the world of realities and tries to adapt themself in real environment.
6. **Formation of sentiments and complexes:** The child at this stage is not in the habit of hiding the feelings and checking his/her emotions. Therefore, no complexes formed at this stage where as in childhood stage it happens. At this stage, preschooler's emotional behavior get itself structured into sentiments. Various sentiments such as those related to religious, moral, patriotic and esthetic aspects begin to develop at this stage.

Physical Development

1. **Biological growth:** Children in preschooler age grow relatively slowly; they become taller and thinner without gaining much weight.
2. **Weight and height:** The preschooler gains approximately 1.8 kilogram per year. At age of 3 years, the child weighs an average of 14.4 kg and at 5 years, the average weight is 18.3 kg.
3. **Baby proportions:** The typical preschooler looks more similar to an adult than does the toddler because of skeletal maturation. The head and neck continue

to decrease in proportion to the size of the rest of the body. The lower extremities grow faster than the head, trunk and arms.

4. **Cardiovascular system:** By age of 4 years, heart size is four times of birth size and is now similar to that of the adult heart. Murmurs may be discovered during the late preschooler period.
5. **Blood values:** During the preschooler years, fat replaces the red marrow of the long bones. The total leukocyte count is slight higher; 5,000–13,000 from 4 to 6 years of age.
6. **Respiratory system:** With growth, the length of structures in the respiratory tract has increased and the incidence of infections decreases.
7. **Gastrointestinal system:** The process of digestion is mature at this time, but the gastrointestinal system is vulnerable to stress, which may be manifested by mild to moderate dysfunction.
8. **Genitourinary system:** The urinary system is nearly mature by age of 5 years. The urine output in the age group is from 600 to 750 mL for a 24-hour period. Daytime bladder control is achieved by the end of the preschooler period with nightmare control still variable.
9. **Immune system:** Adult level of immunoglobulin A (IgA) are reached during the preschool years. Also children develop antibodies to the agents they are exposed to and to the normal flora in their body.
10. **Nervous system:** By 5 years of age, the nervous system comprises one-twentieth of the total body weight. Cerebral dominance is achieved, as demonstrated by the acquisition of handedness.
11. **Motor development:** As children use their muscles, muscle fibers increase in strength and size. Coordination and the ability to voluntary control movements increases significantly, allowing them to refine their skills.

Emotional Development

1. The preschooler watches adults and attempt to imitate their behavior. Imagination and creativity allow them to fantasize, trying out roles and behaviors.
2. Preschool children look forward to become similar to their father and mothers. They learn adult roles from their parents, who serve as role models for behavior.
3. A feeling of conflict may also arise from thoughts; the child realizes actions were not appropriate. Feeling of guilt may also arise from thoughts the child has that are different from expected behaviors.
4. The goal of caregivers during period is to assist children to learn about the world and other people. With this help, preschooler gradually modifies their egocentricity.

Sexual Development

1. Sexual energy, generally, at this stage remains dominant, but merges with great forces at the end of the stage.
2. The sexual behavior of the children at this stage is characterized by the development of an attitude of antagonism and indifference toward opposite sex.
3. While the boys and girls of this stages play together, they wish to play with the members of their own sex.
4. Due to their varied interests they gradually develop a general attitude of antagonism toward the sexes and naturally draws apart. Even when brought together in family gathering, boys and girls of their age are barely civil to one another.
5. Sex antagonism is more pronounced in boys than in the case of girls, the attitude of antagonism, generally takes the form of indifference.

Cognitive Development

1. During Piaget's preoperational stage, between the ages of 2–6 years, the child develops the ability to perform mental operations governed by personal perceptions and linkage to events previously experienced.
2. At this stage, the child acquires new experiences and tries to adopt themself in their environment and prepares themself to solve the problems.
3. The preschooler gains power of reasoning and thinking observation, concentration, perception, imagination, etc. are developed.
4. They develop the concept of length, time and distance, and learn to express themself in various ways.
5. The preschooler uses a personal system for organizing objects and events in his/her mind, and reasons from one particular to another, often by unrelated events, when in reality the particulars are not linked at all.

Moral Development

1. The child's moral development is the most basic level; right and wrong are determined through the rules that parents have established.
2. Preschoolers conform to rules strictly for the purpose self-interest, i.e. to avoid punishment and to have favors returned.
3. According to Kohlberg, moral growth occurs in specific sequences of developmental stages that are called preconventional or premoral stage.

Spiritual Development

1. Preschool children continue in Fowler's stage of intuitive—projective faith.
2. The preschooler has a concrete conception of God, who has physical characteristics and can understand simple religious stories.
3. The preschool children accept the religion of their parents because for them, parents are omnipotent and powerful.
4. Preschool children are old enough to go to Sunday school. Any discussion of religion should be shared experience between parents and their children.

Language and Speech Development

1. Preschool children use language in a symbolic way. They not only imitate sounds at this stage but also use words to represent things.
2. Language is used by preschoolers to communicate their feelings and ideas.
3. They consistently ask questions and learn about the outside world by seeking the meaning of what they experience through sensory stimulates.
4. Preschool children use progressively longer and more complex sentences, and their vocabulary grows rapidly.
5. An analysis of child's questions shows a need for information, for relief from anxiety and for attention.
6. Preschoolers delight in trying out a variety of words. They are unconcerned about the consequences of language and are prone to pick up words that parents may prefer, they not mean to have their vocabulary.

Play Activities

1. Play facilitates the development of an optional self-identity by establishment of an imaginary friend, which helps a child work through a particular different time.

2. Activities that promote small muscle development encourage a child's creativity and fine motor skills.
3. Preschool children play actively; they climb, run, hammer, open doors with a bang and slam them shut.
4. The repetitive play of preschool children is an imitation of the life about them. Many play themes stem from a confusion in children's minds about experiences they have had a real life.
5. The children need to be encouraged to express their own creativity rather than fitting them within a mold of adult expectation. They should be allowed and encouraged to play with toys of their choice independent of gender-role designation.

Nurse's Role in Health Promotion

Nutrition

Preschooler needs to eat only one half as much as adult. The daily requirements range from 1,300 to 1,700 calories, including 30 g proteins. The preschoolers enjoy five meals a day to keep up with energy demand. Food should be selected from the basic four food groups, with a limit of 16 ounces of milk daily.

Accident Prevention

During the preschool years, the child begins to explore outside the home and into the neighborhood. It is also important to remember that the preschool-aged child is less reckless, will listen more to rules and is aware of potential dangers such as hot objects, sharp instruments or dangerous heights.

Hygiene

Many preschoolers enjoy their bath time, but the parental assistance may be needed for hair washing, cleaning finger nails and ears.

Dental Health

The number one dental problem during this time is dental caries, which may cause the premature loss of teeth and a consequent alteration of dental arch, compromising development of the permanent teeth. The preschool child should visit a dentist at least 6 months.

Rest and Sleep

The preschooler sleeps a total of 12 hours a day. Preschoolers may have difficulty sleeping in a dark, a proper parental support and guidance is essential during time.

■ SCHOOL CHILD

1. The phase of development from 6 to 12 years, the school-age years, is crucial to establishing positive self-esteems, a sense of belonging and feeling of competence. The school children gain new ideas from adults outside the family, teacher, parents of their friends, policemen and women, television performers, newspaper writers, and authors of textbooks with those of their parents.
2. School children learn to think of themselves as person in their own right may resent limits that parents continue to improve on their behavior. Parents need help in understanding the normal growth and development of their child when conflicts arise. Today child can experience the world beyond the classroom with the help of the internet, electronic mail, educational videotapes and cable television.

Physical Growth and Development

Biological Growth

Weight and height during the school years show a sex-related difference. Boys tend to gain slightly more weight through 12 years. The yearly height gain is similar in boys and girls, although boys tend to be taller.

Cardiovascular System

The heart assumes a more vertical position in the chest because of left ventricular development and downward placement of the diaphragm. Heart murmur peaks during 6–9 years of age.

Immune System

The immune system continues to develop; response to infection is specific and localized. Normal adult levels of the immunoglobulins are reached during the school years. The increased amount of lymphatic tissue in the nasopharynx continues to cause blockage of the Eustachian tube. As the child reaches puberty and the amount of lymphatic tissue decreases, ear infection decreases in direct proportion.

Nervous System

By 10 years of age, the nervous system is essentially mature. The maturity is evident in the sensory and motor functions as well as in the cognitive process.

Skeletomuscular Development

1. Skeletal growth is particularly noticeable in the long bones of the extremities; growing pain, which occur because the long bone grows faster than the attached muscles.
2. Muscle strength and size also increase at a gradual rate during school-age years, and six basic gross motor skills such as balancing, catching, throwing, running, jumping, climbing, continue to be refined.
3. At the same time, improved balance and coordination enable the school-aged child to explore new physical activities such as bike riding and roller blading.
4. Boys have a greater number of muscle cells than girls, so it is common to find they do well gross motor activities such as throwing and running.

Sensory Development

By the time child reaches the age of 6 years, central visual acuity is established. At age 7 years, visual acuity should be 20/20, which is the adult level. The accommodative and refractive powers of the eye also reach stability. The sense of taste and smell fully mature prior to the school years, allows for greater discrimination.

Motor Development

1. Motor development progress in a cephalocaudal and proximal to distal direction, with reinforcement of both gross motor and fine motor skills occurring as the central nervous system matures.
2. The developmental theory of Erik Erikson identified the major task of the school-age period as identity versus inferiority.
3. During this time, energy is channeled into activities such as school projects, sports and hobbies. The school-age child also develops the ability to work with others on school projects and athletic terms in preparation for becoming a citizen of the world.
4. School children must grow out of the dependency on their family and must find satisfaction in the company of peer groups, and adults outside the home environment.
5. During the school years, the child develops wholesome attitudes toward s a person as set and learns the appropriate masculine or feminine social role.

Psychosexual Development

1. Freud believed that, starting at age 6 years and throughout school age, the child enters a calm period in the development of their sexuality called latency.
2. Freud theorized the school-aged child identified with the same sex parent by modeling the behaviors and emotional of this parent and learned about sex-role behavior, and identify by observing caregiver instructions, the media and friendship with children of the same gender.
3. School-age children become much less eccentric and direct their energies beyond themselves. During the early latency period children associate with same sex peers and tend to ignore members of the same age and tend to draw apart from them.
4. Boys and girls should be informed about the reproductive cycle and their respective roles as they approach puberty.

Spiritual Development

1. In school years, Fowler identified school children as being in the mythic-literal faith stage.
2. During these years, children are learning many specifics about their children that will develop into a religious philosophy to be used in their interpretation of the world.
3. As children reach pubescence, they begin to be less mythical in their thinking and beliefs are more controlled by reason.
4. As the child enters preadolescence, he/she realizes self-centered prayers are not always answered and there is no magic involved in religious beliefs; blind faith that previously existed in the younger child is replaced by reason.

Cognitive Development

1. Piaget suggested that around 6 years of age, children start to move from the egocentric view of the preschool age to the more open and flexible thought of the school-aged child.
2. By 7–11 years, during concrete operational stage characterized by considerable growth in thinking, imagination and language, which allows school-age children to expand and understand their world.
3. School-age children are increasingly able to classify objects in a more complex manner than they could during the preschool years.
4. The school children's mental ability permits them to carry on converse and reverse process. They can solve problems because they can manipulate symbols.
5. During the school-age periods, children think not only of the present but also the past and future. Since children can recall events that happened in the past, they become aware that exist over a period of time.

Moral Development

1. The school-aged child is at the conventional level of moral development, when the conscience develops an internal set of rules that must be followed in order to be good.
2. During third stage of moral development, the child's morality is based on avoiding the disapproval of others and maintaining a positive relationship with friends, family and teachers.
3. Children at this level can also demonstrate rigid behavior in an effort to obey the law. These children can take into account circumstances surrounding and incident rather than just looking at the result.

Language and Speech Development

1. During this period of development, children show tremendous growth in their ability to use words.
2. They extend their vocabulary by 20,000–30,000 words.
3. Their sentence structure and use of grammar continue to improve, and use if adjectives and pronouns increases.
4. Speech proceeds from egocentric to social. The unique culture of the children is reflected in language acquisition and speech patterns.

Play Activities

1. Play activities vary with age; number of play activities decreases with age, whereas the amount of time spent in one particular activity increases.
2. Prefers games with rules because of increased mental abilities.
3. Prefers games of athletic competition because of increased motor ability.
4. Play serves as a learning tool for children and their play changes with developmental needs.
5. Play becomes more formal, more organized, more competitive and to some degree, less physically active.
6. Parent can assist their school children with learning the rules of organized sports. Although parents may not attend sports events and other activities in which their children participate.

Mental Abilities of School Children

Readiness for learning, especially in perceptual organization, such as names of months in year, knows right from left, can tell time and can follow several directions at once. They acquire use of reason and understanding of rules, which needs consistency. Trial and error, problem solving become more conceptual rather than action oriented. Reasoning ability allows greater understanding and use of language.

Common Problems Associated with School Children

School Phobia

School phobia is fear of attending school. It is a type of 'social phobia' similar to agoraphobia (fear of going outside the home). Children who resist attending school this way may develop physical signs of illness such as vomiting, diarrhea, headache or abdominal pain on school days. The causes of resistance to school are the child may be overdependent on the parents or may be reluctant to leave home because he/she feels that younger siblings will usurp the parent affection, while he/she is at school.

Handling school phobia requires coordination among the school, school nurse and healthcare providers who diagnoses the problem. The nurse is the ideal person to coordinate such efforts and to help the parents allow the child some independence not only in going to school but also in other activities.

Stealing

During early school age, most children go through a period in which they steal loose change from their mother's purse or father's dresser. This usually happens at around 7 years of age, when they are learning how to make change and discovering the importance of money. Youngsters, who continue to steal, may require counseling because they should have progressed beyond this normal development step by this age.

Recreational Drug Use

Recreational drug use was once considered as a college or high school problem is now a problem of school age. Illegal drugs are available to children as early as elementary school and certainly by the time they reach the VII or VIII grades.

Alcohol is available in so many homes and often can be purchased in small stores without proof of age; it is a commonly abused drug of this age group. Cocaine is becoming increasingly easy for children to obtain.

Parents should suspect of recreational drug use, if their child regularly appears irritable, inattentive or drowsy. School health personnel should be aware of the increase in this practice among students and look for warning signs.

Children need to be counseled against this because the recreational drug use leads to cardiovascular irregularities, uncontrollable aggressiveness and possible cancer in later life. Both nurses and parents should be role models of excellent health behaviors when earning for school-age children.

Obesity

Many teenagers, particularly boys, become overweight. Some have been overweight since infancy; their prepubertal neutral weight gain makes them obese.

Obese children begin to develop many of the same health problems as obese adults such as hypertension and elevated total cholesterol level with possible atherosclerosis.

A weight reduction program for school-aged children should emphasize long-term life changes such as intake about 1,200 calories, low in fat and designed to reduce weight, active exercise and counseling program.

Role of Nurse in Health Promotion

Nutrition

Children aged 7–10 years require 80 calories per kilogram of body weight. After age in years through adolescence, boys require more protein and iron. Careful meal and physical activity are crucial for the physical and emotional health of the school-aged child.

Accident Prevention

Factors contributing to the high incidence of accidents for this group are their increased independence, desire to have peer approach and increased involvement in physically challenging activities.

Most accidents are related to motor vehicles, but firearm injuries continue to increase in incidence. The second most frequent cause of accidental death is drowning. Accidents also occur when children are skating, skateboarding or riding a bicycle or minibike.

Elimination

School children are old enough to attend school all day; they have learned to control and independently care for their own elimination patterns. Usually stools are well formed and school-aged children have one to two stools per day. The amount of urine passed is dependent on intake, temperature, time of the day and child's emotional state.

Hygiene

Children older than 6 or 7 years of age are capable of carrying out their own personal hygiene practices daily. By the time they are 8 or 9 years of age they can be held responsible for independently bathing, grooming, dressing and properly discarding their soiled clothing. As children become more aware of changes in their bodies as they reach late school age, they begin to take more interest and are more reliable in their own grooming and cleanliness.

Dental Health

Dental caries resulting from poor nutrition is still a significant problem in the school-age population. Raw sugars and candies are common contributors to the development of dental caries. Dental check-ups are recommended every 6 months. The school system should incorporate a dental health educational program into the curriculum.

Sleep and Rest

The 6-year-old child may need 11–12 hours of sleep, whereas the 12-year-old generally needs only 10 hours. Sleep is essential during the school-age years to foster physical growth and academic performance, and failure to receive adequate rest can lead to irritability, and lack of attention span at school. Nightmares and night terrors are less common during the school-age years.

Sex Education

It is important that school-age children be educated about pubertal changes and responsible sexual practices. Sex education should be incorporated into health education throughout the school years in a manner that is appropriate to age and development.

▪ ADOLESCENT

Adolescent is the time period between 13 years and 18–20 years, which serves as a transition period between childhood and adulthood. It is a time of explosion, excitement, discovery, sometimes confusion and despair. Adolescent consist of early, middle and late stages. Each is distinguishing by several aspects of adolescent lives and constitutes the ages 12–14, 15–17 and 18–21 years.

Physical Growth and Development

Weight and Height

Most of the girls are 1–2 inches taller than boys when coming into adolescence and generally stop growing within 3 years from menarche. Thus, those girls who start menstruating at 10 years of age may reach their adult height by age 13.

Musculoskeletal System

1. Significant changes occur in skeletal size, muscle mass, skin and adipose tissue. Full bone length is first reached in the extremities and moves inwards.
2. The skeletal system grows faster than the muscles and muscle mass increases more rapidly than the height.

Teeth

1. Adolescent gains their molars (wisdom teeth) between 18 and 21 years of age. The jaw reaches about size only toward the end of adolescence.
2. Adolescent whose third molars erupt before the lengthening of the jaw is complete may experience pain and may need these molars extracted because they do not fit their jaw line.

Central Nervous System

1. Brain growth continues during adolescence, the cell that support and nourish the nervous system proliferate even though the number of neurons does not increase.
2. Continued growth of myelin sheath allows faster neural processing and is reflected in the adolescent's increasing ability to think abstractly and hypothesize.

Cardiorespiratory System

1. The heart almost doubles in weight and increase in the size by about one half during adolescence.
2. The lung increases in length and diameter during adolescence and the respiratory rate averages 16–20 breaths per minute.
3. Males have greater capacity, volume and rate because of their great shoulder width and chest size.
4. The slower respiratory system growth relative to the growth of other body

system may be another cause of the inadequate oxygenation and fatigue sometimes experienced by adolescents.

Gastrointestinal System

1. Rapid maturation of gastrointestinal system occurs during adolescence and by the 21st birthday, all 32 teeth have erupted.
2. Gastric acid capacity increase up to 1,500 mL to accommodate and facilitate digestion of the increased food intake that occurs in response to rapid growth.

Genitourinary System

1. Secretion of neurohormonal releasing factors by the hypothalamus stimulates the anterior pituitary gland to release follicle-stimulating hormone (FSH) and luteinizing hormone (LH).
2. In females, FSH stimulates growth of ovarian follicle and estrogen production. Estrogen causes breast changes, including enlargement and darkening of the reproductive organs such as vagina, uterus, ovaries, growth and darkening of pubic and axillary hair.
3. In males, FSH is responsible for sperm production and maturation of the seminiferous tubules. LH promotes testicular maturation and testosterone production. Testosterone causes the musculoskeletal system changes and development of the male reproductive system.

Sexual Development

1. Adolescence is the physiological period between the beginning of puberty and cessation of bodily growth.
2. Puberty is the stage of life at which secondary sex characteristics changes begin. Girls began dramatic development and maturation of reproductive organs at approximately age of 10–13 years; for boys 12–14 years.
3. Androgenic hormones are responsible for muscular development, physical growth and increase in sebaceous gland secretions that cause typical acne in both boys and girls.
4. In girls, pubertal changes typically occurs such as growth spurt, increase in the transverse diameter of the pelvis, breast development, growth of pubic hair, onset of maturation, growth of axillary hair and vaginal secretions.
5. The average age at which menarche (the first menstrual period) occurs is 12.5 years. It may occur as early as age 9 or as late as age 17, however, still be within a normal age range.
6. A menstrual cycle can be defined as periodic uterine bleeding in response to cyclic hormonal changes. It is the process that allows for conception and implantation of a new life.
7. Education regarding menstruation is an important aspect of comprehensive sexuality education.

Psychosexual Development

1. According to Frued, the physical changes of puberty reawaken the sexual and aggressive energies felt toward parents during latency of late childhood.
2. Freud argued many psychological issues, which adolescent faces are attributable to physiological changes.

Psychosocial Development

1. **Sense of identity:** According to Erikson, the developmental task of youngsters in early and mid-adolescence is to form a sense of identity. If the young person do not achieve a sense of identity, they develop a sense of role confusion.
2. **Body image:** Adolescents, who developed a strong sense of industry during their school age have learned to solve

problems and are best equipped to adjust to their new body image.

3. **Value system:** Adolescents need to be able to task to peers to develop their values. They dress identically with other members of the group.
4. An important part of adolescent's self-understanding is the value they place on their definition of who they are, which involves self-competency and self-worth.
5. According to Erikson, the youth who is not sure of his identity shies away from interpersonal intimacy or throw himself into acts of intimacy, which may involve in intimate relations.

Cognitive Development

1. The final stage of cognitive development, the state of formal operations, begins at age 12–13 years and grows in depth over the adolescent years.
2. This step involves the ability to think in abstract terms and use the scientific method to arrive at conclusions. Problem solving in any situation depends on the ability to think abstractly and logically.
3. They can create a hypothesis and think through the probable consequences. Thinking abstractly is what allows adolescent to project themselves into the minds of others and imagine how others view them or their actions.
4. Another significant change is cognitive development. Adolescence generally becomes more sophisticated in their ability to understand words and their related concepts.
5. Another important aspect of adolescent's cognitive development is their broadening ability to assume another perspective.

Moral Development

1. Kohlberg's conventional level of moral reasoning, which has been shown to emerge during adolescence and to persist as the predominant stage of moral functioning thought adulthood.
2. Adolescent male would likely reflect judgment-based reasoning of fourth stage thinking, whereas female adolescents would more likely reflect the relationship based on the third stage.
3. Abstract thinking: New level of social communication and understanding can comprehend satire and double meanings. They can say one thing and mean another.

Spiritual Development

1. All most all adolescents question the existence of God and any religious practices they can think.
2. This questioning is a part of forming a sense of identity and establishing a value system at a time in life when they draw away from their families.
3. Religious and scientific views are often compared as teens decide, what is true. More emphasis is placed on internal aspects of religious commitment rather than on attending church.
4. Adolescents become more oriented toward spiritual and ideological matters, and less oriented toward practice, rituals, and strictly observing religious costumes.
5. The late adolescent tends to re-examine and re-evaluate the beliefs and values of childhood and become more personalized less bound to the traditional religious practices compared to younger.

Health Promotion During Adolescence

Nutrition

1. The nutritional objective is to provide nutritional support for demand of rapid growth and high-energy expenditure.
2. Support development of appropriate eating habits through variety of foods, regular pattern and good quality snakes.
3. Nutrition education may be made through association with teenager's concerns about physical appearance, finger control, complexion, physical fitness and athletic ability.

Safety Measures

1. Accidents, most commonly those involving motor vehicles, are the leading cause of death among adolescents.
2. Drowning is one of the chief accident and athletic injuries tend to occur during adolescence because of the vigorous level of competition that occur.
3. Appropriate education regarding sexual maturity, reproduction, sexual behavior, driver education, hazards associated with smoking, alcohol and drug abuse.

Elimination

1. The elimination patterns for adolescents are similar to adults. They should void an average of 700–1,400 mL/day and have stool every day.
2. Constipation in adolescents may be due to a physiological disorder, eating disorder or improper nutritional patterns.

Hygiene

1. Skin care is especially important during this age because of the increased activity of the sebaceous gland, which contributes to acne. Increased sweat gland activity requires careful cleansing as well as the use of deodorant and body powders.
2. For female, menstrual hygiene is especially important and may require extra attention.
3. It is important to remind parents and other adult as well as the adolescent that these are normal physical changes and may require more attention to hygiene.

Dental Hygiene

1. Adolescents are generally very conscious about toothbrushing because of fear of developing bad breath.
2. During adolescents, malocclusion, gingivitis and dental trauma may occur. Malocclusion occurs due to dental crowding or mandibular/facial bone growth changes.
3. The dental teaching should include brushing the teeth at twice a day using a soft-bristled brush and fluoride toothpaste, flossing daily, eating a well-balanced diet and regular dental visits.

Rest and Sleep

1. Protein synthesis occurs most readily during sleep. Because of this, adolescents need proportionately more sleep than school-age children to support the growth spurt during this time, which demands the formation of so many new cells.
2. Nurses need to educate both parents and adolescents on the importance of adequate rest and sleep. Encourage teens to have realistic activity schedules that do not overextend their time.
3. An adolescent's excessive anxiety and fatigue may also result in sleep disturbances, which can continue into adulthood since adult sleep cycles and habits are formed during adolescence.

Health Problems During Adolescence

Alcohol Abuse

1. Alcoholism and alcohol abuse in adolescence are increasing. Many adolescents, who do drink, use it as a mind altering device since it allows participation in risk taking activities they might otherwise avoid.
2. There are numerous hazards of alcohol ingestion. Some may be seen in adolescents, including hepatitis, pancreatitis, gastritis, neuritis, cirrhosis, ulcer of gastrointestinal tract (GIT), cerebellar degeneration and delirium tremors.
3. Parents and nurses with adolescents who abuse or use other mind-altering drugs, and their family members need to be explained about detrimental effects.

Homosexuality

1. Nurses need to recognize that even though many young people explore their own sexual orientation or homosexual attractions, few who engage in homosexual behavior during adolescents, continue the practice into adulthood.
2. Nurses and caregivers recognize that homosexual experimentation is not the same as establishing homosexual orientations, acknowledge same bisexual relationships and attractions, and phrase questions about sexuality and sexual activity carefully.

Suicide

1. The number of adolescents committing suicide has increased dramatically over the last few decades.
2. Stresses related to psychosocial, psychosexual or physiological issues have been identified as cause for the increasing number of adolescent suicides.
3. Risk factors of adolescents are previous history of suicide, family history of psychiatric disorders, living without home, history of physical or sexual abuse and unable to meet scholastic expectations of parents and teachers.
4. Suicide programs for teens should be directed at school staff, community agency personnel and students themselves by providing information relative to warning signs, fact and programs, which can enhance self-esteem and social competence.

▪ ADULTHOOD

The young and middle adulthood is a period of challenges, rewards and crises. Challenges may include the demand of work and raising families, although adult can also be rewarded by success in their carrier endeavors and in their personal lives. Adult development involves orderly changes in characteristics and attitudes. Developmental changes are based on earlier characteristics, which help to shape subsequent behavior and characteristics.

Concepts of Young Adulthood

1. Young adulthood is the period between the late teens and the mid to late 30s.
2. During young adulthood, individuals increasingly separate from their families of origin, establishing carrier goals and decide whether to begin families or remain single.
3. Young adults are active and must adapt to new experiences. The transition into middle age occurs when young persons become aware that changes in reproductive and physical abilities signify the beginning of another stage in life.
4. Middle age is a time of continuing transitions when individuals may reassess their goals in life and add new goals.

5. The adult face such crises as caring for their aging parents, possibilities of job loss in a changing economic environment and dealing with their own developmental needs as well as these of their family members.

Maturity Developmental Tasks

1. People are said to have reached maturity when they have reached a balance of growth in physiological, psychological and cognitive areas.
2. Matured individual feels comfortable with abilities, knowledge and responses that they have developed over the years.
3. They look at the world with a broad view, based on a blend of insight, emotion and imagination. They take problems that can solve, but recognize and learn to live with unsolvable problems.
4. Mature people are open to suggestion and can accept constructive criticism without a major loss of self-esteem.
5. They weigh other person's input and recommendations of making decisions, but are not overly influenced or intimated by others; above all, mature people develop by learning from their own and other experiences.
6. Other characteristics of maturity are related to interpersonal communication and behavior.
7. Mature person acknowledge accomplishments and shortcoming. The mature adults confront tasks openly, use decision-making techniques to solve problems and are accountable/responsible for their actions.

Theories of Young Adulthood

Levinson's Phases of Young and Middle Adult Development

1. **Early adult transition (ages 18–20):** When the person separates from the family and desires independence.
2. **Entrance into the adult world (ages 21–27):** When the persons prepares for and tries out career opportunities and lifestyles.
3. **Transition (ages 28–32):** When the person may greatly modify life activities and thinks about future goals.
4. **Setting down (ages 33–39):** When the person experiences greater stability.
5. **Payoff years (ages 40–65):** A time for maximal influence, self-direction and appraisal.

Gilligan's Intellectual and Moral Development

1. Gilligan's theory (1993) proposes that intellectual and moral development differ between men and women.
2. Women struggle with the issues of care and responsibility, and in turn their relationships progress toward a maturity of interdependence.
3. As women progress toward adulthood, the moral dilemma changes from how to exercise their right without interfering in the right of others and how to lead a moral life, which includes obligations to themselves, their families and people in general.

Gordon (1991)

1. As women entered professional areas, they hoped to develop the caring and nurturing roles in their male colleagues.
2. Women have long recognized that without caring, the perceived quality of life is changed. As a result women maintained caring in the home and education, and frustrated in their development.
3. However, women become frustrated in their development because the responsibility of caring was not shared and frequently nurturing become a gender-specific responsibilities.

Diekelmann's Developmental Tasks

1. They become active independents from parental controls.
2. They begin to develop strong friendship and intimate relationships outside the family.
3. They establish personal set values.
4. They develop a sense of personal identity.
5. They prepare for life work and develop the capacity for intimacy.

Physiological Development

1. The young adult has completed physical growth by the age of 20. The young adult is usually quite active, experience severe illnesses less commonly than older adults.
2. A personal life assessment of the young adult includes assessment of general life satisfaction, hobbies and interests.

Cognitive Development

1. Rational thinking habits increase steadily through the young and middle adult years. Formal and informal educational experiences, general life experiences, and occupational opportunities dramatically increase the individual's conceptual, problem-solving and motor skills.
2. Identifying preferred occupational areas is a major task of young adults. When people known their educational preparation, skills, talents and personality characteristics, occupational choices are easier, and they generally more satisfied with their choices.
3. The young adults are continually evolving and adjusting to changes in the home, work place and personal lives; their decision-making processes should be flexible.

Psychosocial Development

1. The young adult is usually caught between wanting to prolong the irresponsibility of adolescence and wanting to assume adult commitments.
2. The years from 35 to 43 are the time of vigorous examination of life goals and relationships; alterations are made in personal, social and occupational lives.
3. During young adults, people generally give more attention to occupational and social pursuits. During this period, individuals attempt to improve their socioeconomic status.
4. During the young adult, they take major decisions concerning career, marriage and parenthood.

Health Promotion for Young Adult

1. Young adult lifestyles may put them at risk for illness or disabilities during their middle or older adult years. Young adults may also be genetically susceptible to certain chronic disease such as diabetes mellitus and familial hypercholesterolemia.
2. Violence is the greater cause of mortality and morbidity in the young adult population. Death and injury can occur from physical assault, motor vehicle or other accidents and suicidal attempts.
3. Intoxicated young adults may be severely injured in motor vehicle accidents that may result in death or permanent disability to other young adults as well.
4. Sexually transmitted diseases (STDs) have immediate effects such as discharge, discomfort and infection. They may also lead to chronic disorders, which can result from genital herpes, infertility, gonorrhea or even death.

▪ OLDER ADULT

Geriatrics is the care of aged. Aging is a normal process of time-related change that occurs through life. It involves all aspects of the organism and is largely characterized by decline in functional efficiency and decreased capacity to compensate and recover from stress. It does not necessarily occur in an interrelated or synchronous manner, but it does involve physiological, psychological and social changes that interact to influence behavior and adaptation.

Concepts of Old Age

1. Old age is a normal part of human development and is the final phase of the life cycle.
2. Aging is not something that happens to the other person, but is a unique and highly personal experience that affects everyone who lives long enough.
3. Successful adaptation to the aging process probably correlates with the person's previous ability to cope and adopt to change.
4. Other influences include are environmental factors, education and sociocultural determinants as well as the health status of the entire body.
5. Gerontology, the study of the aging process and its effects on older persons, become more important with each passing day.

Developmental Theories of Old Age

1. Certain theoretical models of human development help to point out important turning points during the late years of the cycle.
2. The theories concerning the life cycle incorporate the social, psychological and biological factors of developmental growth, and relate them to age to identity milestones and time development.
3. The theories of Buhler, Jung and Erikson, which are considered to be three of the most prominent theories of adult development have as a common theme, the goal of personal resolution in the second half of life.
4. Buhler's theories perceived that the period from 65 years is one of awareness of the experience of fulfillment or failure and the remaining years are spend in either a continuance of previous activities, or a return to the need satisfying orientations of childhood.
5. Jung suggested that, in the second half of life the individual direct his attention inward, so that through an intensive inner exploration he may find a meaning and totality in life that makes the acceptance of death possible.
6. Erikson's theory explains that the years between 40 and 50 challenge those values that a person places physical power in favor of the value placed on wisdom. People who cling to their waning physical powers becoming more and more depressed, but persons who shift to using their mental abilities as a primary resource appear to age more successfully.
7. The theorists view the first part of life as growth and expansion, and the later part of life as inner withdrawal and contraction.
8. The task of later life involves finding meaning and wholeness in life, and considerations about oncoming death.

Kinds of Aging

Biological Aging

1. Aging occurs with such changes as whitening of the hair, wrinkling of the skin, decline in eye focus and high-register hearing.
2. Biological aging depends on a combination of factors including genetic inheritance, finances and good health.
3. The most serious change for most people is their heightened vulnerability and lessened ability to recuperate from various illnesses.

Psychological Aging

1. Psychological aging refers to role of the individual assigned to themself as they reach a certain chronological age.
2. The two major threat felt by the older persons are the deterioration of his/her concept of self, which results in loss of self-esteem, extensive and continual grief over frequently occurring losses.
3. The plight of the aged in the youth-oriented society continues to receive attention and the process of gerontological counseling is now recognized as a specialized form of helping.
4. The older person should encourage seeing himself/herself as in a dynamic period of growth rather than in a period of rapid deterioration. The older person for the most part, wishes to be treated as a person on worth and dignity.

Sociogenic Aging

1. Society imposes role on people as they reach a certain chronological age. Older persons are seen by many people in our society as either nonpeople or expandable people, merely because they lived longer.
2. Older people have been told by our society that they are supposed to be physically, socially, sexually and intellectually infirm slow in comprehending events going on around them, and rigid in their ways of thinking and behaving.
3. Society also seems to take the attitude that older people should run away and hide until they die. It is important to note the combination of psychological than biological aging for many people.

Physiological Changes During Old Age

Changes in Homeostasis

1. Homeostasis is the body's ability to maintain a stable internal environment. The complex mechanism of homeostasis regulates fluid and electrolyte balance, blood pressure, temperature and food intake.
2. Man is dependent upon the functional integrity of the cell and the stability of the internal environment. If the homeostatic mechanisms are functioning properly, the body is able to adopt or react to stress.
3. However, with aging these mechanisms become less efficient and reserve power is lost. This in turn makes the person more vulnerable to disease. Recovery is also affected since more time is required for the body to return to normal after illness.

Changes in the Nervous System

1. The nervous system is extremely vulnerable to the aging process, as seen in the progressive loss of cells that occurs with advancing years.
2. Here are approximately half as many brain cells in the frontal area at age 80 as at 40 with resulting decrease in brain weight.
3. The steady loss of neurons begins surprisingly early in life and affects both brain and spinal cord. There is also a decrease in the blood flow to the brain.
4. Both physiological changes in the brain and the reduced blood supply may be related to personality changes, sometimes encountered elderly.

Changes in Special Senses

1. The aging process produces varying degree of impairment in hearing, vision, smell, taste and pain perception as well as diminished sensation of touch and slowing reflexes.
2. A decreased sense of smell and in the number of taste buds at times contributes to a loss of appetite.
3. Diminished sensitivity to thirst needs can lead to dehydration and confused behavior as a result of fluid balance.
4. Hearing impairment, which usually is first noticed in the higher frequencies, can result in impairment of speech discrimination and loss of the full sense of background noises.
5. Vision is affected by a decrease in visual acuity and accommodation to glare, and by a marked diminution of night vision and peripheral field of vision.
6. Perception of some types of pain decreases and referral of pain from one part of the body to another seems to become more common with advancing age.
7. The temperature-regulating mechanisms are less reliable and heat-generating activities are reduced.

Cardiovascular Changes

1. In older people, the heart is able to pump effectively under normal circumstances. But because it lacks much of its physiological reserve, it reaches poorly to sudden stress such as blood loss, excessive parenteral fluids or sudden effort.
2. When normal homeostasis is upset, congestive heart failure, arrhythmias and myocardial ischemia may develop.
3. The signs of arteriosclerosis become clinically recognizable when it has reached advanced stage in the elderly people.

Respiratory Changes

1. Most of the changes that occur in pulmonary function in the aged result from loss of elastic tissue surrounding the alveoli and alveolar ducts, and from changes in the anteroposterior of the chest owing to rib and vertebral calcification.
2. There is also changes in the tissues of the lungs and decline in its functional capacity, size and structure as well as weakening of the respiratory muscles.
3. Vital capacity becomes reduced, while there is a concurrent increase in residual volume. Changes in the pulmonary vasculature also occur.

Changes in Kidneys Function

1. Kidneys function decline with age because of a reduction in the number of glomerulus, diminished filtration and tubular function.
2. The blood flow to the kidneys is reduced as a result of decreased cardiac output and increased peripheral resistance.

Metabolic Changes

1. As the body ages, the basal metabolic rate slows and the quantity of oxygen used by the tissue is reduced.
2. As metabolic processes change, the glucose tolerance curve tends toward that of the diabetic. If normal standards for glucose tolerance tests were applied to the aged, 50% of this population would be classified as diabetes.

Musculoskeletal Changes

1. Generally, there is a slow and steady atrophy of muscles that result in muscle wasting, particularly of the trunk and extremities.
2. With loss of muscle power there is a decrease in strength, endurance and agility.

3. Bones gradually lose calcium and form porous and lighter; because bone become more brittle, falls are especially dangerous in the elderly.
4. Ligaments calcify, ossify and joints become stiffened from the erosions of cartilaginous joint surfaces. Changes in the lining of joint cavities can produce degenerative changes.

Skin and Connective Tissue Changes

1. The skin is among the first structures to show the most obvious association with aging.
2. As the person ages, there is loss of subcutaneous supporting tissue and resultant thinning of the skin. With the loss of subcutaneous fat, the skin assumes the characteristic appearance of aging folds, lines, wrinkles and slackness.
3. The dermis become relatively dehydrated and loses strength and elasticity. The skin in general is prone to excess dryness and itching.
4. As a preventive measure, older people should avoid overexposure to the sun, which tends to accelerate aging of the skin and increases the tendency to skin cancer.

Reproductive Changes

1. Physiological changes occurring with menopause can affect sexual function and activity in older women. Atrophy of the vaginal canal and diminished vaginal secretions can lead to local irritation, bleeding and pain with sexual activity.
2. In older male, there may be diminished and delayed ability to achieve a full penile erection, and a reduction in the frequency associated with psychological changes.

Health Promotion Measures for Elderly Population

Health Appraisal

1. Varied health assessment techniques can be implemented to help detect and identify elderly people at risk.
2. Many authorities believe that a comprehensive physical examination, including blood examinations, urinalysis and stool test should be carried out annually.
3. Assessment of health habits is necessary as a basis for health counseling. Positive measures for maintaining health include weight control, exercise, proper nutrition, avoidance of cigarette smoking and protection of accident prevention.

Nutritional Support

1. Dietary inadequacies in the elderly results from such factors as poor nutritional habits, economic constrains and underlying disease condition.
2. Nutrition can have a tremendous impact on health maintenance and disease prevention as well as on the treatment of disease.
3. Older people are vulnerable to low-nutrient intake. Dietary studies show that calcium, thiamine, ascorbic acid and vitamins are the nutrients most commonly lacking in the diets of the aged.
4. The addition of moderate amount of fiber to the diet may alleviate constipation and flatulence. The high incidence of osteoporosis in older women seems to be age related.
5. Other factors contributing to nutritional deficiencies are social isolation, lack of interest in cooking and eating, and problems in food shopping.

Exercise

1. Activity is one key to the prevention of premature aging. Many of the health problems of the aged arise from a lack of conditioning and diminished response to stress.
2. Exercise maintains muscular tone throughout the body and is effective in the prevention and rehabilitation following cardiovascular diseases.
3. Exercise training improves functional capabilities, increase vitality and has psychological benefits.

Temperature Regulation

1. Older people cannot tolerate a cold environment and are very susceptible to hyperthermia. The nursing approach is to provide extra blankets, which may be added for warmth.
2. Efforts are directed to maintain heat and humidity at comfortable levels by fans, air conditioning and humidifiers or dehumidifiers during hot weather.

Hygienic Care

1. With aging, the skin becomes thin and inelastic, predisposing the elderly patient to prevent pressure sores.
2. For elderly people, foot care is essential in order to maintain mobility, physical well-being and independence. A common foot disorder of this age group includes calluses, bunions, toenail problems, corns and fungal infections.
3. The components of dental care for the aging patients include eating a proper diet, maintaining oral health and denture-bearing structure, being motivated to speak proper care and having available adequate dental services.
4. Problems of constipation and bowel incontinence often can be reduced through systematic habit training. Constipation occurs because of altered mobility, decreased mucus secretion and changes in muscle tone and elasticity of the colon, as well as changes in diet.

Recreation

Recreation is more than just having fun; it is fundamental to physical and mental well-being. No matter how old or disabled one becomes, the desire for the dignity that comes only through purposeful activity is never lost.

Common Health Problems of Elderly Population

Disease and Aging

1. The aged are particularly vulnerable to diseases because of such factors as their decreased physiological reserve, a less flexible homeostatic mechanism and lessened defensive mechanism of the body.
2. Chronic diseases have been called the companions of the aged and most persons over 65 are affected by at least one chronic disease.
3. The major disorders of old age include heart disease, malignancy, cerebrovascular disease, influenza and pneumonia.
4. Disease in the aged does not always present with classic signs and symptoms. The usual clinical manifestations may be absent, attenuated or disguised and atypical signs and symptoms may present.

Falls in the Elderly

1. A fall may be a frightening experience that can lead to immobilization and possibly to pneumonia and complete loss of the ability to walk.
2. Falls by the elderly result from age-related physiological decline in postural control and deterioration of the central nervous system or from lightheartedness, postural hypotension, heart block and arrhythmias.

3. Special danger arises from osteoporosis, a condition in which the bones lose calcium and thus become thin and brittle. This condition renders an elderly person susceptible to major fractures.

Depression

1. Depression is the most common emotional disorder in the aged. Depression and grief are common with aged since losses are inevitable.
2. Depression resulting from losses can easily be overlooked and may be mistaken for physical or organic mental illness. The patient may exhibit anger, denial, withdrawal or other maladaptive responses that move him/her further away from reality.
3. Depression in the aged is usually manifested by feelings of apathy, quietness and emptiness, which may be mistaken for senile changes.
4. Treatment in elderly usually referred to community health resources such as the community mental health services can be very beneficial.

Chronic Organic Brain Syndrome (Senile Dementia)

1. The term dementia refers to signs and symptoms of intellectual dysfunction owing to differing etiologies and varying pathophysiologic mechanisms that can occur alone and in combination.
2. It is believed to result from diffuse impairment of brain tissue. The most common long-term disorders of cognitive functions (attention, learning, memory) in the elderly are seen in senile dementia (often called Alzheimer's disease).
3. Senile dementia generally refers to a disturbance of mental status or mental deterioration occurring after the age of 65. There are neuropathological changes associated with changes in the patient's cognitive function, which may include loss of neurons, neurofibrillary tangles, granulovascular changes and neurotic (senile) plaques in the brain.
4. Senile dementia is devastating to the human personality and is a source of anguish and frustration to the patient and loved ones.
5. Senile dementia and related disorders are associated with a high-motility rate and significantly shortened life expectancy.

Acute Brain Syndrome

1. Acute brain syndrome is a temporary psychiatric state caused by a physiologic or an anatomical insult to brain tissue.
2. The disorder have a relatively sudden onset and potentially reversible. They are associated with acute physical illness of physiological disturbances, cardiac and circulatory problems, neurological conditions, cerebrovascular disorders, dehydration, electrolyte imbalance, alcohol or drug toxicity and wide variety of infections.
3. In management of acute brain syndrome, the basic disease must be treated or the etiological toxic agent must be removed.
4. Specific treatment is aimed at alleviating or curing the condition that underlies the confusion. It includes antimicrobials for infection, removal of drugs, removal of fecal impaction, correction of heart failure and treatment of stroke.
5. Appropriate medications such as the phenothiazines, which exert much of their calming action on the lower brain centers may be administered.

▪ BEHAVIOR AND SICKNESS

1. Health in its broadest sense is a dynamic state in which the individual adapts to changes in internal and external environments to maintain a state of well-being.

The internal environment includes many factors that influence health, including genetic and psychological variables, intellectual and spiritual dimensions and disease processes.

2. The external environment includes factors outside the person that may influence health including the physical environment, social relationships and economic variables. Because both environments continuously change, the person must maintain a state of well-being.
3. Health and illness therefore must be defined in terms of individual. Health can include conditions that the client or nurse may have previously considered to be ill. Health is also closely related to an individual's work place and home life, and stressors can be the result of those environments.

Concepts of Health, Illness and Sick Behaviors

1. It is useful for the nurse to be aware of the behavioral components of health, illness and sick-role behavior.
2. Every person develops a system of health beliefs and attitudes; these tend to fall within the framework provided by society or cultural heritage.
3. Health behavior activities a person engages in when feeling well to take measures to prevent disease and illness to detect them before symptom occur.
4. Illness behavior activities a person edges in when feeling ill will lead to the defining of the state of health and that will gain help.
5. Sick-role behavior include activities a person engages in believing himself/herself ill. For any individual, the level of health behavior is determined by the significance of symptoms-danger value, visibility, ambiguity, fear of unknown, the expectations of those from whom help is sought, feeling about dependence and fear of loss of control, the expectorations of the illness position, including past experiences with illness.

Illness Behavior

1. Illness is not merely the presence of disease process. Illness is a state in which a person's physical, emotional, intellectual, social, developmental or spiritual functioning is diminished or impaired compared with that person's previous experiences.
2. Illness behavior involves the ways in which persons monitor their bodies, define and interpret their symptoms, take remedial actions, and use their healthcare system.
3. The important internal values influencing are the way of client's behavior when they are ill or their perceptions of symptoms as the nature the illness. A client's illness behavior can also be affected by the nature of the illness.
4. Acute illness involves symptoms of relatively short duration that are usually severe and may affect functioning in any dimension.
5. Chronic illness persists, usually longer than 6 months and can affect functioning in any dimension.
6. External variables influencing a client's illness behavior include the visibility of symptoms, social groups, cultural background, economic variables, accessibility of the healthcare system and social support.

Stages of Illness Behavior

1. **Symptom experience:**
   a. During the initial stage, a person is aware that something is wrong. A person usually recognizes a physical sensation or a limitation in functioning, but does not suspect a specific diagnosis.

   b. The person's perception of symptoms includes awareness of a physical change such as pain, a rash or a lump.
2. **Assumption of the sick-role:**
   a. The assumption of the sick-role results in emotional changes such as withdrawal or depression and physical changes.
   b. Emotional changes may be simple or complex, depending on the severity of the illness, the degree of disability and anticipated length of the illness.
3. **Medical care contact:**
   a. If symptoms persist despite home remedies, become severe or require emergency care, the person is motivated to seek professional health services.
   b. In this stage, the client seeks or expects acknowledgement of the illness, as well as treatment. In addition, the client seeks an explanation of the symptoms, the cause of the symptoms and the course of the illness for future health.
   c. Client's illness can be validated at any point on the health-illness continuum. A health professional may determine that they do not have an illness or that illnesses are present and may be life threatening.
4. **Dependent client role:**
   a. After accepting the illness and seeking treatment, the client enters the fourth stage of illness behavior.
   b. In this stage, the client depends on healthcare professionals for relief of symptoms. The client accepts care, sympathy and protection from the demands and stresses of life.
   c. It is socially permissible for clients in the dependent role to be relieved of normal obligations and tasks.
5. **Recovery stage:**
   a. The final stage of illness behavior, recovery and rehabilitation, can arrive suddenly such as when a fever subsides.
   b. The recovery is not prompt; long-term care may be required before the client is able to resume an optimal level of functioning.
   c. In the case of chronic illness, the final stage may involve an adjustment to a prolonged reduction in health and functioning.

Impact of Illness on Family

1. **Behavioral and emotional changes:**
   a. People react differently to illness. Individual behavioral and emotional reactions depend on the nature of the illness, the client's attitude towards it, the reaction of others to it and the variables of illness behavior.
   b. Severe illness, particularly one that is life-threatening can lead to more extensive emotional and behavioral change, such as anxiety, shock, dental, anger and withdrawal.
2. **Impact of family roles:**
   a. When an illness occurs, the roles of client and family may change. Such a change may be subtle and short term, or drastic and long term.
   b. An individual and family generally adjust more easily to subtle short-term changes. In most cases they know that the role change is only temporary.
   c. Long-term changes, however, require an adjustment process similar to the grief process. The client and family often require specific counseling and guidance to assist them in coping with role changes.

3. **Impact on body changes:**
   a. Some illness result in changes in physical appearance; clients and families react differently to these changes.
   b. When changes in body image occur such as that result from a leg amputation, the client generally adjusts in the following phases, i.e. shock, withdrawal, acknowledgment, acceptance and rehabilitation.
   c. Withdrawal is an adaptive coping mechanism that can assist the client in making the adjustments.
4. **Impact of self-concepts:**
   a. Self-concept is individual's mental image of themselves, including how they view their strengths and weaknesses in all aspects of their personalities.
   b. Self-concepts depend on part of body image and roles, but also include other aspects of psychological and spiritual self.
   c. Self-concept changes because of illness may no longer meet the expectations of the family, leading to tension or conflict.
5. **Impact of family dynamics:**
   a. Family dynamics is the process by which the family functions, makes decisions, give support to individual members and copes with every day changes and challenges.
   b. If a parent in a family becomes ill, family activities and decision-making often come to halt as the other family members wait for the illness to pass or they delay action because they are reluctant to assume the ill person's roles or responsibilities.

Health and Illness Continuum

1. According to Neumann (1990), health on a continuum is the degree of client wellness that exist at any point in time ranging from an optimal wellness condition with available energy at its maximum to death, which represents total energy depletion.
2. According to the health-illness continuum model, health is a dynamic state that continuously alters as a person adapts to changes in the internal and external environments to maintain a state of physical, emotional, intellectual, social, developmental and spiritual well-being.
3. The continuum is thought of a complex, dynamic process that includes physical, psychological and social components. There are adoptive or maladaptive behavioral responses to internal and external stimuli.
4. Health and illness tend to merge, but may represent patterns of adoptive change along the continuum. The direction of change may be reversible, depending on the quality of the individual's adoptive efforts.
5. The individual at the illness end of the continuum is characterized by feeling of uncertainty, helplessness, loss of control, loss of identity and incapacity for problem solving.
6. As the patient is in the sick role, there is incapacity to meet other social roles, the person has sought diagnosis and get treatment.
7. Less far along the illness end of the continuum, as illness behavior are brought into play, the person may be tired, run down and irritable with complains of loss of sleep, appetite, dependence, self-absorption, minor illnesses such as colds, infections, headaches and backaches.
8. Between illness and wellness, there is the ambiguous area where no symptoms are present and the person is neither especially well nor especially ill.

9. At the health end of the continuum, as health behaviors are utilized, the persons is not only unaware of disease and without pain, fatigue or somatic complications but also tends to be resistant to infections, industrious, vigorous and physically agile with a strong sense of identity and autonomy, caring out usual social roles and needing no health care.
10. The goal in preventive health care is to maintain equilibrium between health and illness with balance in favor of maximum wellness for the individual.

Models of Health and Illness

1. **Health-wellness model:**
   a. Health-wellness model was developed by Dunn (1997), the high-level wellness model is oriented toward maximizing the health potential of an individual.
   b. Health-wellness model requires the individual to maintain a continuum of balance and purposeful direction within the environment.
   c. It involves progress toward a higher level of functioning, open ended and expanding challenges to live at the fullest potential.
2. **Agent-host environmental model:**
   a. The agent-host environmental model of health and illness originated in the community health work of Leavel et al.
   b. According to this approach, the health or illness of an individual, or group depends on the dynamic relationship of the agent, host and environment.
   c. The agent is any internal or external factors that its presence or absence can lead to disease or illness.
   d. The host is the person or persons who may be susceptible to a particular illness or diseases.
   e. The environment consists of all factors outside the host. It includes physical environment, social environment and biological environment.
3. **Health belief model:**
   a. Rosenstoch's/Bakerand's (1794) and Maiman's (1975) health belief model addresses the relationship between a person's belief and behavior.
   b. It provides a way of understanding and predicating how clients will behave in relation to their health and how they will comply with healthcare therapies.
   c. The first component in this model involves the individual's perception of susceptibility to an illness.
   d. The second component is the individual's perception of the seriousness of the illness. This perception is influenced and modified by demographic and sociopsychological variables, perceived threats of the illnesses, and cues to action.
   e. The third component, the likelihood that a person will take preventive action, is the person's perception of the benefits of taking action.
4. **Health promotion model:**
   a. The health promotion model was proposed by Pender (1996). It was designed to be a complementary counterpart to models of health protection.
   b. Health promotion is directed at increasing a client's level of well-being. The model focuses on three functions.
   c. The model also organizes cues into a pattern to explain the likelihood of a client's participation in health-promotion behavior.
   d. The focus of this model is to explain the reasons that individuals engage in health activities. It is not designed for use with families or communities.

Biopsychosocial Aspects of Health and Illness

Physical, social, cultural and psychological factors interact dynamically and have an important influence on patient care needs. There are needs, common to everyone no matter their sociocultural background, so called human needs. These needs when not met create tensions and these tensions may give rise to anxiety that can hamper recovery, if not relieved.

Developmental needs

Prenatal: This stage determines many characteristics of the person and to some extend the requirements for use of adaptive resources throughout life.

Neonatal: Developmental tasks are mostly physical; foundations are begun at this time for later personality responses.

Infancy: This is a time of much physical, but foundations are begun at this time for future developments.

Childhood: Marked physical growth continues during this time. There is the beginning of role identification and moving out from the family to the peer group and community.

Adolescence: Many physical and emotional changes occur as growth and maturation continues; changing hormonal activity and search for identity are major stresses for the adolescent.

Young adulthood: Physical maturation is completed. There are many psychosocial stresses related to family and community roles during this stage.

Middle adulthood: Developmental tasks are mostly psychosocial, relating to reassessment of goals, physical stamina and hormone output beginning to decline.

Older years: Physical conditioning is generally declining and decreased sensory acuity may be noticeable. Developmental tasks are related to sharing accumulated experiences and evaluating achievements.

Cultural influences

1. Culture may be thought of as the total way of life of people, social legacy the individuals acquire from his/her groups.
2. The culture concept is cardinal to understand ourselves and our world.
3. Custom and group habits are referred to as folkways and mores. Folkways are the accustomed and time-honored ways of doing things, the social habits that become routine and are often performed without thinking.
4. The patient's cultural background helps to determine the way the relationship with the physician or nurse is perceived and facilitates or impedes interaction or communication.

Religious aspects

1. Religion traditionally has focused on God beyond the individual and has concentrated itself with relating the individual, and has concerned itself with relating the individual to that God.
2. Religious beliefs are seldom held to oneself, but are part of group processes, so that there is immediate family or group support for the patient.
3. It helps the patient's own attitude or belief that recovery is possible and that there are forces available to facilitate the healing process.
4. It is important, if the nurse is to help, to understand not only the spiritual needs of the patient but also the means and methods that organized religion has for meeting those needs.

■ CONCLUSION

Life span developmental psychology is the field of psychology, which involves the examination of both constancy and change in human behavior across the entire life span, i.e. from conception to death. Developmental psychologists are concerned with diverse issues ranging from the growth of motor skills in the infant, to the gains and losses observed in the intellectual functioning of the elderly. The goal of study in developmental psychology is to enhance our knowledge about how development evolves over the entire life span, developing knowledge of the general principles of development, and the differences and similarities in development across individuals.

■ REVIEW QUESTIONS

Long Essays

1. Define developmental psychology. Explain the need and issues in developmental psychology.
2. Describe physical, physiological and psychological development during infancy.
3. Enumerate the growth and development of school-going child. Explain the role of nurse in health promotion.

Short Essays

4. Explain the nurse's role in health promotion of infancy.
5. Describe psychosexual development and health promotion methods in toddler.
6. Discuss the emotional and cognitive development of preschooler.
7. Explain the physical growth and development, and sexual development of adolescent.
8. Describe the concepts and theories of adulthood.
9. Describe the developmental theories in old age.
10. Enumerate the physiological changes and health promotion measures in old age.
11. Describe whether behavior and sickness are interrelated. Explain the stages of illness behavior.
12. Discuss the impact of illness on family.
13. Describe the models of health and illness.

Short Answers

14. Cerebral palsy.
15. Characteristics of preschooler.
16. School phobia.
17. Obesity.
18. Recreational drug use.
19. Health promotion in adolescent.
20. Kinds of age.
21. Common health problems in old age.
22. Health-illness continuum.
23. Health promotion model.
24. Biopsychosocial aspects of health and illness.

■ BIBLIOGRAPHY

1. Adele Pilliteri. Maternal and Child Health Nursing, Care of the Childbearing and Childrearing Family. Philadelphia: Lippincott company; 1999.
2. Alphonsa Jacob. Paediatric Nursing. Indore: NR Brothers Publishers; 2003.
3. Annamalai University MA Psychology Study Material. Life Span Psychology. Chidambaram; 2000.
4. Arunasree S. Play and Children. College Souvenir Government College of Nursing. Hyderabad; 2005.
5. Arvind Saili. Challenges in Neonatology: A Compendium of Management Protocols. New Delhi: Jaypee Brothers Medical Publishers; 1997.
6. Basic Guide to Reproductive Child Health Programme. Department of Family Welfare, Government of India.
7. Behrman. Textbook of Pediatrics. Bangalore: Prism Books (P) Ltd; 1996.
8. Boedecker. Women's Life Patterns. Role Involvement and Satisfaction at Midlife. Doctoral dissertation abstract. Pennsylvania State University; 1979.
9. Bullo Vern G, Bannie Bullough. The Emergency of Modern Nursing. New York: Macmillan; 1969.

10. Carlin ME. Large group treatment of severely disturbed/conduct-disordered adolescents. Int J of Group Psychother. 1996;46(3):379-97.
11. Davis Fred. The Nursing Profession, Five Sociological Essays. New York: Wiley; 1966.
12. Fox CO. Toward a sound historical basis for nurse-midwifery. Bull Am Coll Nurse Midwives. 1969;14(1):76.
13. Parulekar V, Shashank. Textbook for Midwives, 2nd edition. Mumbai: Vora Medical Publishers; 1995.
14. Smith EA, Palen LA, Caldwell LL, et al. Substance use and sexual risk prevention in Cape Town, South Africa: an evaluation of the HealthWise program. Prev Sci. 2008;9(4):311-21.

CHAPTER 21

Educational Psychology

■ INTRODUCTION

Educational psychology provides a base to education. It studies the problem, which crop up in the education of the children. Educational psychology has it primary concern with a viewpoint, with the organization of information and with group of techniques and activities for a sound education. It is an area of experiment, not a collection of specific subject matter. Through this subject the contents, techniques and ways of functioning of psychology are applied in the solution of the problems of the classroom. It may be remembered that educational psychology is not merely general psychology applied to educational problems. The number of researches in various areas connected with educational psychology is increasing at a phenomenal rate.

■ NATURE OF EDUCATIONAL PSYCHOLOGY

1. Psychology is a science, which studies all the aspects of human behavior. It is concerned with the reasons of human behavior and with those principles, which may predict a behavior and bring modifications in it.
2. Education is mainly a social process. The chief aim of it is to modify behavior. In this sense both education and psychology are similar. From the fusion of psychology and education, we get that branch of psychology, which is known as educational psychology.
3. Educational psychology is the study of human behavior as it is influenced by the social process. It also studies those processes, which provide an understanding of the way in which the modifications are brought in the behavior.
4. Educational psychology has its own applied theory. This theory is as basic as the theory underlying the discipline of psychology.

■ DEFINITION

1. Educational psychology is that special branch of psychology concerned with the nature, conditions, outcome and the evaluation of school learning and retention. —*Anusubel*
2. Educational psychology is that branch of psychology, which deals with teaching and learning. —*Skinner*
3. Educational psychology describes and explains the learning experiences of an individual from birth through old age. —*Crow and Crow*

■ SCOPE OF EDUCATIONAL PSYCHOLOGY

Scope of the subject implies its field of study. Speaking in specific terms, it means the areas of study that are included in a particular subject. The scope of educational psychology is securing greater and greater importance in the field of education. Educational psychology is the combination of two, i.e. educational and psychology. So, educational psychology is the study of behavior of the teacher, taught and persons connected to educational environment. Educational psychology is a branch of educational content, which deals with human behavior and its modification. The following are included in the scope of educational psychology (Fig. 21.1).

Human behavior: It studies human behavior in educational situations. Psychology is the study of behavior and education deals with the modification of behavior and hence, educational psychology pervades in whole field of education.

Growth and development: It studies growth and development of the child. How a child passes through various stages of growth and what are the characteristics of each stage are included in the study of educational psychology.

Learning process: It studies the law of learning. Learning is a major phenomenon in education. It studies how learning can take place most effectively and economically.

Heredity and environment: To what extent heredity and environment contribute toward the growth of the individual and how this knowledge can be used for bringing about the optimum development of the child and form a salient feature of the scope of educational psychology.

Personality: Educational psychology deals with the nature and development of the personality of an individual. In fact, education has been defined as an all-round development of the personality of an individual; personality development also implies a well-adjusted personality.

Individual difference: Every individual differs from another and it is one of the fundamental facts of human nature, which has been brought to light by educational psychology. This one fact has revolutionized the concept and process of education.

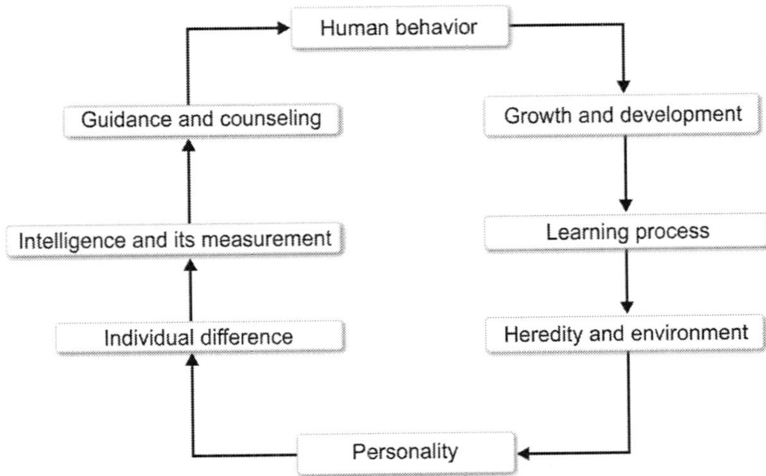

Figure 21.1: Scope of educational psychology

Intelligence and its measurement: The scope of educational psychology includes the study of the nature of intelligence as well as its measurement. This is of great importance for a teacher or an educator.

Guidance and counseling: This is one of the most important fields or areas of study included in the field of educational psychology. Education is nothing, but providing guidance to the growing child. Thus, guidance forms an important aspect of educational psychology.

The following five areas were named by American Psychological Associations:

1. Human growth and development including the effect of heredity and environment on various aspects of individual.
2. Learning: The nature of learning process, factors influencing the learning process, etc.
3. Personality and adjustment: It include many subtopics such as mental health of the students and teachers character.
4. Measurement and evaluation statistics.
5. Techniques and methods of educational psychology.

Thus, educational psychology describes and explains the learning experience of an individual from birth to old age. Its subject matter is concerned with the conditions that affect learning.

IMPORTANCE

- Educational psychology helps in the realization of education aims
- Offers new viewpoints
- Ensures proper discipline in the proper manner
- Sets forth proper techniques and methods of teaching
- Keeps the educator informed about individual differences
- It helps in the understanding of group behavior
- Asks the teacher to teach according to the stages of development of the child
- Emphasizes the role of the learner.

AIMS AND OBJECTIVES

- Developing proper attitudes in the teacher
- Assisting the teacher to set up appropriate educational situations
- Helping the teachers in teaching their pupils sympathetically and impartially
- Helping them in the organization of the subject matter
- Helping them to have a clear understanding of social relationships
- Assisting the teacher to understand his/her own job
- Making the teacher conversant with methods and techniques for the analysis of his/her and other's behavior
- Organizing the proper guidance programs
- Guiding the administrators
- Helping them in planning out the proper evaluation techniques
- Furnishing the teacher with proper method available.

GENERAL CATEGORIES

1. Learning, which is the most frequent topic in the field by far.
2. Readiness of learning, which includes the phenomena of interest, aptitudes and motivation.
3. Mental health and social adjustment, which focus on the non-cognitive purposes of the school and correlates intellectual learning.
4. Measurement and evaluation, which comprises the techniques for assessing the education growth of learners, diagnosing of learning problems and clarifying the criteria to be used in an evaluation of the school.

CONCEPT OF EDUCATION

1. Education modifies the behavior. It brings such changes in the behavior of a child, which is for his/her good. In the past, the education of a child meant the filling up of the child's mind with stuffed knowledge.

2. The modern education aims at the harmonious development of the personality of the child. The schools and the teachers are to create such situation were the personality can be developed freely and fully.
3. Education is a social process; its main concern is the modification of behavior. Thus, educational psychology studies the human behavior as it is influenced by the social process of education.
4. It also studies and investigates those processes that lead to the understanding of the way in which behavior is modified through education.
5. Education psychology constitutes the foundations of education. It provides an approach to educational problems and set up techniques for studying children, and problems that arise in their function.

■ PSYCHOLOGICAL BASIS OF EDUCATION

1. Psychology deals with response to any and every kind of situation of the life presents. Educational psychology deals with the behavior of the human being in educational situations.
2. To make an estimate of the value of educational psychology, it is necessary to understand the modern concept of education.
3. Education provides both experience to the individual and his/her adjustment to the environment. It is also a process, which is individualistic as well as social in its nature.
4. The bringing of psychological basis in education has resulted in completely overhauling our outlook on education. Now, education is a much more pleasant process than what it was. Information and instructions are replaced by the word help and guidance. Love, sympathy and play are considered most important in the educational process.

■ VALUES OF EDUCATIONAL PSYCHOLOGY

1. The study of educational psychology should develop the student's interest in people, both children and adults, and help to understand them.
2. The study on educational psychology should have a favorable effect on the attitudes, behaviors and psychological understanding of students in the both personal and professional relationship.
3. The study of educational psychology should enable the students to use the body of knowledge that is derived from research studies in this field and that helps to explain the way in which learning occurs.
4. The study of educational psychology should improve the effectiveness of the prospective teacher's ability to learn.
5. The study of educational psychology should foster the student's appreciation and understanding of research on education.

■ MAJOR SUBDIVISIONS OF EDUCATIONAL PSYCHOLOGY

- Psychology and education
- Human growth and development
- Learning
- Personality and adjustments
- Group psychology
- Measurement and evaluation
- Statistical and research methods.

■ ELEMENTS OF EDUCATIONAL PSYCHOLOGY (Fig. 21.2)

Learner

In educational process, the learner occupies the most important place. There can be no teaching without there being a learner. By the learner, we mean the pupils who individually or collectively comprise the classroom group. The teaching is the classroom to a great extent

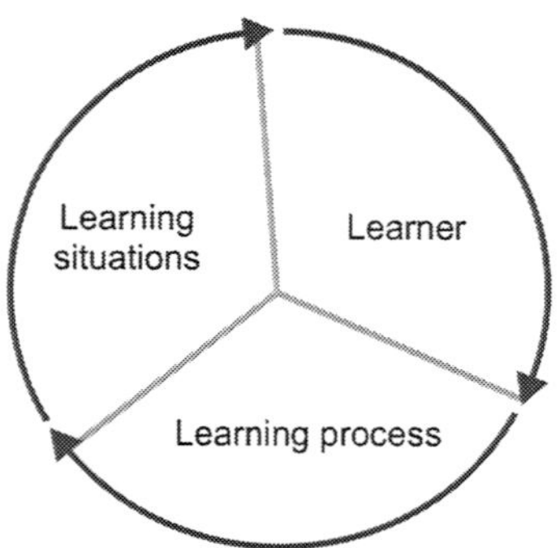

Figure 21.2: Elements of educational psychology

depends on the personality's developmental stages and psychological problems of the students.

Learning Process

Learning process is the process by which people acquire changes in their behavior, improve performance, recognize their thinking or discover new ways of behaving and new concepts and information. This process may be directly observable as while the pupils learn writing, computing, talking, etc. or may be indirectly observable as in perceiving, thinking and remembering. The concern of the educational psychologist is with the way in which the learning process takes place.

Learning Situations

Learning situations refers to the environment in which the learner find himself/herself and in which the learning process takes place. The teacher's attitude, the classroom setting, the emotional climate of the school and the interest the community takes in the school affairs may all form the part of the learning situations.

■ LIMITATIONS

The application of educational psychology can be made in a limited manner keeping in view the nature of teaching. In accordance with the nature of teaching, the experience, interest, attitude, etc. are as essential for a teacher as the knowledge of psychology. The educational psychology is limited to the extent that the testing of facts or search of new facts is only helpful in arriving at a decision. They do not lead automatically to ultimate decisions or judgments. The educational psychology is bound by the boundaries of psychology.

■ CONCLUSION

Educational psychology is nothing, but one of the branches of applied psychology. It is an attempt to apply the knowledge of psychology to the field of education. It consists of the application of the psychological principles and techniques to human behavior in educational situations. In other words, educational psychology is the study of the experiences and behavior of the learner in relation to educational environment.

■ REVIEW QUESTIONS

Long Essays

1. Define educational psychology. Explain the nature and scope of psychology.
2. Describe the major elements of educational psychology.

Short Essays

3. Describe the aims and objectives of educational psychology.
4. Explain the values of educational psychology.

Short Answers

5. Importance of educational psychology.
6. Psychological basis of education.
7. Limitations of educational psychology.
8. Learning process.
9. Concept of education.

■ BIBLIOGRAPHY

1. Aggarwal JC. Educational Research: An Introduction. New Delhi: Arya Book Depot; 1975.
2. Aggarwal JC. Essentials of Educational Technology. New Delhi: Vikas Publications; 1996.
3. Ausubel DP, Robinson FG. School learning: An Introduction to Educational Psychology. New York: Hott Rinehart & Winson Inc; 1969.
4. Best JW. Research in Education. New Jersey: Prentice Hall; 1970.
5. Dandapani S. Advanced Educational Psychology. New Delhi: Anmol Publications Pvt Ltd; 2000.
6. Garrett HE. Statistics in Psychology and Education. Bombay: Vakils, Feffer and Simons Ltd; 1996.
7. Hilgard ER, Atkinson RL, Athinson RC. Introduction to Psychology, 7th edition. New York: Harcourt Brace Jovanovich Inc; 1979.
8. Kasinath HM. Advance Educational Psychology. Gadag: Vidyanidhi Prakashan; 2000.
9. Koul Lokesh. Methodology of Educational Research. New Delhi: Vikas Publishing House Ltd; 1984.
10. Richmond Kemmeth. The Concept of Educational Technology. London: Kogan Page Ltd; 1970.
11. Sampath Kumar K, Pennirselvam A Santhareme. Introduction to Educational Technology. New Delhi: Sterling Publishers; 1981.
12. Seetharamu AS. Philosophies of Education. New Delhi: Ashish Publication House; 1987.
13. Sodhi, Sandhu, Singh. Philosophies of Education. Ambala Cantt: The Indian Publication; 1987.
14. Srivastava SK. Tradition and Modernization Process and Change in India. Allahabad: India International Publication; 1976.
15. Tuckman Bruce W. Conducting Educational Research. New York: Harecourt Brace; 1972.

CHAPTER 22

Social Psychology

■ INTRODUCTION

Social psychology is one of the latest extensions of the great movement of scientific thought that achieved its most striking results in the investigation of physical phenomena. The advances of natural science were the indispensable conditions for a study of psychology. In the study of man, psychology occupies a unique and commanding position. One may say that what physics is to the natural sciences, psychology is to the sciences of man. All activities in society such as economic, political, artistic have their center in individuals, in their strings, needs and understanding. The individual is the point of intersection of nearly all that is of consequence in the social sphere. For purpose of convenience one may divide the interest and concentrate on a particular phase of social process.

With the increasing variety of courses offered in psychology and education, it is inevitable that social psychology will trespass upon related fields. In spite of possible overlapping, it has been decided that social psychology as an independent discipline that is required today because of several transformations, with the growth of mass industrialization, the concentration of great populations in cities and spread of rapid communication have altered the human situation in definite ways.

■ MEANING AND NATURE OF SOCIAL PSYCHOLOGY

Psychology and sociology each often claims the whole domain of human behavior as its individual bailiwick. The history of these two disciplines reveals basic differences in their approaches to the understanding of human behavior. These differences have generally been the result of varying approaches to the types of problems posed for different levels of behavior being analyzed by the two disciplines. One has emphasized one level of obstruction and the other has some differences stemmed from differing definitions in describing the significant problems. For example, in the early psychology, psychologists tended to emphasize the physiological bases of behavior and minimized social and cultural experience, while sociology tends to minimize the physical bases, and emphasized social processes and conditions.

■ DEFINITION

Glance at representative topics of social psychology, its ground rules and the converging trends in the present state of its development was preparation for definition of social psychology. The definition of any class of objects or events requires specification of what it is and what it is not. This is not an easy matter in the complex subject matter. Major generalizations are implied in defining a discipline such as the claim that one knows its scope and how to go about studying its problems. There has been disagreement on these matters since the first two books appeared under the label of 'social psychology' in 1908. One was written by the psychologist William McDougall and the other by the sociologist Ross EA. Since then several textbooks on Social Psychology have appeared. The definition of Social Psychology offered here is suggested by three converging trends in contemporary social psychology that were noted above, namely:

1. Increased adherence to the ground rules of the scientific approach and utilization of scientific methods and techniques.
2. Awareness of the need for checks to guard against ethnocentric conclusions.
3. Conception of behavior within its appropriate frame of reference as a product of interacting influences coming both from the individual and his/her social surroundings. Social psychology is the scientific study of the experience and behavior of the individual in relation to social stimulus situations.

Let take the terms in the definition one by one as an orientation to the principal theoretical issues in social psychology and its relation to the social sciences.

▪ PRINCIPLES (Fig. 22.1)

Scientific Study

Specifying that social psychology is a scientific study underscores the task of adhering closely to the ground rules of science and their ramifications in the actual operations of research. Policy makers, religious leaders, novelists and commentators on the social scene cannot be held accountable for adhering to the ground rules of communicability and reproducibility of methods that permit verification, but social psychologists are. In this book, the scientific ground rules, their associated methods and the techniques are presented on the whole, through the summaries of significant research studies that exemplify their use.

Study of the Individual

The phrase of the individual specifies that the unit of analysis in social psychology is the individual. Because the field is social psychology and not psychological sociology, its concepts refer to the individual's perception. The individual is the unit of analysis for social psychology whether the investigator happens to be stationed in a university's department of psychology or sociology (the field's twin parents). Social psychologists today do not

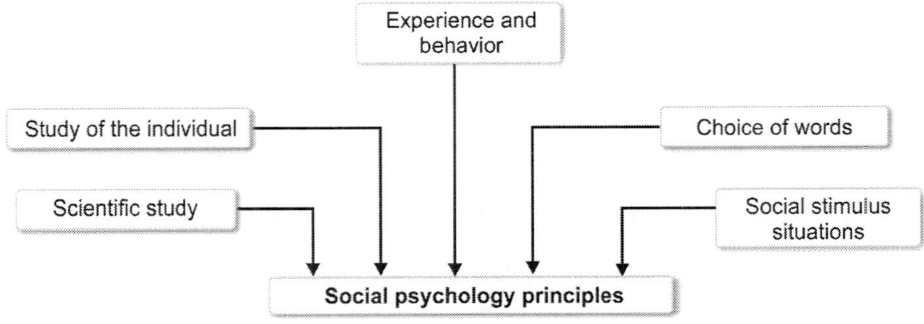

Figure 22.1: Principles of social psychology

use concepts such as 'group mind.' A group cannot perceive or feel, or think. The designation 'social' in the label refers to the fact that particular task is to study the individual's behavior in relation to those aspects of his/her surroundings that are interpersonal or sociocultural. When the individual has traffic first with these aspects of his/her environment, they are external, on the stimulus side of the familiar stimulus organism response (SOR) scheme for analysis.

Experience and Behavior

Experience is a general term that refers to the awareness of the individual and not just to past experiences, as conveyed in expressions such as "My experience has shown that...," what a person perceives, feels, learns or remembers. In a word, his/her experience is inferred from his/her behavior, i.e. his/her deeds and words as well as subtle expressions and movements. For this reason, some psychologists refer to all psychological phenomena as behavior. The terms 'consciousness and mind' and 'awareness' were for a time almost banished from academic psychology.

Choice of Words

In any definition the choice of words is important. The importance of these particular words reflects controversies during the earlier development of social psychology. The phrase 'determined by' was deliberately avoided in the definition. The individual is not merely a passive recipient, a tabula rasa, reflecting the imprints of his/her environment, whether social or not. Anything that impinges on the individual from the social world around him/her is processed and his/her motives, desires, attitudes and ideas enter into processing. The processing reflects selectivity in what he/she reacts to and whom they transacts with. The processing is also affected by what he/she confronts. Hence, experience and behavior that count for the individual and in the social process is always a joint product of influences in the social environment and those from within themselves, whatever they may be at a given time with all of his/her past learning, enduring and momentary motives, and viewpoints toward the issue at hand.

Social life is the natural habitat of the human individual. It is not alien to his/her nature. Therefore, how an individual learns the requirements and values of his/her group and culture, how he/she responds to pressures from them, and the molding of his/her behavior within these requirements are not the sole problems of social psychology.

Social Stimulus Situations

The final phrase in the definition of social psychology is social stimulus situations. The phrase seems self-explanatory. To show that it is not, will consider more seriously what constitutes a social situation for the individual at a given time. This analysis will enable us to indicate the scope and variety of social stimuli that an individual may encounter in his/her surroundings.

■ RELATIONSHIP BETWEEN SOCIAL PSYCHOLOGY AND EDUCATION

Social psychology is an attempt to understand and explain how the thought, feeling and behavior of individuals are influenced by the actual, implied or imagined presence of others. —*Allport YK*

There is an increasing complexity in social life and also personal life of an individual in the society because of explosion of population, explosion of knowledge and industrialization. This has greater impact on the education field. Because of this, the educationists, administrators, parents, teachers and the persons involved in the educational activities are confronting many problems in the execution of educational programs in spite of their knowledge of psychology and sociology. This might have happened because psychology deals with individual behavior as a separate entity apart from the society, whereas sociology deals with society group behavior without emphasizing the individual. It is from this angle, it is very significant to deal with social psychology in relation to education because social psychology studies the behavior of the individual in a social context.

Social psychology begins with the individual and looks at political, social and cultural systems through the eyes of the individual, whereas political science, sociology and cultural anthropology begin as the larger systems and look at the individual through the eyes of this system in all.

■ SCOPE OF SOCIAL PSYCHOLOGY

It is very difficult to restrict the scope of social psychology. It is inclusive of many of the aspects as its subject matter for the study. This idea becomes clearer by Krech and Crutchfield's saying that social psychology is concerned with every aspect of the individual's behavior in the society. Therefore one can define social psychology as the science of behavior of the individual in the society. Newcomb's (1900) contention is that interaction constitutes subject matter of social psychology. Therefore, one can say that it encompasses all types of interaction processes for its study.

The subject matter of social psychology is composed of two psychologically important aspects of the individual. One is directly observable, the overt behavior, what the individual does and the second one is not directly observable, but determines behavioral and psychological dynamics, what the individual experiences. The first is referred to as the phenotypic self and the second as genotypic self. It deals with mass communication and the social structure, intergroup attitudes, interpersonal attraction, interpersonal perception, social power, prejudice and stereotypes, group norms and social control, social roles, leadership, group productivity and satisfaction, self and personality, social motivation, social interaction, socialization, affiliation, social organization, attitudes, etc. which are social psychological approaches to the problem of human nature.

Scope of Education

It is once again difficult to explain the scope of education because it is an open system and a very comprehensive discipline. In the real sense of the term, it is a process, which goes on from birth to death, encompassing each and every aspect of human life. Pestalozzi's conception of education is that it reforms and elevates society, it involves a natural and harmonious development of all the faculties of the individual and it requires an active cooperation between home and school.

Education is Joint Endeavor

Education is joint endeavor of home, school and society to bring about a desirable behavioral change among children, so that they become contributing citizens of the society. Education as a discipline is concerned biological, physical, mental, intellectual, emotional, cultural and spiritual development of the individual.

Scope of education is very broader because it stretches its hands toward different directions as vocational education technical education, adult education, non-formal education, and guidance and with social, counseling, etc. Its scope ranges from teaching three R's, through development of values, attitudes, etc. to the all-round development and self-realization of the individual. By observing the scope of social psychology and of education one can say that both of them concentrate, emphasize and deal with the individual for his/her harmonious development and in turn make the society a place suitable for human existence. As such it is very significant to study the relationship between social psychology and education.

Social Psychology and Education

Social psychology deals with the behavior of the individual in a 'social context.' School is a miniature 'society' where deliberately planned educational programs are executed. Therefore education and social psychology are interrelated. Formulation of social objectives for education, incorporation of social objectives into curricular or design of classroom social process as a means of achieving social goals, etc. require the helping from social psychologists to educationists. Educators often face a series of social problems such as prejudice, pupil's dislike of school and conflicts among students, and also among staff members that can be solved easily with the help of social psychology.

Education refers to school-related behavior and related variables. Education is fundamentally an interpersonal process, carried out through the interdependent cooperation of two roles educator and learner, requires for its elucidation precisely the kinds of analytical tools and data provided by social psychology. The knowledge of social psychology provides the understanding about individual and group differences, which provide a basis for developing alternative educational treatment of different individuals or groups that would benefit all, more than teaching everyone the same way would.

Schools are complex social environments, where in addition to learning, social interaction takes place. Therefore, social psychology, which focuses its attention and discusses elaborately on 'social interaction' helps the education field, particularly school program to a large extent. In the same way education also helps in social interaction, understanding the group norms, which leads to minimizing group conflicts, developing right types of attitudes, inculcation of values, better interpersonal relationship, etc. Therefore in conclusion educational problems provide sophisticated and complex issues to challenge social psychologists to utilize the best available theory and methods and to challenge the field to develop new approaches. In a parallel way, the social psychological perspective is important for educators and significantly improves educational practice.

From the above discussion one can see how intimately social psychology and education are related. Discussing this, Eradsick and High shall argue that educational psychology must be fundamentally not cognition or a developmental or a personality psychology, but a social psychology.

Though this much of intimate relationship is there between social psychology and education, educational issues were ignored by social psychologists previously say up to 1954–1955. Only after this period, the educational issues drew attention of social psychologists and led to the development of social psychology of education. From this points of view, will discuss largely the development of social psychology of education.

Development of Psychology of Education

There were many reports and textbooks containing laboratory experiments mainly in psychology and educational psychology up to 1935. Among them, very few of them contained about social factors. In 1941 Trow complained that most of the educational psychologists were limiting their investigation to the psychology of the individual neglecting the social aspects of individual behavior.

In 1954, Geizels complained in his book *The Handbook of Social Psychology* that usually textbooks contain chapters on the social psychology of industry and politics. Social psychologists have tended to ignore educational issues.

From the views of the above two authors, one can observe that though there was a change in the attention from educational psychology to social psychology emphasizing on the social aspects of the individuals behavior, there was very little or no attention of social psychologists towards the educational issues. At the same time, it reveals that initiation and awareness about the necessity of knowledge of social psychology to the educational field. Because of this, there was initiation to the development of social psychology of education. Some of the more successful texts by Bichies (1981), Jrander (1957) and Perkins (1969) contained some of the aspects of educational issues viewed from the social psychological perspective. Though the work started in social psychology of education since 1959 to bridge the gap between social psychology and education the work was geared up in 1970s, and then social psychology of education became a subdiscipline finding clearly its scope.

Social psychology for education merely uses social psychological principles to explain educational problems. Here, mostly the researches are carried out in laboratory setting (not educational settings). In contrast, the social psychology of education defines its scope according to a problem focus on educational issues. The topics in social psychology of education are those social psychological issues that concern the social functioning of individuals and groups in educational systems, i.e. the topics of social psychology of education does not necessarily correspond to the standard topics of social psychology. Here, researches are carried out on the educational setting itself.

■ CONCLUSION

The scope of social psychology and education are vast and inclusive of many of the aspects, and they are intimately related to a larger extent. The knowledge of social psychology helps to a greater extent in solving the educational problems. This intimate relationship of mutual contribution led to the development of a new discipline, namely social psychology of education. This deals mainly with the educational issues from the social psychology perspective, which helps in achieving educational goals.

■ REVIEW QUESTIONS

1. Define social psychology. Explain the nature and meaning of social psychology.
2. Describe the principles of social psychology.
3. Enumerate the differences between social psychology and education.
4. Explain the scope of social psychology.
5. Discuss the need and importance of social psychology.

■ BIBLIOGRAPHY

1. Abram Kardiner. The Psychological Frontier of Society. New York: Columbia University Press; 1945.
2. Alfred R, Lindesmith Anseim L, Strauss. Readings in Social Psychology. Chicago; Holt, Rinehart and Winston; 1969.
3. Allport FH. Social Psychology. Boston: Houghton Mifflin; 1924.
4. Allport GW. Kramer BM. Some roots of prejudice. J Gen Psychol. 1946;22:9-39.
5. Allport GW. Personality: A Psychological Interpretation. New York: Holt, Rinehart and Winston; 1937.
6. Allport GW. The Nature of Prejudice, Reading, Mass. Addison Wesley Publishing Company; 1954.
7. Argyris C. Interpersonal Competence and Organizational Effectiveness. Homewood, IL: Irwin-Dorsey; 1962.
8. Argyris C. Personality and Organization. New York: Harpercollins Publishers; 1954.

Section VI

Mental Health Process

CHAPTER 23

Mental Health and Hygiene

■ INTRODUCTION

Mentally healthy person is the one who is able to make adjustments, fully mature, able to evaluate him/her, leading a regular life, having balanced behavior and satisfied with his/her job, etc. Mental health is the ability of a person to make personal and social adjustments. Actually, it is essential to be mentally healthy for optimum health and well-being. Mental health is an important constituent of optimum health. Mental health is essential for a healthy and successful life. Mental health and physical health are interrelated and that is the reason behind the popularity of saying healthy mind lives in healthy body. Ancient saints of India have stressed the importance of emotional balance. It means, mental health is the balanced department of a person's personality and emotional attitudes because of which he/she becomes capable of living happily with his/her friends, relatives and environment.

■ MENTAL HEALTH

Definition

1. A mentally healthy person is the one who is comfortable with himself/herself, lives peacefully with his/her neighbors, brings up his/her children to be healthy civilians and after completing basic duties, he/she has the energy and strength to do something for the welfare of society. *—Luken PV*
2. Mental health is a process of adjustment, which involves compromise, adaptation, growth and continuity. *—Bhatia and Craig*
3. Mental health is defined as the capacity in an individual to form harmonious relations with others and to participate in or contribute constructively to the changes in his/her social and physical environment. *—World Health Organization (WHO)*
4. Mental health concerns with the development of wholesome balanced personality, one who does not comfort himself/herself such as a series of compartmentalized selves, honest on Sunday, dishonest on Monday, generous today, crabbed tomorrow, reasonable and logical at times, at other times confused and inconsistent. *—Walton JEW*
5. Mental health is the full and harmonious functioning of the personality as a whole. *—Hadfield JA*
6. Mentally healthy person is one who is happy lives peacefully with his/her neighbors, makes his/her children healthy citizens and after fulfilling such basic responsibilities is still empowered with sufficient strength to serve the cause of the society in any way. *—Lewkan PB*

7. Mental health is defined as the adjustment of human being to the world and to each other with a maximum of effectiveness and happiness. It is the ability to maintain even temper an alert intelligence, socially considerate behavior and a happy disposition.

   —Menninger KA
8. Mental health is the ability, which helps us to seek adjustment in the different situations of life.

   —Cutts and Mosley
9. Mental health is defined as simultaneous success at working, living and creating the capacity for mature and flexible resolution of conflicts between instincts and conscience.

   —American Psychiatric Association
10. Mentally health is defended as a positive, but relative quality of life. It is a condition, which is characteristic of the average person who meets the demands of life on the basis of his/her own capacities and limitations.

    —John, Sutton and Webster

Nature and Meaning

1. Mental health is influenced by both biological and social factor.
2. Major importance of mental health is related to the ability of a person to develop pleasant relations with other. Also, it stresses the constructive and positive contribution or participation in the changes of both physical and social environment.
3. Mental health is the ability of a person to establish personal and social balance.
4. Mental health is the balanced development of a person's personality and attitudes, which makes persons capable of living in harmony with themselves and their relatives.
5. Mental health is a state of the individual's mind, where he/she can adjust and adapt to the situations in a harmonious manner, body and mind work together in same direction in order to lead a happy and protective life.
6. A good mental health is the ability to respond to many varied experiences of life with flexibility and sense of purposes.

Characteristics of Mentally Healthy Person (Fig. 23.1)

Mental health is a state similar to physical health. This condition can be recognized by its following characteristics.

Self-evaluation

A mentally healthy person is aware of his/her limits, accepts his shortcoming and tries to overcome these. He/She also introspects to reduce his/her problem and is able accurately estimate his/her potential.

Adjusting Capacity

A mentally healthy two person lives in present not in the past dreams or future. He/She adjusts with the new condition with minimum of pain and sorrow. He/She is well acquainted with the fact change is the rule of life. Therefore, he/she is ready for every change.

Maturity

A mentally healthy person exhibits emotional maturity. He/She behaves in a responsible manner and expresses his/her feelings and thoughts clearly. His/Her sexual behavior is also mature.

Nonextremist

Excess of everything is bad, is the right principle for mental health. Excess of any behavior or desire has adverse effect on health. Being excessively courageous, excessive speaking,

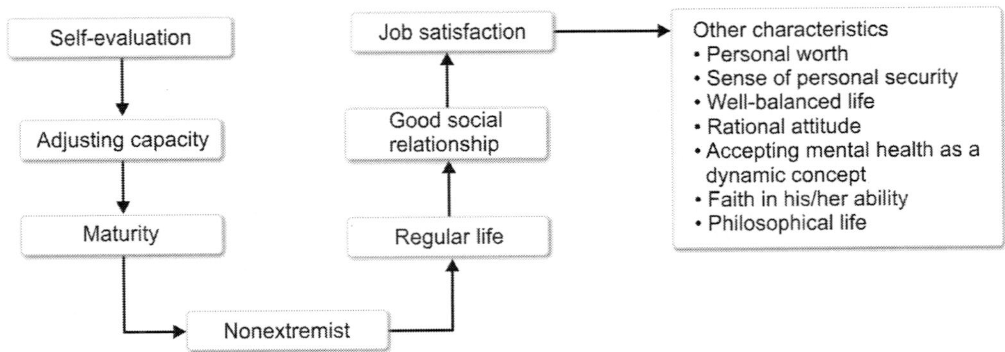

Figure 23.1: Characteristics of mentally healthy person

Mental Health in Different Age Groups (Table 23.1)

Table 23.1: Different age group and mental health

Sl No.	Age group	Description
1.	Prenatal and postnatal period	Emotional level of pregnant mother affects the mental behavior of child. Some women are much tensed during pregnancy or pregnancy can be an existing and frightening experience for them. Therefore, along with the physical care of mother, she should also be given due emotional support. Maintaining a healthy and creative mental level by mother during pregnancy is very important for the mental hygiene of child. The psychiatric nurse should give health education to mother during antenatal and postnatal period about the importance of healthy living for healthy baby. After birth, the baby needs mother protection, food and love for normal growth.
2.	Infancy (1 month to 1 year) and childhood	In the womb, the fetus feels more comfortable and enjoys warmth. But the newborn is full of fear when he/she comes to this open world. Primary childhood is the foundation of mental health.
3.	Toddler to 12 year	It is essential that during this period, parents should have loving and close relations with other children. Any incident that occurs in school is imprinted in child mind. Therefore, behavior of other children in the school, student-teacher relations and environment of school should be friendly and assisting in providing the emotional satisfaction to the child. Parent responsibility is to provide happy and conductive environment for the child to grow. Understanding and sympathetic approach in meeting child's need, is essential as adequate satisfaction of physical needs, which forms a basis for adequate mental health.
4.	Adolescence (13–18 year)	Adolescence is the most sensitive period from the point of normal health. Mental illnesses arising in adolescences can be prevented by recognizing the needs of adolescence, proper adjustment with opposite sex, giving due importance to the freedom of teenagers and the balanced and understanding behavior of parents.

Contd...

Contd...

Sl No.	Age group	Description
5.	Adulthood (20–60 year)	Adulthood is a period in which person should be complete mentally healthy, but the tensions of the responsibility of family, social beliefs, financial limitations and other environment-generated stresses affect the mental health of the person.
6.	Old age (60 and above)	Mental problems of elderly have increased significantly owing to various factors. These include reduction in the importance of joint family system, changing moral and life values, industrialization and urbanization, financial dependence, physical disabilities and diseases, etc.

lewd or ambitious does not let the person relax, which has an ill effect on health. Therefore excessive (extremism) should be avoided for the development of mental health.

Regular Life

Healthy habits are the basis of mental health. Regularity of habits, as those of living, eating, sleeping and walking, etc. are essential. Regular habits save time and energy. Mentally healthy people are able to accomplish all works of life in a natural and mature manner without any problem.

Good Social Relationship

A mentally healthy person maintains good social relations with the people of society, colleagues and family members. Mutual cooperation helps in the building and development of personality. Goodwill and good behavior is more important for such people. Balanced relations in society help in the development of mental health.

Job Satisfaction

Being satisfied with one's job or occupation is essential for mental health. Dissatisfaction with work gives birth to frustrations. Hence, one should increase interest in his/her job by making adjustments to achieve satisfaction and thus the standard of mental health can be increased.

Other Characteristics

Mentally healthy person do not daydream, they are expert in social etiquettes. They exhibit the capacity to tolerate stress and ability to take decisions as per the situation. Mentally healthy person pay attention to make balance in every aspect of life, work and behavior. They take responsibility of their actions.

Personal worth: He/She has a sense of personal worth, feels worthwhile and important. He/She has self-respect and feels secure in a group.

Sense of personal security: He/She has sense of personal worth, feels worthwhile and important. He/She has self-respect and feels secure in a group.

Well-balanced life: He/She has a variety of interests and generally lives a well-balanced life of work, rest and recreation. He/She has the ability to get enjoyment and satisfaction out daily routine job. According to Fromm, a mentally healthy person has developed a zest of living that includes a desire for activity, which is reflected in an attitude of utilizing wherever possibilities he/she possesses in productive forms of behavior.

Rational attitude: He/She has a rational attitude toward problems of his/her physical health. He/She maintains a daily routine of health practices, which promote healthful living. He/She practices good health habits with regard to nutrition, sleep, rest, relaxation, physical activity, personal cleanliness and protection from disease.

Philosophical life: He/She has developed a philosophy of life that gives meaning and purpose to his/her daily activities. This philosophy belongs to this world and discourages the tendency to withdraw or escape from the world. It makes him/her to something concrete about his/her problems as they rise. He/She does not evade responsibility or duty.

Faith in one's ability: He/She has faith in his/her ability to succeed; person believes that he/she will do reasonably well whatever he/she undertakes. He/She solves problem largely by his/her own initiative and effort. He/She feels confident of everyday life, more or less effectively.

Accepting mental health as a dynamic concept: Mental health denotes a state of balance or equilibrium of the mind. This balance is not static, it is quite dynamic. The circumstances in the life are never static, they are changeable and so is to adjustment.

Factors Influencing Mental Health

Heredity

Heredity provides raw material or the potentialities of the individual. It sets the limits for person's mental health. What individual inherits are the potentialities in relation to growth, appearance, intelligence and the life. The development and utilization of these potentialities is determined to a large extent by environmental opportunities. Investigations show that hereditary may predispose a person to the development of a particular type of mental illness, which the person is placed under extensive stress. In the words of Wallin, defective heredity may furnish a fertile soil for the development of mental and nervous diseases, but so far as minor personality maladjustments are concerned, heredity supplies only a predisposing condition (Fig. 23.2).

Physical Factor

Physical health factors make a significant contribution to mental health. One will agree that an erect posture, a winning smile, color in the cheeks, a feeling of exhilaration promote a sense of personal security and have a marked influence on other people. People with greater strengths, better looks and robust health enjoy a social advantage in the development of personality characteristics. An individual with a feeling of physical well-being ordinarily a good disposition and is enthusiastic and intellectually alert. Sick people find it more difficult to make adjustments to new situations than healthy people. Vitamin deficiencies have been found to be the causative factors in many personality difficulties.

Social Factor

Social factor pertains to the individual's society in which he/she lives, the interactional process and his/her social functioning with other persons. It is the social environment, which shapes the knowledge, skills, interests, attitudes, habits, values and goals that he/she acquires. Every individual is born into a society, which influences the content of his/her behavior. Of the social factors, the most important are home, school and community.

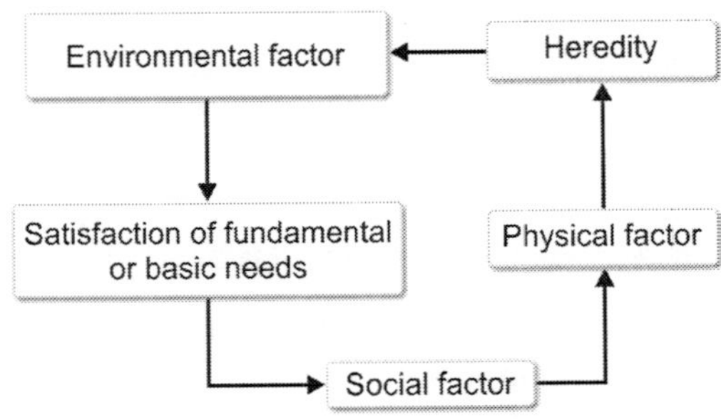

Figure 23.2: Factors influencing mental health

Satisfaction of Fundamental or Basic Needs

From the discussion of the physical and social factor, it will be clear that mental health in childhood and later depends very much on the adequate satisfaction of fundamental or basic needs. The basic needs are physical, organic as well as emotional or psychological. The organic needs are to be satisfied for maintaining physical well-being. Hunger, thirst, fatigue, lack of sleep, physical pain, exercise, heat or cold and the like set up certain tension in the individuals, which must be relieved.

Environmental Factor

Environmental factor has now been established account of various researches in the field of mental hygiene that environmental forces such as family, school and society are more responsible for bringing mental illness than the hereditary or constitutional forces.

Principles Contributing to Mental Health

1. One should respect his/her own and other's personality.
2. One should be aware of the limitations of the self and others, and should also have the knowledge of other's abilities.
3. This fact should be understood that every behavior has some reason.
4. Person should be evaluated according to his/her total behavior.
5. Important needs or drive should be recognized and efforts should be made to fulfill these.

Needs of Mental Health

To develop ideal mental health, one should pay attention to the important needs, which are given below:

- Need for love and attachment
- Desire for being independent and self-sufficient
- Desire for achievements
- Need for recognition and respect
- Need for self-actualization
- Need for the identification of personality. Major foundations of mental health are:
- Sound physical health
- Fulfillment of the basic needs of a person such as physical, psychological and social
- Development of healthy habits, education, philosophy of life, etc.
- Various components related to hereditary and environment.

Skills Needed for Positive Mental Health

World Health Organization has recommended some life skills, which may be used for promotion of mental health. These skills should teach every person to maintain the positive mental health:

1. **Problem solving:** Learning steps of problem solving and generating solutions to difficult problems.
2. **Decision-making:** Learning basic steps for decision-making.
3. **Creative thinking:** Developing creativity in thinking and adaptation behavior.
4. **Critical thinking:** Through making objective judgment about risks and choices.
5. **Effective communication:** Developing positive communication skills during the stress period.
6. **Interpersonal relationship:** Learning importance of interpersonal relations, making support groups for the need of time.
7. **Self-awareness:** Identifying one's own qualities, strengths and weaknesses.
8. **Coping mechanisms:** Understanding the emotions, their affects and coping with emotional distress and stressful situations.

9. **Empathy:** It is through caring of people and avoiding prejudices and discriminations.

Nurses' Responsibilities in Promotion of Positive Mental Health

Nurses are responsible to provide mental health care to all sections of the people, community and hospitals. In this regard, some important activities of community health nurse (CHN) are given:

1. Educating the community about mental health, its importance and needs.
2. Educating the parents and other specific sections of society, this may be responsible for psychological development of children. It is necessary to caution against overprotection.
3. Preventing infection, trauma and poisoning before, during and after birth, which may lead to various mental health problems in the life span of a person.
4. Providing anticipatory guidance and counseling to prevent psychological problems.
5. Providing school mental healthcare services.
6. Avoiding misconceptions, superstitions about mental illness.
7. Educating the individuals about coping mechanisms.
8. Providing counseling services to parents of mentally and physically handicapped children.
9. Identifying the high-risk groups in the community and preventing them from forthcoming mental problems.
10. Providing mental healthcare services to sufferer of mental diseases.
11. Implementing the National Mental Health Program.

Importance of Mental Health

Health is rightly said wealth. It involves one's physical as well as mental health. As said earlier, mental health has much wider scope than physical health as it aims for the development of wholesome balanced and integrated personality:

1. **Mental health helps in the development of desirable personality:** A wholesome, well-balanced and integrated personality.
2. **Mental health helps in proper emotional development:** There is a close relationship between one's mental health and emotional behavior. The individual who enjoy good mental health are supposed to demonstrate proper emotional maturity in their behavior.
3. **Mental health helps in proper social development:** One's mental health helps one in becoming quite sociable and establishing proper social relationships in the society.
4. **Mental health help in proper moral development:** The individuals who enjoy sound health are usually found to behave as a man of integrity and character by following the ethical standards of the society.
5. **Mental health helps in proper esthetic development:** Proper mental health helps the individual in the development of appropriate aesthetic sense, artistic tastes and refined temperament.
6. **Mental health help in actualizing one's potentialities:** Every one of us has a fund of natural abilities and potentialities that can be actualizing through proper efforts. Exercising such effort and striving toward the actualization of one's mental health.
7. **Mental health helps in seeking proper adjustment:** A mentally healthy individual is an adjusted person. He/She is able

to seek adequate adjustment 'with the self and environment'. He/She is able to adjust his/her needs to the demands of the situations and well-being of the society.

8. **Mental health helps in seeking goals of life:** Mental health helps the individual to strive properly for the realization of the goals of his/her life. These goals may differ from person to person depending upon their lifestyles and philosophy of life.
9. **Mental health helps in the progress of the society:** Mental health helps the individuals to develop as well balance useful citizens who are conscious not only for their rights, but for their responsibilities also. They take essential from the society for their proper development and living, but also ready to give something to the society for its progress and development.
10. **Mental health helps in the prevention of mental illness:** Mental health helps the individual in protecting him/her against abnormalities of behavior, maladjustment, illness and mental diseases in the same ways as physical health is helpful in saving him/her from the physical illness, ailments and diseases. A sound mind and balanced personality has enough resistance for fighting with the odds of life and bearing the accidental stresses and strains of life in comparison to the people having impaired mental health.

Symptoms of Poor Mental Health

- Emotionally unstable and easily upset
- Apprehensive, suspicious and insecure
- Lack of self-confidence and willpower
- No adequate adjustment with the self and environment—physical, social and professional
- The failure in setting a proper level of aspiration
- Suffering from frustrations, unresolved conflicts, strains and stresses
- Always remains in the state of over anxiousness and tension
- Lack of enduring power and tolerance
- Lack of decision-making ability
- Poor self-concept and achievement motivation
- Unrealistic attitude toward the life and people
- Suffering from mental disturbances, disorder, ailments and diseases
- Always dissatisfied with his/her achievements and tries to seek over perfection in his/her or other's work
- Lives in the world of his/her own imagination and fantasy.

■ MENTAL HYGIENE

Mental hygiene is concerned with realization and maintenance of mind's health and efficiency or in other words it deals with healthfulness of mind. Mental hygiene is concerned with the study of factors, which go against mental health and efficiency. Mental hygiene means the balanced and integrated development of personality. It is a science that deals with human welfare and pervades all fields of human relationships. The aim of mental hygiene is to aid people to achieve more satisfying and more productive lives through the preventing anxieties and maladjustments. According to dictionary, mental hygiene is the science or arts of maintaining mental health and preventing the development of maladjustment and neurosis.

Professor Beers W is called Father of mental hygiene. Once, when he was suffering from some ailments, he realized that various ailments are caused due to failure of the individual to adjust him with situation and requirement of environment. This maladjustment also leads to the development of various mental ailments. It is necessary to do away with them. With this aim in view an international mental health society was established in 1908. The society believed in the slogan sound mind resides in sound body.

Definition

1. It is concerned with the principle and practice in promotion, maintenance of the mental health and prevention of mental disorders. —*Hadfield JA*
2. The means by the process of mental health is related it is a way of life and involves that influences what one feels, says and does. —*Bernard HW*
3. Mental health is defined as the realization and maintenance of the mind's health and efficiency. —*Klein DB*
4. Mental hygiene is defined as the science and art of preserving and maximizing the mental health. —*English and English*
5. It is organized attempts to effort human adjustment through the application of principles and practices of living. —*Bhatia BD and Craig M*
6. Mental hygiene means establishment of environmental conditions, emotional attitudes and habits of thinking that will resist an onset of personality maladjustments. It is the study of principles and practices in the promotion of mental health and the prevention of mental disorder. —*Dictionary of education*
7. Mental hygiene is defined as the application of a body of hygienic information and technique called from sciences of psychology, child study, education, sociology, psychiatry, medicine and biology, (a) for the purpose of observation and improvement of mental health of the individuals and the community, (b) for the prevention and care of minor or major mental diseases and defects, and mental, educational and social maladjustments. —*Wallace Wallin*

Spheres of Mental Hygiene

There are two spheres of mental hygiene, prophylactic hygiene and meliorative hygiene.

1. **Prophylactic mental hygiene:** It is oriented toward the prevention of diseases, breakdown, weakness, disaster and death.
2. **Meliorative mental hygiene:** It is oriented toward the acquisition of better health, more energy and abundant life. It stresses the normal and the ideal as opposed to the abnormal and pathological.

Promotive and Preventive Mental Health

The terms mental health promotion and prevention have often been confused. Promotion is defined as intervening to optimize positive mental health by addressing determinants of positive mental health before a specific mental health problem has been identified with the ultimate goal of improving the positive mental health of the population. Mental health prevention is defined as intervening to minimize mental health problems by addressing determinants of mental health problems before a specific mental health problem has been identified in the individual, group or population of focus with the ultimate goal of reducing the number of future mental health problems in the population. Mental health promotion and prevention are at the core of a public health approach to children and youth mental health, which addresses the mental health of children focusing on the balance of optimizing positive mental health as well as preventing and treating mental health problems.

Promotion

Mental health promotion attempts to encourage and increase protective factors and healthy behaviors that can help prevent the onset of a diagnosable mental disorder and reduce risk factors that can lead to the development of a mental disorder. It also involves creating living conditions and environments that support mental health and allow people to adopt and maintain healthy lifestyles or a climate that respects and protects basic civil, political, socioeconomic and cultural rights is fundamental to mental health promotion. Without the security and freedom provided by these rights, it is very difficult to maintain a high level of mental health. Specifically, mental health can be promoted through:

1. Early childhood interventions (e.g. home visits for pregnant women, preschool psychosocial activities).
2. Providing support for children (e.g. skills building programs, child and youth development programs).
3. Programs targeted at vulnerable groups including minorities, indigenous people, migrants and people affected by conflicts and disasters (e.g. psychosocial interventions after disasters).
4. Incorporating mental health promotional activities in schools (e.g. programs supporting ecological changes in schools and child-friendly schools).
5. Violence prevention programs.
6. Community development programs.

Positive youth development is defined by the interagency working group on youth programs as an intentional, prosocial approach that:

1. Engages youth within their communities, schools, organizations, peer groups and families in a manner that is productive and constructive.
2. Recognizes, utilizes and enhances youths' strengths.
3. Promotes positive outcomes for young people by providing opportunities, fostering positive relationships and furnishing the support needed to build on their leadership strengths.

It provides a lens for promoting the mental health of youth by focusing on protective factors in a young person's environment and on how these factors could influence one's ability to overcome adversity. Learn more about positive youth development.

Prevention

Prevention efforts can vary based on the audience they are addressing, level of intensity they are providing and the development phase they target. The different types of prevention as defined by the Institute of Medicine, United States of America are depicted in Figure 23.3. As prevention efforts move from universal prevention interventions to treatment they increase in intensity and become more individualized.

Interventions may vary not only based on level of intensity but also on the development phase of the youth. Figure 2 provides examples of preventive interventions for each of the developmental stages through young adulthood.

■ ROLE OF NURSE IN MENTAL HEALTH/HYGIENE

Primary mental health care is an essential role of the Psychiatric-mental Health Nurse Practitioner (PMHNP), who can also help manage co-existing physical conditions with physical assessment, differential diagnosis and drug assessment. Although, most PMHNPs work in psychiatric settings, PMHNPs are beginning to provide mental health intervention in primary care settings. A PMHNP can provide significant benefits to patients in the primary care setting. Even though in 2002, the President's Commission on Mental Health documented that primary medical providers deliver about half of the care for common mental disorders and prescribe most of the psychotropic drugs, they are not

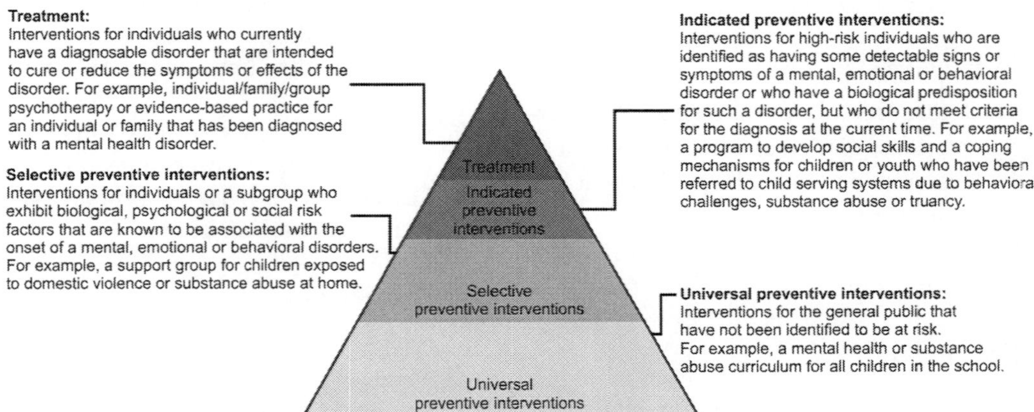

Figure 23.3: Promotive and preventive aspects of mental health

specifically trained to assess and treat psychiatric conditions, and they may be limited by time constraints. The onsite support and collaboration offered by a PMHNP can address both of these problems.

The interventions of a PMHNP in a primary care setting can increase patient participation in treatment plans of medical patients referred to mental health services, though up to 50% do not follow through with their referrals. Typical barriers to seeking mental health treatment include inconvenience, transportation problems, stigma and cost. Scheduling appointments in the same facility is more convenient and has less stigma attached. Early detection of mental disorders and evidence-based treatment approaches delivered by PMHNPs increases recovery rates, can improve physical health and in turn, reduces overall healthcare costs.

The PMHNP can also help integrate medical and psychiatric care. Patients with chronic mental illness are at high risk for multiple physical problems. The prolonged mood, anxiety and psychotic disorders often results in detrimental health behaviors such as a sedentary lifestyle, poor eating and sleeping habits, strained personal and professional relationships, and poor lifestyle choices and coping skills (smoking, substance abuse physical or emotional abuse and anger outbursts). In addition, common newer antipsychotic drugs (called atypical antipsychotics) have a lower risk of some adverse reactions than older drugs, but they put patients with chronic mental illness at greater risk for obesity, cardiovascular disease and diabetes. Some examples of these newer drugs are clozapine (Clozaril), risperidone (Risperdal) and olanzapine (Zyprexa). Psychiatric mental health nurse practitioners in the primary care setting can implement evidence-based interventions. With immediate access to medical records, onsite laboratory and primary care providers, they can easily screen for co-existing problems.

■ CONCLUSION

Mental health is defined as a state of wellbeing in which every individual realizes his/her own potential, can cope with the normal stresses of life, can work productively and fruitfully and is able to make a contribution to his/her community. The positive dimension of mental health is stressed in WHO definition of health as contained in its constitution.

■ REVIEW QUESTIONS

Long Essays

1. Define mental health. Explain the characteristics of mentally healthy person.
2. Describe mental health of different age group of people in detail.
3. Discuss the role of nurse in promotion and prevention of mental health.

Short Essays

4. Enumerate the factors influencing mental health.
5. Skills needed for positive mental health.
6. Discuss the principles contributing to mental health.
7. List out the importance of mental health.
8. Explain the nurse's responsibility in promotion of positive mental health.
9. Define mental hygiene. Explain symptoms of mental health.

Short Answers

10. Well-balanced life.
11. Needs of mental health.
12. Spheres of mental hygiene.
13. Primary mental health care.
14. Mental health promotion.

CHAPTER 24

Defense Mechanisms and Adjustments

■ INTRODUCTION

The human individual is as much equipped with mental capacities to protect himself/herself against conflicts and frustrations as with physical energy and powers to safeguard against physical dangers or distress. These mental capacities give rise to protective devices known as mental mechanisms or adjustment mechanisms or defense mechanisms. This adjustment mechanism helps the individual in overcoming threats to his/her ego and thus in maintaining inner balance or harmony. Mental mechanisms interact and overlap in our behavior. They are not mutually exclusive, nor do they generally operate as separate entities. Both well-adjusted and maladjusted individuals make use of these mechanisms in their daily behavior.

■ DEFINITIONS

1. Defense mechanism is a pattern of adjustment through which an individual relieves or decrease anxieties caused by an uncomfortable situation that threatens self-esteems.
2. Ego defense mechanisms are consciously or unconsciously operating devices to keep confliction issues out of consciousness of the individual to bring some protective measures.
3. Ego defense mechanisms are learned, usually during early childhood and are considered to be maladaptive when they become the predominant means of coping with stressors.
4. When psychological equilibrium is threatened by severe emotional trauma, frustrations or conflicts, the mind resorts to a variety to protective subterfuges and detours called mental mechanisms or dynamisms. —*Page*
5. An adjustment mechanism is a device resorted in order to achieve an indirect satisfaction of a need so that tension will be reduced and self-respect maintained. —*Carroll*
6. Certain patterns of behavior that are employed for protection against threat or anxiety are called defense mechanisms or adjustments mechanisms. Sometimes they are referred to as ego defense mechanisms since they are serve to defend the ego or the self from threat. —*Arkoff*
7. A defense mechanism is a strategy, unconsciously utilized that serves to protect the ego from anxiety. —*Davison and Neale*

■ DEFENSE MECHANISMS

Meaning

Ego defense mechanisms are learned, usually during early childhood and are considered to be maladaptive when they become the predominant means of coping with stressors. Ego psychology comprises a related set of theoretical concepts about human behavior that focus on the origins, development, structure and functioning of the executive arm of the personality the ego and its relationship to other aspects of the personality and to the external environment. The ego is considered to be a mental structure of the personality responsible for negotiating between the internal needs of the individual and the outside world.

Functions

1. **Reality testing:** The accurate perception of the external environment of one's internal world.
2. **Judgment:** An individual must not only develop the capacity to test reality accurately but also act upon the outside world.
3. **Sense of reality of the world and of the self:** It is possible to perceive inner and outer reality accurately, but to experience the world and the self in distorted ways.
4. **Regulation and control of drives, affects and impulses:** The ability to modulate, delay, inhibits or control the expression of impulses and affects (fallings) in accord with reality is the hallmark of adaptive functioning and is essential to living among others.
5. **Object (or interpersonal) relations:** Within contemporary ego psychology, the concept of object relations has assumed a more central position than it held previously.
6. **Thought processes:** Mature thinking generally is taken for granted in the most individuals can perceive and attend to stimuli, concentrate, anticipate, symbolize, remember and reason.
7. **Adaptive regression in the service of the ego:** The concept of regression originated in Freud's writings as a defense in which an individual literally goes backward, returning to a previous phase of development.
8. **Defensive functioning:** Because of the significance of defense in normal and abnormal development.
9. **Stimulus barrier:** All living organisms are responsive to internal and external stimuli as a result of their sensor motor apparatus.
10. **Autonomous functions:** Hartmann originally proposed that certain ego functions such as attention, concentration, memory, learning, perception.
11. **Mastery competence:** The degree to which one is and feels competent originates early in childhood as a function of one's innate abilities.
12. **Synthetic-integrative function:** Many authors including Freud, have emphasized the ego's organizing role in addition to its more discrete functions.
13. Protecting from dangerous situation.
14. To deal with inner hurt, pain, anger, anxiety, sadness and self-devaluation.
15. Removing anxiety and hurt.
16. Play an important role in normal adjustment mechanism.

Characteristics

1. The purpose of defense mechanism is to reduce anxiety.
2. Defense mechanism is the compromise solution.
3. The pattern of defense mechanism depends on one's stability.
4. The same individual may use varied mechanisms as his/her need.

5. Defense mechanisms may be used consciously, but usually act at unconscious or subconscious level.
6. Defense mechanisms are devised in the forms of a certain pattern of behavior.
7. These mechanisms provide protection against whatever threatens our ego or self-esteem.
8. There are many situations in our environment and also within us which threaten our psychological equilibrium.
9. Defense mechanism may be evolved by anything in conflict with minimum ideal of what the self must be.
10. Defense mechanisms are quite temporary defense against anxiety and inadequacies. By resorting to them one tries to deceive himself/herself more than somebody else.
11. Defense mechanisms are largely unconscious. They do tend to operate in a machine-like or automatic way. In fact, they are always in corresponding degree, self-deceptive and thus aim at softening or disguising what is unaccepted to us in terms of our failure or inadequacies.
12. Defense mechanisms should not be confused with symptoms of neuroses or other abnormal conditions. These mechanisms are purely psychic or mental devices, or ways of perceiving and desiring.

Types

Psychotic (Level I) Defense Mechanism

Denial: It is protecting self from unpleasant reality by refusal to perceive it or face it. It is a defense mechanism in which a person is faced with a fact that is too painful to accept and reject it. The individual may deny the reality of the unpleasant fact altogether, admit the fact, but deny its seriousness or admit both the fact and seriousness but, denies responsibility.

Distortion: A gross reshaping of external reality to meet internal needs. For example, mentally ill patients have no intact contact with reality. These patients are suffering with psychosis.

Delusional projections: Gross frank delusions about external reality, usually of persecutory nature. The delusions are the false beliefs of the person, which are not shared by race, age, educational background, etc.

Immature Defense Mechanism (Level II)

Fantasy: It is gratifying frustrated desire by imaginary achievements. It is the defense mechanism involving tendency to retreat into fantasy in order to resolve inner and outer conflicts.

Projection: It is unconscious denial of unacceptable feelings and emotions in one, while attributing to others. It is primitive form of paranoia.

Hypochondriasis: The transformation of negative feeling toward others into negative feelings such as self, pain, illness and anxiety. Hypochondriasis sometimes referred to as health phobia, refers to an excessive preoccupation or worry about having a serious illness.

Passive aggression: Aggression toward others expressed indirectly or passively. Passive aggressive defense create or disorder known as passive aggressive. Personality disorder is said to be marked by a pervasive pattern of negative attitudes and passive, usually resistance in interpersonal or occupational areas.

Acting out: Direct expression of unconscious wish or impulse without conscious awareness of the emotion that derives the expressive behavior. This behavior is very common in children with temper tantrum, oppositional defiant disorder, truancy, etc.

Regression: It is returning to an earlier stage of behavior when stress creates, problem at the present stage, involving less mature responds and usually lower level of aspiration. For example, regression mechanism of going from the present pattern to the past level of behavior. The individual returns to patterns of behavior that were successful in earlier stages of development.

Idealization: Subconsciously choosing to perceive another individual as having positive qualities he/she may actually have.

Neurotic Defense Mechanism (Level III)

Displacement: Defense mechanism that shifts sexual or aggressive impulses to a more acceptable, or less threatening target; redirecting emotion to a safer outlet; separation of emotion from its real object.

Dissociation: It is temporary drastic modification of one's personal identity or character to avoid emotional distress; separation or postponement of a feeling that normally would accompany a situation or thought.

Isolation: It is separation of feelings from ideas and events. For example, describing a murder with graphic details with no emotional response.

Intellectualization: It is avoiding unavoidable emotions by focusing on the intellectual aspects. It is separating from emotional contents of an event, focusing instead on the facts.

Reaction formation: Converting unconscious wishes or impulses that are perceived to be dangerous into their opposites; behavior that is completely the opposite of what one really wants or feels; taking the opposite belief because the true belief causes anxiety.

Repression: It acts to keep information out of conscious awareness. Repression is more complicated mechanism in which unpleasant or unacceptable experiences, emotions or motivations are actively forced into the unconscious and kept there. Repression operates wholly on an unconscious level. Unacceptable feeling is unconsciously kept out of awareness. A man is jealous of his good friend's success, but is unaware of his feelings or jealously.

Mature Defense Mechanism (Level IV)

Altruism: This is constructive service to others that brings pleasure and personal satisfaction. Altruism loves others as oneself, behavior that promotes the survival chances of others at a cost to one's own. In other words, it is self-sacrifices for the benefit of others.

Sublimation: The transformation of negative emotions or instincts into positive actions, behavior or emotion is sublimation. Sublimation is a defense mechanism that allows us to act out unacceptable impulses by converting these behaviors into a more acceptable form.

Suppression: It is a device where a conscious effort is made by the individual to dismiss the impulses, feelings and thoughts that are unpleasant to the preconscious mind. So the unacceptable feelings and thoughts are consciously kept out of awareness.

Humor: Overt expression of ideas and feelings (especially those that are unpleasant to focus or too terrible to talk about) that gives pleasure to others.

Identification: The unconscious modeling of one's self upon another person's character and behavior. Some individuals try to resemble with another person's character, e.g. a lonely teenager being copying the clothes and action of a popular peer.

Introjections: It is identifying with some ideas or objects so deeply that it becomes a part of that person. It is complete acceptance of another's opinion and values as one's own.

■ PSYCHOLOGICAL TECHNIQUES

Among the psychological techniques used in ego-supportive intervention, are those that are more sustaining, directive, educative and structured, in contrast to those that are more nondirective, reflective, confronting and interpretive.

Eight Main Groups of Psychological Techniques

1. **Sustaining techniques** consisting of sympathetic listening and receptiveness, conveying an attitude of acceptance of the client's worth and uniqueness, and providing reassurance and encouragement.
2. **Direct influence** consisting of suggestion and advice to the client.
3. **Exploration, description and ventilation** consisting of eliciting the client's subjective and objective feelings.
4. **Person-situation reflection** consisting of focusing on the client's current situation and relationships. The client is helped in:
   a. His/Her perceptions or understanding of others or of any other objective situation external to him/her.
   b. His/Her understanding of the nature of his/her behavior and its effects on others.
   c. His/Her understanding of why he/she behaves in certain ways in specific situations.
   d. His/Her evaluation of his/her inner feelings, his/her self-concept, attitudes, values and so on. Person-situation reflection may involve rational discussion or thinking through the pros and cons of taking certain actions.
5. **Pattern-dynamic reflection,** consisting of helping the client to identify and consider his/her pattern of behavior including his/her defenses and their impact. The goal is to help the client to develop greater dynamic understanding of the nature and reasons for his/her behavior. This may involve the worker's pointing out (confronting) maladaptive, contradictory, but often ego-syntonic behavior as well as interpretations of the underlying reasons for it.
6. **Developmental reflections** consisting of helping the client to think about his/her past and the way it is affecting his/her current behavior. As with pattern-dynamic reflection, the goal is to help the client gain greater insight into the dynamics of his/her maladaptive behavior that may stem from irrational feelings and fears from past situations of conflict or from development arrests.
7. **Educative techniques** consisting of providing the client with information essential to his/her functioning in his/her various roles or in negotiation of external systems; helping him/her to gain understanding of the effects of his/her behavior on others; and helping him/her to gain understanding of others' needs and motivations. Education techniques also involve modeling, role-playing and rehearsal, anticipatory planning, and the promotion of new behavior within the client-worker relationship.
8. **Structuring techniques** consisting of partializing problems, focusing intervention on key areas, using time limits flexibly, assigning homework tasks and planning activities. Many of these techniques have arisen out of crisis-oriented, planned short-term or task-centered intervention.

Work With the Social Environment

Environmental intervention has not been well conceptualized in the social work literature. It is critical, however, to intervene efforts within an ego psychological perspective. For example, it may be important to mobilize resources and opportunities that will enable the individual to use his/her inner capacities. It may be necessary to restructure the environment, so that it nurtures or fits better with individual needs and capacities. Environmental work also may be essential to modifying maladaptive patterns within an individual. For example, it may be utilized where the family system is perpetuating, reinforcing or aggravating a family member's difficulties.

■ ADJUSTMENT

The word adjustment means to fit, make suitable, adapt, arrange, harmonize, correspondence with. Adjustment is defined as the series of techniques, methods or processes by which an individual tries to meet the environmental, spatial or psychological changes and maintains a satisfactory equilibrium (balance) with his/her world. It is also called adaptation. There are different types of changes to which a person has to adjust himself/herself. These changes can be environmental, e.g. change in temperature, humanity, oxygen level, etc. Spatial (e.g. change of a place) and psychological (e.g. the husband leaves the job; family members face a problem of change of job of the head of the family).

Definitions

1. Adjustment can be defined in that form of social process in which two or more people, or groups interact to end or reduce conflict. —*Fitcher*
2. Adjustment is that special process through which a person is able to develop the tendency of cooperation in his environment. —*MacIver and Page*
3. Any operation whereby an organism becomes more favorably related to the environmental and internal. —*Warren*
4. It is the establishment of satisfactory relationship, as representing, harmony, conformance, adoption, etc. —*Webster*
5. A continual process in which a person varies his behavior to produce a more harmonious relationship between himself and his environment. —*Gates and Jersild*
6. The process of finding and adopting modes of behavior suitable to the environment or the change in the environment. —*Cater V Good*
7. An individual's adjustment is said to be adequate, wholesome or healthful to the extent that he/she has established harmonious relationship between himself and the conditions, situations and persons who compromise his physical or social environment. —*Crow and Crow*
8. Adjustment is psychological survival. —*von haller*

Nature of Adjustment (Fig. 24.1)

Continuity: The process of adjustment is continued throughout life. Individual from birth to death has to adjust in one or the other way. The individuals who are able to adjust themselves to the changing situations in their environment can live a harmonious, happy and continued life.

Mental peace: Conflict upsets a person, whereas adjustment provides peacefulness.

Universality: Adjustment is prevalent in all the aspects of life, e.g. social, economic, political, religious, etc.

Social necessity: Adjustment is necessary to prevent society.

Harmonious relationship: This is between individual, their needs and environment is essential. The individual meets demands either by adopting, modifying previous ways of doing or facing the challenges.

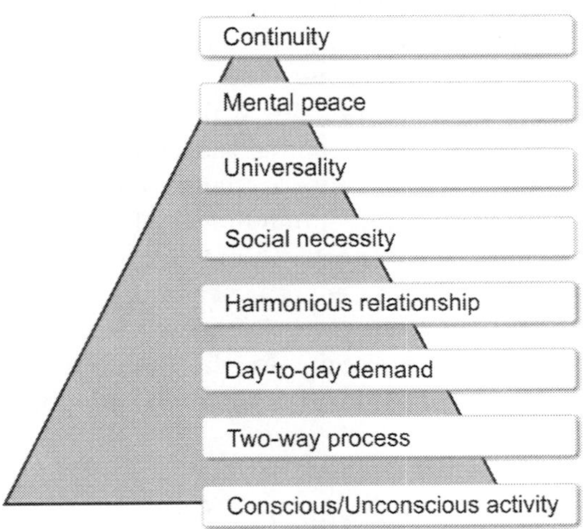

Figure 24.1: Nature of adjustment

Day-to-day demand: Adjustment will help the individual to change his/her way of life according to the demand of the situation and gives strength, ability to bring about the necessary changes in the environment conditions.

Two-way process: Adjustment is a process of fitting oneself into available circumstances, but also the process of changing the circumstances to fit one's own needs. In majority of cases, adjustment is compromise between two extremes.

Conscious/Unconscious activity: To adjust in a society, the individual learns morals, traditions, etc. from birth to death in conscious and unconscious manner to adjust and accommodate to the needs and demands of self and society.

Aims of Adjustment

- To maintain harmonious and active relationship between structural components of society
- For social reform and social construction
- To lead a harmonious social life
- To perform functions effectively in relation to their culture customs, values and beliefs
- To provide good interpersonal relationship
- To promote character building
- To develop orderly social unity
- To manifest collective behavior in terms of state, religion, economic agencies, organization and social group.

Measurement of Adjustment

1. **Testing techniques:** To assess the individual characteristic at the unconscious level.
2. **Projective techniques:** To assess the individual's characteristics at the unconscious level.
3. **Sociometric techniques:** To measure social relationships and provide clues to the level of social adjustment.
4. **Scaling techniques:** Opinions or views are collected from other person about the adjustment pattern of a particular interval known to the respondents.
5. **Inventory techniques:** They may have many advantages to the techniques.

Methods of Adjustment

Direct Method

1. **Improving efforts:** To improve the behavioral process and to solve difficult situations in the environment, he/she will increase his/her efforts to improve efficiency.
2. **Compromising methods:** Individual changes his/her efforts in a different direction to fulfill his/her aspiration.
3. **Withdrawal and submissiveness:** Accepts his/her own defeat and surrounding himself/herself to the powerful environmental forces.
4. **Making proper choices and decisions:** A person adapts himself/herself and to serves harmony with his/her environment by making use of his/her intelligence for the proper choices and wise

decision particularly when faced with conflicting situations and stressful moments/situations.

Indirect Method

By using defense mechanism/coping strategies, the individual will try to adopt themself to the changing situation and accommodating new lifestyles.

Improving Adjustments

Improving adjustments is very important to establish positive adjustment by finding out reasons of stress, hopelessness, frustration and maladjustments:

1. **Find patterns of behavior that satisfy** basic needs and solve problems effectively.
2. **Assume conscious control** of behavior.
3. **Use problem solving** to find the best possible solution for a problem situation instead of acting impulsively.
4. **Use emotion constructively** when appropriate; express feelings at the time they are experienced.
5. **Self-evaluate** in a constructive sense. Look for ways to improve, but avoid feelings of guilt or inadequacy.
6. **Avoid burnout:** Perform effective stress management techniques such as yoga, meditation, exercises, etc.
7. **Adapting to new situation:** When a change occur in your life situation or your patterns of behavior in order to achieve a state of good adjustment in new situations.

▪ CONCLUSION

Ego psychology embodies a more optimistic and growth-oriented view of human functioning and potential than do the earlier theoretical formulation. It generated changes in the study and assessment process and led to an expansion and systemization of interceptive strategies with individuals. It fostered a reconceptualization of the clinic worker relationship, of change mechanisms and of the intervention process. It helped to refocus the importance of work of with the social environment as well as work with the family and the group. Moreover, it has important implications for the design of service delivery, large-scale social programs and social policy.

▪ REVIEW QUESTIONS

Long Essays

1. Define defense mechanism. Explain the meaning and functions of defense mechanism.
2. Describe the different types of defense mechanisms.

Short Essays

3. Explain the characteristics of defense mechanism.
4. Describe psychological techniques used in ego-supportive intervention.
5. Define adjustment and explain the maturity of adjustments.
6. Describe the direct and indirect methods of adjustments.
7. Enumerate the aims of adjustment.

Short Answers

8. Reaction formation.
9. Sublimation.
10. Repression.
11. Mental peace.
12. Positive adjustments.
13. Id, ego and superego.
14. Measures to avoid burnout.

CHAPTER

25 Mental Illness

■ INTRODUCTION

Mental health problems range from the worries we all experience as part of everyday life to serious long-term conditions. The majority of people who experience mental health problems can get over them or learn to live with them, especially if they get help early on. Mental health problems are usually defined and classified to enable professionals to refer people for appropriate care and treatment. But some diagnoses are controversial and there is much concern in the mental health field that people are too often treated according to or described by their label. This can have a profound effect on their quality of life. Nevertheless, diagnoses remain the most usual way of dividing and classifying symptoms into groups. Mental illness is maladjustment in living. It produces a disharmony in the person's ability to meet human needs comfortably or effectively and function within a culture. Mentally ill person loses their ability to respond according to the expectations they have for themselves and the demands that society has for them.

■ DEFINITION

Mental and behavioral disorders are understood as clinically significant conditions characterized by alterations in thinking, mood (emotions) or behavior associated with personal distress and/or impaired functioning. —*WHO, 2001*

■ CAUSES OF MENTAL ILLNESS

Mental disorder is not a disturbance in the function of a single organ as the brain. It means the maladapted and disordered psychobiological functioning of the organism. Mental disorder brings about conditions of behavior, which hinder adequate adjustment of life situations. The modern tendency is to regard a mental disorder as a mode of behavior or of living rather than as a disease entry. Often people confuse mental disorder with deficiency.

Mental health and mental illness can be viewed as being on opposite ends on a mental health continuum on the illness and the person is rarely touched by reality. On healthy side of the continuum, the person demonstrates high-level wellness. The midpoint on the continuum can be regarded as normal mental health. Health illness results from an individual ability to cope with a situation that he/she finds overwhelming often maladaptive behavior in a response to acute anxiety.

■ FACTORS CAUSING MENTAL ILLNESS

Many factors are responsible for the causation of mental illness. These factors may predispose an individual to mental illness, precipitate or perpetuate the mental illness (Fig. 25.1).

Predisposing Factors

Predisposing factors determine an individual's susceptibility to mental illness. They interact with precipitating factors resulting in mental illness. These are:
- Genetic makeup
- Physical damage to the central nervous system
- Adverse psychosocial influence.

Precipitating Factors

Precipitating factors are events that occur shortly before the onset of a disorder and appear to have induced it. These are:
- Physical stress
- Psychosocial stress.

Perpetuating Factors

Perpetuating factors are responsible for aggravating or prolonging the diseases already existing in an individual. Psychosocial stress is an example. Thus, etiological factors of mental illness can be:
- Biological factors
- Physiological factors
- Psychological factors
- Social factors.

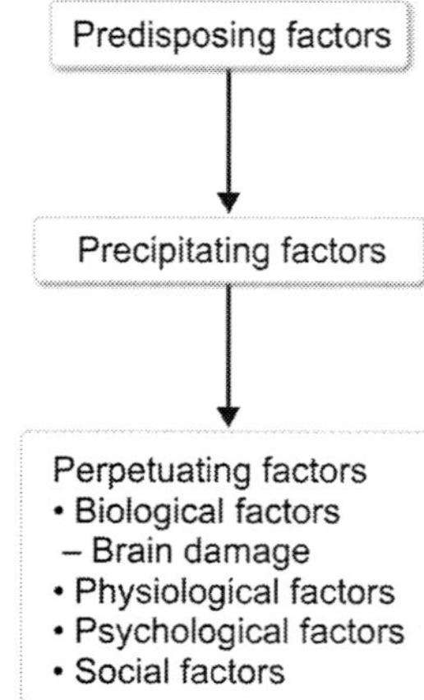

Figure 25.1: Factors causing mental illness

Biological Factors

Heredity

What one inherits is not the illness or its symptoms, but a predisposition to the illness, which is determined by genes that we inherit directly. Studies have shown that three fourth of mental defectives and one third of psychotic individuals owe their condition mainly to unfavorable heredity.

Biochemical factors

Biochemical abnormalities in the brain are considered to be the cause of some psychological disorders. Disturbance in neurotransmitters in the brain is found to play an important role in the etiology of certain psychiatric disorders.

Brain damage

Any damage to the structure and functioning of the brain can give rise to mental illness. Damage to the structure of the brain may be due to one of the following causes:

1. **Infection:** Neurosyphilis, encephalitis, human immunodeficiency virus (HIV) infection, etc.
2. **Injury:** Loss of brain tissue due to head injury.
3. **Intoxication:** Damage to brain tissue due to toxins such as alcohol, barbiturates, lead, etc.
4. **Vascular:** Poor blood supply, bleeding (intracranial hemorrhage, subarachnoid hemorrhage and subdural hemorrhage).
5. **Alteration in brain function:** Changes in blood chemistry that interfere with brain functioning such as disturbance in blood glucose levels, hypoxia, anoxia and fluid/electrolyte imbalance.

6. **Tumors:** Brain tumors.
7. **Vitamin deficiency and malnutrition,** in particular deficiency of vitamin B complex.
8. **Degenerative diseases:** Dementia.
9. **Endocrine disturbances:** Hypothyroidism, thyrotoxicosis, etc.
10. **Physical defects and physical illness:** Acute physical illness as well as chronic illnesses with all their handicapping conditions may result in loss of mental capacities.

Physiological Factors

It has been observed that mental disorders are more likely to occur at certain critical periods of life namely puberty, menstruation, pregnancy, delivery, puerperium and climacteric. These periods are marked not only by physiological (endocrine) changes but also by psychological issues that diminish the adaptive capacity of the individual. Thus, the individual becomes more susceptible to mental illness during this period.

Psychological Factors

1. It is observed that some specific personality types are more prone to develop certain psychological disorders. For example, those who are unsocial and reserved (schizoid) are vulnerable to schizophrenia when they face adverse situations and psychosocial stresses.
2. Psychological factors such as strained interpersonal relationships at home, place of work, school or college, bereavement, loss of prestige, loss of job, etc.
3. Childhood insecurities due to parents with pathological personalities, faulty attitude of parents (overstrictness, overleniency), abnormal parent-child relationship (overprotection, rejection, unhealthy comparisons), deprivation of child's essential psychological and social needs, etc.
4. Social and recreational deprivations resulting in boredom, isolation and alienation.
5. Marriage problems such as forced bachelorhood, disharmony due to physical, emotional, social, educational or financial incompatibility, childlessness, too many children, etc.
6. Sexual difficulties arising out of improper sex education, unhealthy attitudes towards sexual functions, guilt feelings about masturbation, pre- and extramarital sex relations and worries about sexual perversions.
7. Stress, frustration and seasonal variations are sometimes noted in the occurrence of mental diseases.

Social Factors

1. Poverty, unemployment, injustice, insecurity, migration and urbanization.
2. Gambling, alcoholism, prostitution, broken homes, divorce, very big family, religion, traditions, political upheavals and other social crises.

■ WARNING SIGNS OF MENTAL ILLNESS

Children

1. **Mood changes:** Look for feelings of sadness or withdrawal that last at least 2 weeks or severe mood swings that cause problems in relationships at home or school.
2. **Intense feelings:** Be aware of feelings of overwhelming fear for no reason, sometimes with a racing heart or fast breathing, or worries or fears intense enough to interfere with daily activities.
3. **Behavior changes:** This includes drastic changes in behavior or personality, as well as dangerous or out of control behavior.

4. **Fighting frequently,** using weapons or expressing a desire to badly hurt others also are warning signs.
5. **Difficulty in concentrating:** Look for signs of trouble focusing or sitting still, both of which might lead to poor performance in school.
6. **Unexplained weight loss:** A sudden loss of appetite, frequent vomiting or use of laxatives might indicate an eating disorder.
7. **Physical harm:** Sometimes a mental health condition leads to suicidal thoughts or actual attempts at self-harm or suicide.
8. **Substance abuse:** Some kids use drugs or alcohol to try to cope with their feelings.
9. Changes in school performance.
10. Poor grades despite strong efforts.
11. Excessive worry or anxiety (i.e. refusing to go to bed or school).
12. Hyperactivity.
13. Persistent nightmares.
14. Persistent disobedience or aggression.
15. Frequent temper tantrums.

Older Children/Preadolescents

- Substance abuse
- Inability to cope with problems and daily activities
- Changes in sleeping and/or eating habits
- Excessive complaints of the physical ailments
- Defiance of authority, truancy, theft and/or vandalism
- Intense fear of weight gain
- Prolonged negative mood, often accompanied by poor appetite or thoughts of death
- Frequent outbursts of angel.

Adults

- Confused thinking
- Prolonged depression leads to sadness or irritability
- Feelings of extreme highs and lows
- Excessive fears, worries and anxieties
- Social withdrawal
- Dramatic changes in eating or sleeping habits
- Strong feelings of anger
- Delusions or hallucinations
- Growing inability to cope with daily problems and activities
- Suicidal thoughts
- Denial of obvious problems
- Numerous unexplained physical ailments and substance abuse.

To learn more about symptoms that are specific to a particular mental illness, refer to the Mental Health America brochure on that illness.

Warning Signs and Symptoms of Drug/Alcohol Abuse in Teens

Someone with alcohol dependence may suffer serious withdrawal symptoms, such as trembling, delusions, hallucinations and sweating, if he/she stops drinking suddenly (cold turkey). Once alcohol dependence develops, it becomes very hard to stop drinking without outside help.

Symptoms

Symptoms of an alcohol problem include:

- Personality changes
- Blackouts
- Drinking more and more for the same 'time'
- Denial of the problem.

A person with an alcohol problem may:

- Gulp or sneak drinks
- Drink alone or early in the morning
- Suffer from the shakes
- He/She may also have family, school or work problems, or get in trouble with the law because of drinking.

Physical Signs

- Loss of appetite, increase in appetite, any changes in eating habits, unexplained weight loss or gain

- Slowed or staggering walk, poor physical coordination
- Inability to sleep, awake at unusual times and unusual laziness
- Red and watery eyes, pupils larger or smaller than usual, blank stare
- Cold, sweaty palms, shaking hands
- Puffy face, blushing or paleness
- Smell of substance on breath, body or clothes
- Extreme hyperactivity, excessive talkativeness, runny nose, hacking cough
- Needle marks on lower arm, leg or bottom of feet
- Nausea, vomiting or excessive sweating
- Tremors or shakes of hands, feet or head
- Irregular heartbeat.

Behavioral Signs

- Change in overall attitude/personality with no other identifiable cause
- Changes in friends, new hangouts, sudden avoidance of old crowd, does not want to talk about new friendsm friends are known drug users
- Change in activities or hobbies
- Drop in grades at school or performance at work, skips school or is late for school
- Change in habits at home, loss of interest in family and family activities
- Difficulty in the paying attention and forgetfulness
- General lack of motivation, energy, self-esteem, "I do not care" attitude
- Sudden oversensitivity, temper tantrums or resentful behavior
- Moodiness, irritability or nervousness
- Silliness or giddiness
- Paranoia
- Excessive need for privacy, unreachable
- Secretive or suspicious behavior
- Car accidents
- Chronic dishonesty
- Unexplained need for money, stealing money or items
- Change in personal grooming habits
- Possession of drug paraphernalia.

The key is change; it is important to watch for any significant changes in your child's physical appearance, personality, attitude or behavior.

▪ FEATURES OF MENTAL ILLNESS (Fig. 25.2)

The features of mental illness are classified under four headings:

1. Disturbances in bodily functions.
2. Disturbances in mental functions.
3. Changes in the individual and social activities.
4. Somatic complaints.

Disturbances in Bodily Functions

Sleep: Disturbed sleep throughout the night or no sleep at all, or difficulty in falling asleep or waking up in the middle of night and failing to fall asleep again. In addition, the individual may experience lethargy and lack of freshness in the morning.

Appetite and food intake: Increased appetite or decreased appetite, weight loss or weight gain, nausea and vomiting.

Bowel and bladder movement: Diarrhea or constipation, increased micturition and bed-wetting.

Sexual desire and activity: Decreased interest in sex, premature ejaculation, impotence or lack of sexual satisfaction. In some conditions

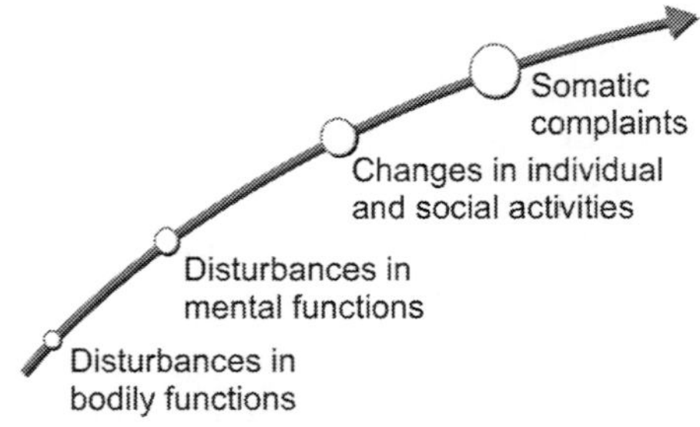

Figure 25.2: Features of mental illness

there can be excessive sexual desire or lack of social inhibitions.

Disturbances in Mental Functions

Behavior: The patient may exhibit over activity, restlessness, irritability, may be abusive to others for trivial or no reasons at all, or the patient may become dull, withdrawn and not respond to external or internal cues. At times the patient may behave in a bizarre way, which the family members may find irritating. Sometimes the patient's behavior can be dangerous to self or others.

Speech: Patient talks excessively and unnecessarily or talks very little or stays mute. The talk becomes irrelevant and understandable (incoherent).

Thought: Patient expresses peculiar and wrong beliefs, which others do not share.

Emotions: Patient may exhibit excessive emotions such as excessive happiness, anger, fear or sadness. Sometimes emotions can be inappropriate to situations. They may laugh to self or weep without any reason.

Perception: The patient may perceive without any stimulus. There can be misinterpretation of perception. For example, a mentally ill person can see things or hear sounds, or feel objects, which do not exist or which others do not see. This is known as hallucinations. A patient who is hallucinating is seen talking to self, laughing or weeping to self, wandering in the streets and behaving in a manner, which others may find abnormal.

Attention and concentration: Patient may have decreased attention and concentration; may get distracted easily or have selective inattention.

Memory: Patient may lose memory and start forgetting important matters.

Intelligence and judgment: In some mental illnesses, intelligence and the ability to take decisions deteriorate. Patient loses reasoning skills and abilities, may not be able to perform simple arithmetic or commits mistakes in routine work.

Level of consciousness: In some mental illnesses due to possible brain damage, there may be changes in the level of consciousness. Patient fail to identify relatives. They can be disoriented to time and place, may remain confused or become unconscious.

Changes in Individual and Social Activities

Patients may neglect their bodily needs and personal hygiene. The patient may also lose social sense. They behave in an inappropriate manner in social situations and embarrass others. They behave strangely with their family members, friends, colleagues and others. They may insult, abuse/assault them.

Somatic Complaints

Patient may complain of aches and pains in different parts of the body, fatigue, weakness, involuntary movements, etc.

■ COMMON SIGNS AND SYMPTOMS OF MENTAL ILLNESS (Fig. 25.3)

1. **Disturbances in motor behavior:** Motor retardation, stupor, stereotypes, negativism, ambitendency, waxy flexibility, echopraxia, restlessness, agitation and excitement.
2. **Disorders of thought, language and communication:** Pressure of speech, poverty of speech, dysarthria, flight of ideas, circumstantialities, loosening of association, tangentiality, incoherence, preservation, neologism, clang association, thought block, thought insertion, thought broadcasting, echolalia, delusions, obsessions and phobias.

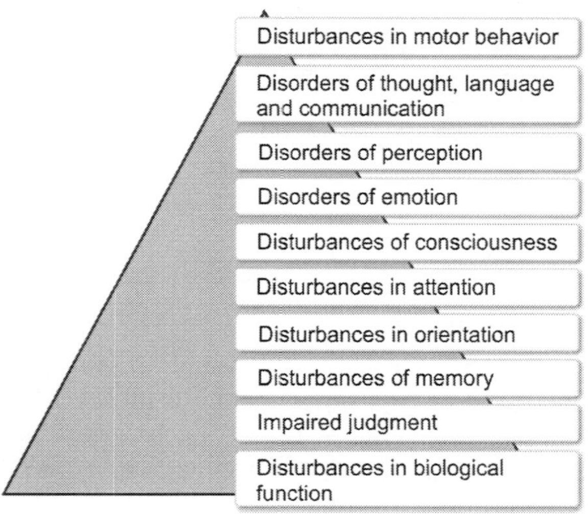

Figure 25.3: Common signs and symptoms of mental illness

3. **Disorders of perception:** Illusions, hallucinations, depersonalization and the derealization.
4. **Disorders of emotion:** Blunt affect, labile affect, elated mood, euphoria, ecstasy, dysphoric mood, depression and anhedonia.
5. **Disturbances of consciousness:** Clouding of consciousness, delirium and coma.
6. **Disturbances in attention:** Distractibility, selective inattention.
7. **Disturbances in orientation:** Disorientation of time, place or person.
8. **Disturbances of memory:** Amnesia, confabulation.
9. **Impaired judgment:** This is also a common sign.
10. **Disturbances in biological function:** Persistent deviations in temperature, pulse and respiration, nausea, vomiting, headache, loss of appetite, increased appetite, loss of weight, pain, fatigue, weight gain, insomnia, hypersomnia and sexual dysfunction.

■ CONCEPT OF NORMAL AND ABNORMAL BEHAVIOR

Psychiatry as evident from the above is concerned with abnormal behavior in its broadest sense, but defining the concepts of normal and abnormal behavior as such has been found to be difficult. These concepts are much under the influence of sociocultural factors. Several models have been put forward in order to explain the concept of normal and abnormal behavior (Fig. 25.4). Some of them are:

1. **Medical model:** It considers organic pathology as the definite cause for mental disorder. According to this model abnormal people are the ones who have disturbances in thought, perception and psychomotor activities. The normal are the ones who are free from these disturbances.
2. **Statistical model:** It involves the analysis of responses on a test or a questionnaire or observations of some particular behavioral variables. The degree of deviation from the standard norms arrived

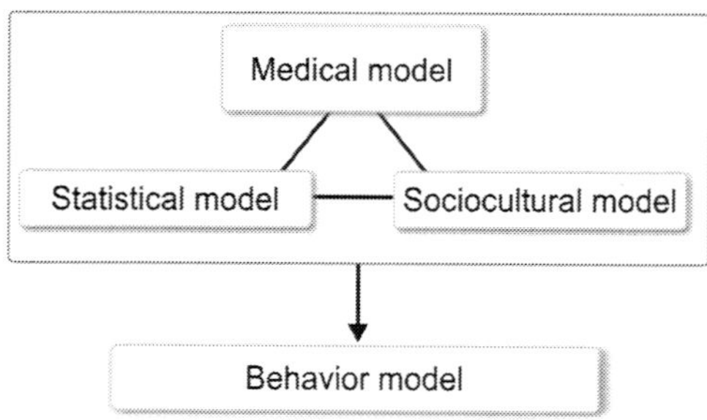

Figure 25.4: Concept of normal and abnormal behavior

at statistically, characterizes the degree of abnormality. Statistically normal mental health falls within two standard deviations (SDs) of the normal distribution curve.

3. **Sociocultural model:** The beliefs, norms, taboos and values of a society have to be accepted and adopted by individuals. Breaking any of these would be considered as abnormal. Normalcy is defined in context with social norms prescribed by the culture. Thus, cultural background has to be taken into account when distinguishing between normal and abnormal behavior.
4. **Behavior model:** Adaptive behavior is normal and maladaptive is abnormal. The abnormal behavior is a set of faulty behaviors acquired through learning.

PROBLEMS OF MENTAL DISORDERS

1. Self-care limitations or impaired functioning related to mental illness.
2. Significant deficits in biological, emotional and cognitive functioning.
3. Disability, life process changes.
4. Emotional problems such as anxiety, anger, sadness, loneliness and grief.
5. Physical symptoms that occur along with altered psychological functioning.
6. Alteration in thinking, perceiving, communicating and decision-making.
7. Difficulties in relating to others.
8. Patient's behavior may be dangerous to self or others.
9. Adverse effects on the well-being of the individual, family and community.
10. Financial, marital, family, academic and occupational problems.

BURDENS OF MENTAL DISORDERS

Mental disorders are common, affecting more than 25% of all people at some time during their lives. They are also universal, affecting people in all countries and societies, individuals of all ages, women and men, the rich and the poor, from urban and rural environments. They have an economic impact on societies and on the quality of life of individuals and families:

1. Mental disorders at any point of time are present in about 10% of the adult population. Around 20% of all patients seen by primary healthcare professionals have one or more mental disorders.
2. During the last two decades many epidemiological studies have been conducted in India, which show that mental disorders prevail in 18–207 per 1,000, with median 65.4 per 1000 at any given time. About 2.3% of the population suffers from seriously incapacitating mental disorders or epilepsy. A large number of adult patients (10.4–53.0%) coming to the general outpatient department are diagnosed as mentally ill.
3. It is estimated that in 2000, mental disorders accounted for 12% of the total disability adjusted life years (DALYs) lost due to all diseases and injuries. Common disorders, which usually cause severe disability, include depressive disorder, substance use disorders, schizophrenia, epilepsy, Alzheimer's disease, mental retardation and disorders of childhood and adolescence.

4. More than 450 million people today suffer from mental and behavioral disorders. Within the next 20 years depression will have the dubious distinction of becoming the second biggest cause for global burden of disease.
5. Worldwide 70 million people suffer from alcohol dependence, 50 million from epilepsy, 24 million from schizophrenia and another 20 million people attempt suicide every year.
6. Global Burden of Disease (GBD) 2000 estimates show that mental and neurological conditions account for 30.8% of all years lived with disability (YLD). Depression causes the largest amount of disability, accounting for almost 12% of all disabilities. Six neuropsychiatry conditions figured in the top 20 causes of disability worldwide, which include:
   - Unipolar depressive disorders
   - Alcohol use disorders
   - Schizophrenia
   - Bipolar affective disorders
   - The Alzheimer's disease and other dementias
   - Migraine.
7. Mental illnesses cause massive disruption in the lives of individuals, families and communities. Individuals suffer the distressing symptoms of disorders. They also suffer because they are unable to participate in work and leisure activities often as a result of discrimination. They worry about not being able to shoulder their responsibilities towards their family and friends and are fearful of being a burden to others. Mental illnesses are common to all countries and cause immense suffering. People with these disorders are often subjected to social isolation, poor quality of life and increased mortality. These disorders are thus the cause of staggering economic and social costs.
8. It is estimated that one in four families has at least one member currently suffering from a mental illness. These families are required not only to provide physical and emotional support but also to bear the negative impact of stigma and discrimination present in all parts of the world.
9. Families in which one member is suffering from a mental disorder make a number of adjustments and compromises that prevent other members of the family from achieving their full potential in work, social relationships and leisure. These are the human aspects of the burden of mental disorders that are difficult to assess and quantify.
10. The impact of mental disorders in communities is large and manifold. There is the cost of providing care, the loss of productivity and certain legal problems associated with some mental disorders.

■ MISCONCEPTION ABOUT MENTAL ILLNESS

Beliefs about mental illness have been characterized by superstition, ignorance and fear. Although, time and advances in scientific understanding of mental illness have dispelled many false ideas, there remain a number of popular misconceptions. Some of them are as detailed below:

1. **Mental illness is caused by supernatural power and is the result of a curse or possession by evil spirit.** Many people do not consider mental illness as an illness, but possession by spirits or curse that has befallen on the patient or family because of past sins or misdeeds in previous life.
2. **Mentally ill people show bizarre behavior.** Patients in mental hospitals and clinics are often pictured as a weird lot, who spend their time exhibiting useless bizarre behavior such as twisting of hands, etc.

3. **Mentally ill people are dangerous.** People who have or had a mental illness are viewed with suspicion and as dangerous persons.
4. **Mental illness is something to be ashamed of.** This idea arouses an unsympathetic, cruel attitude towards a mentally ill person. This is the reason why many people hide mental illness in the family.
5. **Mental illness is not curable.** People object to have normal relationship with mentally ill people or to give them employment even after being cured, or even to accept them as neighbors.
6. **Mental illness is contagious.** The fear that it is contagious is the main false notion, which leads people to view suspiciously or object to marital relations with a person belonging to the household of the mentally ill.
7. **Mental illness is hereditary.** It is not a rule that children of mentally ill patients should become mentally ill.
8. **Marriage can cure mental illness.** Mentally ill persons can get worse if they get married when they are ill, as marriage can become an additional stress. A patient who has recovered can get married and live a normal life similar to any other person.
9. **Mental hospitals are places where only dangerous mentally ill individuals are treated and restraint is a major form of treatment.** People hesitate to take their relatives to mental hospitals for treatment because of fear. Further, as ex-patient of a mental hospital, he/she, as well as his/her family members is often isolated. Therefore, people seek help from mental hospitals only as a last resort.

GENERAL ATTITUDE TOWARD THE MENTALLY ILL

1. In general the community responds to the mentally ill through denial, isolation and rejection. There is also a lack of understanding of mental illness as any other illness, and a lack of tendency to reject both the patients and those who treat them.
2. Mentally ill are viewed as people with no capacity for understanding.
3. People feel mental illness cannot be cured and even if the patient gets better, complete physical rest is considered essential.
4. The mentally ill are by and large perceived as aggressive, violent and dangerous.

An individual's values and personal beliefs affect his/her attitude about mental illness, the mentally ill and treatment of mental illness. There still exists a stigma surrounding individuals who need to use psychiatric mental health services. The need continues for public education to modify or alter misconceptions about mental illness and people with mental disorders.

MENTAL HEALTH TEAM

Multidisciplinary approach refers to collaboration between members of different disciplines who provide specific services to the patient. The multidisciplinary team includes (Fig. 25.5):

- A psychiatrist
- A psychiatric nurse
- A clinical psychologist
- A psychiatric social worker
- An occupational therapist or an activity therapist
- A pharmacist and a dietitian
- A counselor.

Psychiatrist

A psychiatrist is a medical doctor with special training in psychiatry. He/She is accountable for the medical diagnosis and treatment of patient. Other important functions are:

- Admitting patient into acute care setting
- Prescribing and monitoring psychopharmacologic agents

- Administering electroconvulsive therapy
- Conducting the individual and family therapy
- Participating in interdisciplinary team meetings
- Owing to their legal power to prescribe and write orders, psychiatrists often function as leaders of the team.

Psychiatric Nurse

A psychiatric nurse is a registered nurse with specialized training in the care and treatment of psychiatric patients. He/She may have a Diploma, MSc, MPhil or PhD in psychiatric nursing and is accountable for the biopsychosocial nursing care of patients and their milieu. Other functions include:

- Administering and monitoring the medications
- Assisting in numerous psychiatric and physical treatments
- Participate in interdisciplinary team meetings
- Teach patients and families
- Take responsibility for patient's records
- Act as patient's advocate
- Interact with patients' significant others.

Clinical Psychologist

A clinical psychologist should have a Masters Degree in Psychology or PhD in clinical psychology with specialized training in mental health settings. He/She is accountable for psychological assessments, testing and treatments, and offers direct services such as individual, family or marital therapies.

Psychiatric Social Worker

A psychiatric social worker should have a Masters Degree in Social Work or PhD with specialized training in mental health settings. He/She is accountable for family case work, community placement of patients, conducts group therapy sessions and emphasizes intervention with the patient in social environment in which he/she will live.

Occupational Therapist

An occupational therapist or an activity therapist is accountable for recreational, occupational and activity programs. He/She assists the patients to gain skills that help them cope more effectively to gain or retain employment and to use leisure time.

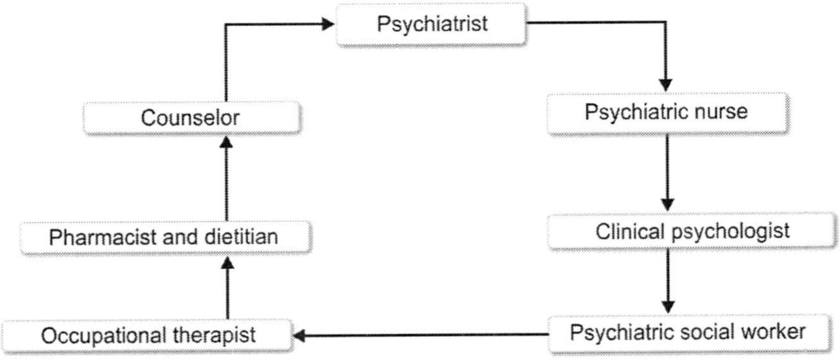

Figure 25.5: Mental health team

Counselor

A counselor provides basic supportive counseling and assists in psychoeducational and recreational activities.

▪ ROLE OF NURSE IN MENTAL ILLNESS

Mental health nursing is often complex, demanding and very rewarding. As many as one in three people are thought to suffer some form of mental health problem. However, dealing with the human mind and behavior is not an exact science. Mental ill health is often brought on by a crisis in life such as depression after the death of a partner. However, depression is just one of the ranges of conditions that come under the heading of mental ill health. There are also neuroses, psychoses, psychological and personality disorders. Therapeutic relationships between the mental health nurse, those with mental ill health and their families are critical to successful mental health nursing. Helping people back to mental health is also every bit as valuable and satisfying as caring for those with a physical illness.

Mental health nurses work with people suffering from various mental health conditions and their family and careers to offer help and support in dealing with the condition. The work involves helping the patient to recover from their illness or to come to terms with it in order to lead a positive life. The nurses may specialize in working with children or older people, or in a specific area such as eating disorders. Mental health nurses often work in multidisciplinary teams, liaising with psychiatrists, psychologists, occupational therapists, general practitioners (GPs), social workers and other health professionals. As a registered mental health nurse (RMN), you may work with patients in a variety of settings including their own homes, community healthcare centers, hospital outpatients departments or specialist units, or secure residential units.

Typical Work Activities

The work carried out by a mental health nurse can vary depending on the setting and specialist group they are working with. But the role typically consists of:

1. Caring for patients experiencing acute mental distress or who have an enduring mental illness.
2. Assessing and talking to patients about their problems, and discussing the best way to plan and deliver their care.
3. Building relationships with patients to encourage trust, while listening to and interpreting their needs and concerns.
4. Ensuring the correct administration of medication, including injections and monitoring the results of treatment.
5. Responding to distressed patients in a non-threatening manner and attempting to understand the source of distress.
6. Applying 'de-escalation' techniques to help people manage their emotions and behavior.
7. Preparing and participating in group and/or one-to-one therapy sessions, both individually and with other health professionals.
8. Providing evidence-based individual therapy, such as cognitive behavior therapy for depression and anxiety.
9. Encouraging patients to take part in art, drama or occupational therapy where appropriate.
10. Organizing social events aimed at developing patients' social skills and helping to reduce feelings of isolation.
11. Preparing and maintaining the patient records.
12. Producing care plans and risk assessments for individual patients.
13. Ensuring that the legal requirements appropriate to a particular setting or group of patients are observed.

14. Working with patients' families and careers, helping to educate them and the patient about their mental health problems.
15. Promoting a recovery-based approach to care.

In community, the role may also involve:

1. Coordinating the care of patients.
2. Liaising with patients, relatives and fellow professionals in the community treatment team. Attending regular meetings to review and monitor patients' care plans.
3. Visiting patients in their home to monitor progress and carrying out risk assessments with regard to their safety and welfare.
4. Assessing patients' behavior and psychological needs.
5. Identifying whether and when patients are at risk of harming themselves or others.

■ CONCLUSION

Mental illness leads to maladjustment in living. It produces a disharmony in the person's ability to meet human needs comfortably or effectively and function within a culture. A mentally ill person loses his/her ability to respond according to the expectations one has from himself/herself.

■ REVIEW QUESTIONS

Long Essays

1. Define mental illness. Explain causes and factors that influence mental illness.
2. Enumerate the normal and abnormal behavior in detail.
3. Explain the roles and responsibilities of a nurse in caring mentally ill patient.

Short Essays

4. Describe the warning signs of mental illness.
5. Discuss the features of mental illness.
6. Disturbances of bodily and mental functions.
7. Explain the common signs and symptoms of mental illness.
8. List out the misconceptions of mental illness.
9. Enumerate in brief about mental health team.

Short Answers

10. Alcohol dependence.
11. Medical model.
12. Behavior model.
13. Problems of mental disorders.
14. General attitude towards mentally ill person.
15. Psychiatric social worker.

CHAPTER 26 Guidance and Counseling

■ INTRODUCTION

The guidance is one of the major applications of psychology. It enables or assists the individuals to solve educational, vocational and psychological problems to guide means a sort of help, assistance or suggestions for progress. In the field of psychology and education, the word guidance is having a specific meaning. It refers to a process of helping the individuals to discover themself, which means, their potentialities and propensities, capacities and capabilities, abilities and aptitudes, interests and natural endowments and to help them in achieving maximum advantage and state.

■ CONCEPT/FEATURES OF GUIDANCE

1. Guidance refers to a process of assisting the individuals to develop their body, mind, personality and character, and to help them in achieving maximum educational, vocational and personal or psychological adjustments.
2. Guidance is regarded as a kind of specialized service provided to the individual to solve problems of crucial nature.
3. Guidance is regarded as any form of assistance given to children who makes their best development of personality.
4. Guidance is not confined to a professional setting, since it is a continuous process starting from early childhood extending up to sometimes old age.
5. Guidance is the educational context. For example, assisting students to select courses of study appropriate to their needs and interests, achieve academic excellence to the best possible.
6. Guidance is not just providing direction, imposition of one's view point on another, making decision for another individual and carrying burden of another's life.

Definition

1. 'Guidance' involves personal help given by someone, it is designed to assist a person to decide where he/she wants to go, what he or she wants to do or how he/she can best accomplish his/her purpose; it assists him/her to solve problems that arise in life. —*Jones, 1951*
2. Fundamental of all guidance is the help or assistance given by a competent person to an individual, so that the latter may direct his/her life by developing own point of view to make own decision and carry out those decisions.

   —*Crow and Crow*

3. The purpose of guidance is to help the student to make more favorable adjustments. —*Fowler*

Principles of Guidance

1. The debility of the individual is supreme.
2. Each individual is different from every other individual.
3. The primary concern of guidance is the individual in one's social setting.
4. The attitudes personal perceptions of the individual provide the basic for action.
5. The individual generally acts to enhance one's perceived self.
6. The individual has the innate ability to learn and therefore can be helped to make choices that will lead to self-direction consistent with reality.
7. The individual needs a continuous guidance process from childhood onwards.
8. Each individual may at times need the information and personalized assistance given by competent professional personal.

Elements of Guidance

1. Guidance focuses our attention on the individual and not the problem.
2. It helps to the discovery of abilities of an individual.
3. It is based on interests, abilities, assets, needs and limitations of the individual.
4. It gives rise to self-development and self-direction.
5. It makes the individual to plan wisely for the present and future.
6. It makes the individual to become adjusted in the new environment.
7. Guidance is helpful in achieving success and happiness.

Characteristics

1. The basis of guidance is individual differences, it is a known fact that no two individual are alike. Individuals are different in capacities, capabilities, potentialities, propensities, abilities, aptitude and variations within the individual.
2. Guidance is the basis of rigid code of ethics, it is important to follow a rigid code of ethics in guidance programs.
3. The basis of guidance is on educational and vocational objectives, it means that guidance realization of educational and vocational aims and objective.
4. Guidance is able to develop the insight of an individual; the counselor is helpful to the individual in such a way that he/she gains insight to make own decisions and choices.
5. Guidance regards most of the individuals as average normal persons; it must be known to all the students that the services of guidance workers are available to all.
6. Guidance is slow, but a continuous process; individuals need considerable time to make suitable adjustments and are unable to make wise decisions choices and adjustments in a day or so.
7. Guidance is universal, it is essential for all the pupils of all the stages. It is for those who seek it and also for those who do not seek it.
8. Guidance is planning: Guidance personnel attempts to review the entire situation and gives plans for future in educational, vocational and social field.
9. Guidance is developmental as well as comprehensive: Guidance is developmental because it is dealing with the month to month, year to year and stage to stage.
10. Guidance is practical side of education; education sets the goal, while guidance makes the realization of that goal.
11. Guidance is mainly child-centered, guidance workers or counselors do not impose anything on individual, but they to find out the needs of the trying

children and provides them only their suggestion.

12. Guidance is considered as an organized service and not incidental, i.e. it is a service, which is having a specific purpose.
13. Guidance is specialized and generalized service; many persons such as the teacher, the parent, the Headmaster, the counselor and the career master play their specific role.

Basic Assumptions of Guidance

1. The differences between individuals in native capacities, abilities and interests are quite significant.
2. Variations within the individual are quite significant.
3. The native abilities are not generally specialized.
4. Abilities and aptitudes do not depend upon race, color and sex.
5. There is always need for assistance to certain crisis.
6. The school is in a strategic position to provide the needed assistance.
7. Guidance is progressive self-directive, but not prescriptive.

Purposes of Guidance (Fig. 26.1)

1. **Understanding the individual:** The main purpose of guidance is to discover and understand capacities and potentialities of the individual, and to make evaluation of the self in relation to personal and social experience, and to use the self more efficiently in everyday living.
2. **Help the individual in making adjustments:** Another aim of guidance is to assist the individual so as to be making satisfactory and maximum adjustments to home, school, teachers, pupils and to society.
3. **Develop personal abilities and potentialities:** Another purpose of guidance is to help the individuals to develop their abilities, potentialities and points of view, to develop their body, mind, personality and character.
4. **Improve school activities:** The guidance programmer helps the school staff to solve problems and improve all the activities of the school.
5. **Coordinating home, school and society:** Erickson as correctly said that one of the important purposes of guidance has been coordinating home, school and community influences on the child.

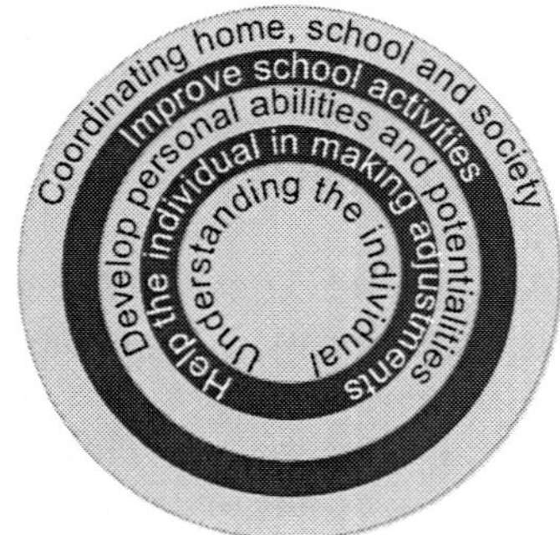

Figure 26.1: Purposes of guidance

Need for Guidance (Fig. 26.2)

1. **Educational need:** Guidance has given to the students to select of subjects of counsel, to select of books, to select of hobbies, to select of co-curricular activities, to develop study habits, to organize time and work, to concentrating on studies, to building social relationship and to make satisfactory progress and adjustments in school.
2. **Psychological need:** Guidance is required from psychological and social point of view. Youth of 20th century is subjected too much great emotional strain in the home and in the community. The number of children having problems, delinquent children, backward children and maladjusted children has been increasing in our schools.

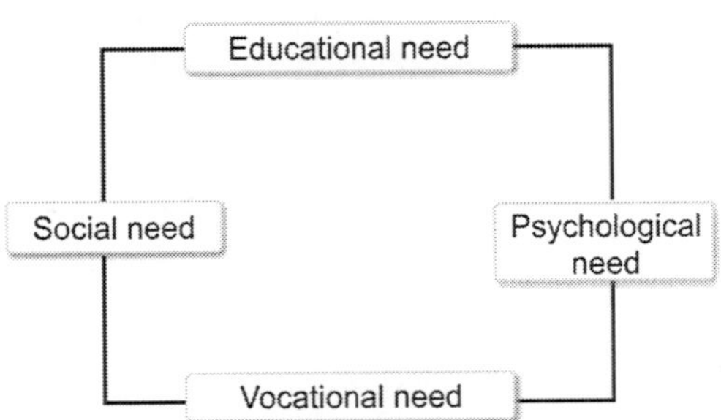

Figure 26.2: Need for guidance

3. **Vocational need:** The vocational guidance is essential for helping the individuals to know themself, for knowing the world of work, adequate information about jobs, skills and opportunities for making a right choice in the vocation according to their abilities, interest and aptitudes and to obtain suitable jobs in their chosen fields.
4. **Social need:** Society is becoming complex, starting changes have occurred in the entire structure of our economic, social and political system.

■ TYPES OF GUIDANCE

- Educational guidance
- Vocational guidance
- Individual guidance service:
  - Religious guidance
  - Guidance for home relationship
  - Guidance for citizenship
  - Guidance for leisure and recreation
  - Guidance for personal well-being
  - Guidance in right doing
  - Guidance in the thoughtfulness and cooperation
  - Guidance in wholesome and cultural action.

Educational Guidance

Guidance services are meant to help students make proper adjustments with the environment in which they are living and also make the best possible contributions commensurate with one's strengths and limitations. Educational guidance refers to guidance to students in all aspects of education.

The emphasis is on providing assistance to students to perform satisfactory in their academic work, choose the appropriate course of study, overcome learning difficulties foster creativity, improve levels of motivation and utilize institutional resources optimally such as library, laboratory, etc.

Definitions

1. The educational guidance deals with assistance or support given to pupils in their choices and adjustments with relation to schools, curriculum, courses and school life. —*Jones*
2. Educational guidance refers to a process, which is concerned with bringing about an individual pupil with distinctive characteristics on the one hand and differing group of opportunities and requirements on the other, a favorable setting for the individual's development or education. —*Myer*

Objectives of Educational Guidance

1. To monitor the academic program of students.
2. To identify special learners such as academically backward, gifted and creative.
3. To assist students in further education.
4. To provide assistance to special learners by catering to their educational needs.
5. To diagnose the learning difficulties of students in different subjects.
6. To help students in their adjustments to curriculum and co-curricular demands of the educational programs.
7. To provide career information.

Need of Educational Guidance

1. **Wastage and stagnation:** There occurs a lot of wastage and stagnation in education. The number of failures in the examination is responsible for much wastage to the nation.
2. **Diversified curriculum:** The curriculum is being diversified in the higher secondary and multipurpose schools. Therefore, the need for guidance in the selection of subjects of studies is becoming an almost necessity.
3. **Decision for further education:** Educational guidance is needed in order to help the pupil to make the best use of their potentialities and resources.
4. **Preparation for future vocation:** There is an urgent need required for preparing and helping the pupils for further vocation, while keeping in view their potentialities, interests and aptitudes, and the demands of the society.

For balanced life simple vocational education is not sufficient, children must be educated to live and help together.

Purposes of Educational Guidance

1. **Wise selection of the curriculum:** It is known that the pupil's success in the field of education depends upon the wise selection of curriculum. Hence, an important purpose of education assists in selecting a curriculum in accordance with their abilities, aptitudes and interests.
2. **Improvement in methods of study:** Another aim of educational guidance is to improve the methods of study. The methods of study includes such factors as made of reading mode of taking notes, methods of memorizing and summarizing.
3. **Providing special methods of education to backward students:** Guidance is mainly given to evolve special methods of education for pupils who usually fail at examinations, show signs of delinquency indiscipline or run away from classes. The methods of education for backward children are evolved by keeping in view the causes of backwardness; include special schools and specialists, and special curriculum and special methods of teaching.
4. **Making special arrangements for gifted students:** Another specific aim of educational guidance is to arrange special educational program for the gifted students.
5. **Taking into account the failures at examination:** A large number of failures at various examinations is responsible for much wastage and stagnation. Many students lose their mental equilibrium as a result of failure.
6. **Educational guidance**:
   a. To help the students to secure information concerning the possibility and desirability of further schooling.
   b. To help them to know the requirements for entrance into the school of their choice.
   c. To help the students to find the purpose and functions of different types of schools.
   d. To guide them for the selection of vocations.

Stages of Educational Guidance

At elementary stage

1. To help pupils to develop good habits, right attitudes and basic skills.
2. To help pupils to make a good beginning.
3. To help pupils to plan intelligently.
4. To help pupils to obtain the best out of their education.

At secondary stage

1. Helping the child to know himself/herself.
2. Helping the child to understand about the environment.

3. Helping the child to make the right choice of subjects.
4. Helping the child to know about the college education.

At college stage

1. Providing library facilities for broadening the mental horizon of the students.
2. Providing special guidance for certain subjects and preparation for examination.
3. Providing special guidance for selection of books and reference books.
4. Guiding the individual to learn how to read books, make notes, summarize and organize the materials, and how to make use of quotations.

Factors Involved in Educational Guidance

1. Secondary schools become less selective.
2. Emphasis upon individual difference.
3. Growing complexity of the world of work.
4. Expansion of the school programs.
5. Concept of the child growth and their development.
6. Beneficial effects of group testing.
7. Influences of social and economic conditions.

Basic Principles of Educational Guidance

1. Guidance should be provided to all.
2. Standardized tests should be employed.
3. Selection of curriculum should be done.
4. Remedy should be given in the beginning.
5. Relevant information has to be obtained.
6. Follow-up study must be there.
7. Relationship between school and parents should be set up.

Vocational Guidance

In this scientific and technological age, one of the most important aspects of man's life is vocation. Therefore, one has to choose vocation for himself/herself. One of the main aims of education is to give maximum help is one's professional life. If vocational aim of education is not fulfilled, then education becomes worthless.

Vocational guidance is fundamentally an effort for conserving the priceless native capacities of youth and the costly training provided for youth in the school. It conserves these riches of all human resources by the individuals to invest and use them, will bring greatest satisfaction and success to them and greatest benefit to society.

Definitions

1. According to International Labor Organization, vocational guidance as assistance given to an individual in solving problems related to occupational choices and progress with due regard for the individuals characteristics and their relation to occupational opportunity.
2. According to vocational guidance association, vocational guidance is the process of assisting the individual to choose an occupation, prepare for it, and enter upon and progressing in it.

Need of Vocational Guidance

1. To increase the number of occupations.
2. Vocational guidance to maintain the health.
3. To promote personal and social values.
4. To discover and utilize the individual potentialities.
5. To meet the needs of an individual and complex nature of the society.
6. To promote the financial growth of an individual and society.

Special Aims of Vocational Guidance

1. To assist the student to acquire suck knowledge of the characteristics and functions, the duties and rewards of the group of occupations.

2. To enable them to find what general and specific abilities, skills, etc. are required for the group of occupations.
3. To give opportunity for experiences in school that will give much information about conditions of work as will assist the individual to discover his/her own abilities, which help in the development of wider interests.
4. To help the individual to develop the point of view that all honest labor is worth and that the most important bases for choice of an occupation.
5. To assist the individual to acquire a technique of analysis of occupation information and to develop the habit of analyzing such information before making a final choice.
6. To assist the individuals to secure such information about themselves, their abilities, i.e. general and specific, their interest and powers, as they may need for wise choice.
7. To assist economically handicapped children who are above the compulsory attendance age to secure through public or private funds, scholarships or other financial assistance.
8. To assist the student to secure knowledge of the facilities offered by various educational institutions for vocational training and the requirements for admission to them, the length of training offered and the cost of attendance.
9. To keep the workers to adjust themselves to the occupation in which, they are engaged; to assist them to understand their relationship with workers in their own related occupations and with society as a whole.
10. To enable the student to secure reliable information about the danger of alluring shortcuts to fortune.

Characteristics of Vocational Guidance

1. It helps the children to develop their potentialities to all optimum level.
2. It is a process, which helps the persons to impart occupational information, broadening occupational horizon and including their interest in vocational self-help.
3. It is a process, which helps the individuals to select an occupation for life, to prepare for it and to place them against a suitable job. Also, their progress in the job is to be watched.
4. It is a process, which helps in the persons to develop and accept an integrated and correct picture of themselves, and their role in the economy of the society to which they belongs.
5. It is a process, which helps the individuals to evaluate their role in term of reality or practicability.
6. It is a process, which helps the individuals to achieve the vocational goal. The process of achieving the vocational goal should be useful to society.
7. It is a process, which helps the individuals to make adjustments in relation to their occupation or job.

Stages of Vocational Guidance

At elementary stage

1. In this period the habits, skills and attitudes develop.
2. For developing basic skills and attitudes.
3. For developing the habit of doing the work in a neat and systematic manner.
4. For developing the good interpersonal relationships.

At secondary stage

1. To help pupil to appraise or know their vocational assists and liabilities.
2. To make pupils to be familiar with various occupations and their requirements.
3. To help pupils to make a right choice.
4. To help pupils to make a right choice.
5. To help pupils to prepare themselves for entering into the occupations of their choices.

6. To help pupils to get suitable jobs in their chosen field.
7. To help pupils to think seriously whether to go to college or not.

At college stage

1. To help people for making a comprehensive study of the cancer, which they would like to pursue.
2. To help pupils to relate their studies to vocations, i.e. open to them.
3. To help pupils for acquainting themselves with different avenues of work.
4. To help pupils to acquainting themselves with avenues for higher studies and various programs for financial assistance, scholarships, stipends, grants, fellowship, etc.
5. To help pupils to make contacts that would help in putting their plans into successful operation.

Individual Guidance Service

Individual guidance service is some type of help, which is provided to individual to understand develop and potentialities, make the best use of potentialities and solve his/her problems. Individual problems are concerned with physical health, home problems, school problems, leisure time problems, sex problems, other emotional and psychological problems, and vocational problems.

Stages of Individual Guidance Service (Fig. 26.3)

At elementary stage

1. The childhood period refers to the period of growth and development.
2. During this stage the basic foundations of physical, intellectual, emotional, social and other type of personality development are laid.
3. It is considered to be the most impressionable period of life, when the character, traits, attitudes, values and habits get developed.

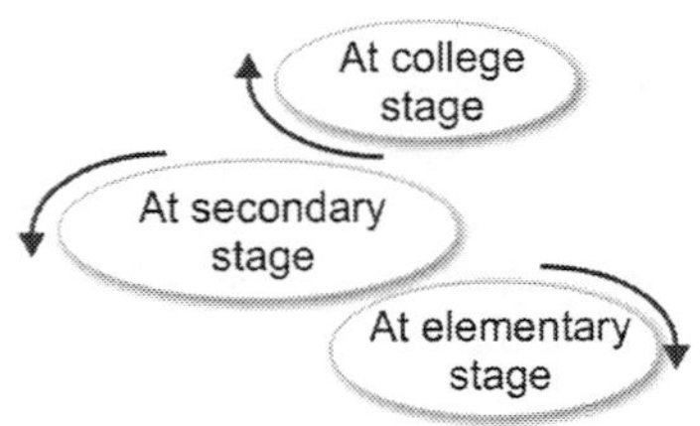

Figure 26.3: Stages of individual guidance service

4. Some of the task or purposes of individual guidance service at this stage are to make a right start in the school, to build good physique and to make emotional adjustments.

At secondary stage

Secondary stage is regarded as the most critical stage of individual's developments, because it is the stage of stress and strain, storm and strife, heightened emotionality and hypersuggestibility, anxieties and worries, conflicts and frustrations. The main aims of individual guidance at this stage are as follows:

1. To make the individual to solve problems concerning physical health.
2. To make the individual to solve problems concerning sex, emotionally and mental health.
3. To guide the individual in making family adjustments.
4. To advise the individual in making social adjustments including adjustment with school.
5. To guide the individual in making suitable progress in the school.

At college stage

The main purpose, aims or functions of individual's guidance at college stage are as follows:

1. Guidance is essential to help the individual in solving all types of the emotional problems, sex problems and other personal problems.
2. It is also needed to help the individual in making adjustment with new environment.

3. It is also needed to help the individual in developing healthy ideas and building a new philosophy of life.
4. Guidance is also essential to help them in participating in social activities.
5. It is also essential to help the individual in making suitable educational progress.
6. It is also essential to help the individual in getting suitable job.

Needs for Individual Guidance Service (Fig. 26.4)

1. **Problems concerning physical health:** The advice and treatment of an expert may be required by an individual for curing physical ailment and building up the physique.
2. **Family problems:** There are many family problems such as the strained relationship between child and parents, between husband and wife, between brothers and sisters, constant quarrels between the father and mother, presence of stepfather or stepmother in the house. Jealousy among various siblings in the family may contribute another factor in home environment, which may become a potent cause of maladjustments.
3. **Utilization of leisure time:** In order to utilize the leisure time profitably individual might require guidance in sports, games and hobbies.
4. **Personal problems:** Sometimes, the main cause of maladjustments are personality problems such as bullying, teasing, frightened, anxiety, nail biting, thumb sucking, grinding of teeth and inferiority complex these difficulties require competent guidance.
5. **School problems:** The individual may be unable to make progress in various academic, physical, social and recreational activities of school, and thus require guidance.
6. **Vocational problems:** The individual might require guidance for selecting the occupation, for adequate training for particular occupation or for the change of an occupation.

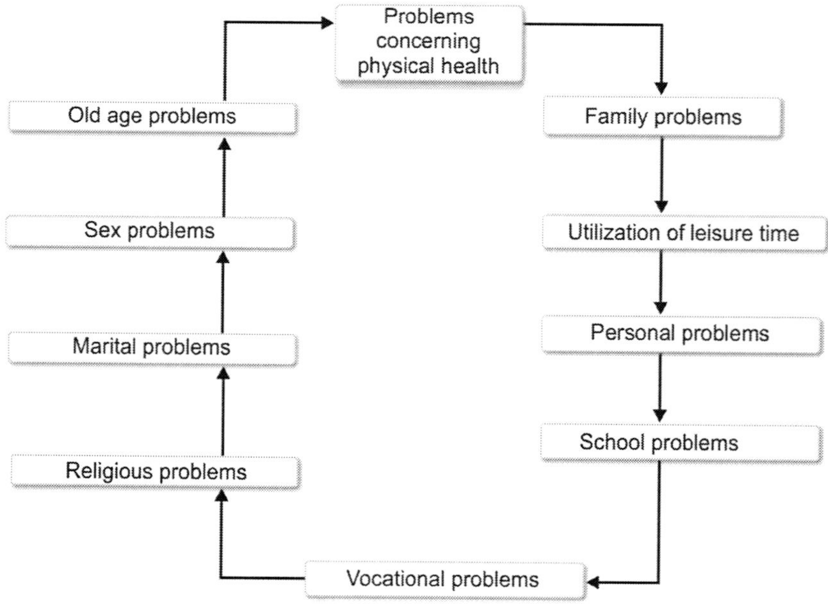

Figure 26.4: Needs for individual guidance service

7. **Religious problems:** The individual might be having certain religious doubts or wrong philosophy of life for which he/she might require guidance.
8. **Marital problems:** Happy man is one who has got the good life partner. For carrying out the right choice of a partner the person might require guidance.
9. **Sex problems:** Sometimes individuals have sex problems due to menstruation, nightmares, excessive sex curiosity, heterosexual interests and activities. In order to help the individual in solving sex problems and in leading a healthy sexual life, individual guidance becomes essentials.
10. **Old age problems:** Old age brings its own problems. At this age various organs of the body loses their strength and the various senses such as eyesight, hearing and smell, etc. will start growing feeble day by day. Such an age group requires guidance regarding proper utilization of time and for keeping the body in strength.

Steps Involved in Individual Guidance Service (Fig. 26.5)

Collection of facts

1. Most of all physical details such as age, sex, physical health and defects such as defect in eyesight, defect in hearing, defect in nose, throat, etc. are to be noted.
2. Then family details such as family background, size, education, income of parents, order of birth in the family, other members in the family, discipline in the home and mutual relations between different members of the family are to be noted.
3. Then details regarding attitude towards school, classmates, teachers, subjects, cocurricular activities, achievements in examinations and sports. Failure and promotions, positions and distinction in the class and main difficulties in school or college subjects are to be noted.

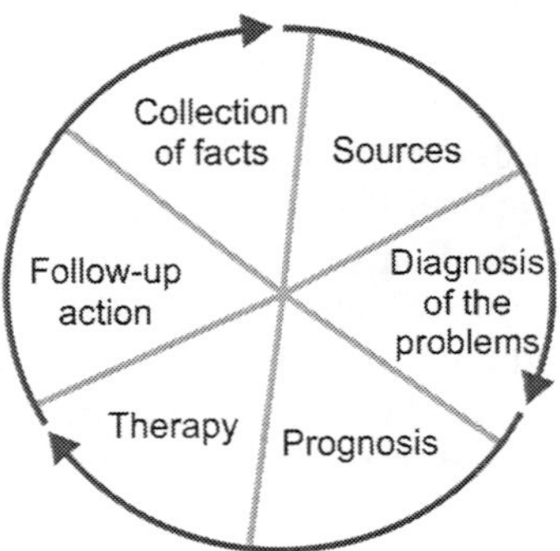

Figure 26.5: Steps involved in individual guidance service

4. The details concerning vocational choices, special skills, vocational interests and ambitions, jobs held in the past, satisfied or dissatisfied during the job, reasons of dissatisfaction, relation with the employer, etc. are to be noted.
5. Then, the details of social development such as individuals relations with parents, brothers and sisters, other relatives, playmates, class fellows, teachers, friends, neighbors, etc. are to be noted.
6. Then, the details concerning mental abilities such as intelligence, aptitudes and other mental abilities should be collected with the help of various tests and examinations intended for the purpose are to be noted.
7. Finally, the details concerning other qualities of personality such as individual's emotional maturity, interests, motives, ambitions and ideals are to be noted.

Sources

1. **Parents:** They can provide quite useful information about the child. This information can be obtained by inviting parents to school on special occupations or contacting them at their homes.
2. **Teacher:** They are also able to provide much information about the student. This information has been based on

observation, individual records, marks secured in examinations, interview and home visits.

3. **Students:** The primary sources of student's (individual's) data have been students themselves and other individuals in the schools. Also their friends and companions can also provide much useful information about them.
4. **Guidance worker:** A guidance worker can obtain information about students from many sources. They may able to collect this information from family doctors, social workers and members of the community.

Diagnosis of the problems

1. After collecting relevant information concerning individual the guidance worker would like to analyze the information so as to find out the ways and means of solving the problem.
2. This process involving the analysis of information and efforts to find out ways and means of solving the problem is called diagnosis of the problem.
3. The guidance worker is unable to impart individual guidance to the individual without proper diagnosis of the problem.

Prognosis

1. Prognosis involves the visualizing the extent to which the guidance workers will be successful in solving person's problem.
2. Guidance workers visualize the result to the guidance, which they offer, to the individual so as to solve his/her problems.
3. For example, by observing a person's past performance in mathematics and by measuring their mental abilities, it is possible to make some tentative estimate of what they will achieve after the guidance is rendered.

Therapy

1. Here the guidance workers offer a satisfactory solution of the problem. They will make the individual gain inspirit to solve his/her problem.
2. Various techniques used in therapy include suggestion, sublimation through substitution, rational persuasion, re-education, play therapy and change in environment, psychoanalysis, group therapy, occupational therapy and non-directive therapy.

Follow-up action

After providing guidance it becomes essential to know that up to what extent the problem is solved. Hence, follow-up becomes essential. Individual guidance is more or less incomplete without follow-up. The following methods find use in follow-up study:

1. **Card file method:** In this method, details of interview such as name of the interview, his/her age, sex, address, purpose of interview and details of the problems have been indicated.
2. **Questionnaire method:** Guidance workers give questionnaire to counselee. In the questionnaire those items are included that deals with various aspects of the progress of problems concerning which the advice was provided.
3. **Contact through letters:** In this method, counselee is contacted through letters, which can be used even to provide further guidance to the person.

■ COUNSELING SERVICE

We have quite often heard the term counseling used in newspaper in the context of counseling for engineering, demission computer-related admissions and so on. Counseling forms the heart of all guidance programs. As we know that proper functioning of the heart, similarly the success or failure of the guidance programs could be determined by counseling service.

Meaning of Counseling

1. Counseling refers to a progress in which the people are made to approach or an

individual level. People get help in educational, vocational or psychological field only at problem points.

2. In counseling, the subject matter would be pupil's needs, abilities, aims, aspirations, plans, decisions, actions and limitations.
3. Counseling may be referred to a sort of specialized, personalized and individualized service, which makes effective use of information gathered about any individual.
4. This information provides self-insight, self-analysis and self-direction. This self-direction helps individual to make maximum education, vocational and psychological adjustments.

Definitions

1. Counseling is a process involving an interaction between a counselor and a client in a private setting, with the purpose of helping the client to change his/her behavior, so that satisfactory resolutions of needs may be obtained.

   —*Pepinsky, 1954*
2. Counseling or assisting an individual in the solution of his/her problems. The interview has an important place in guidance, but is only one stage in the whole process of counseling.

   —*Crow and Crow*
3. Basically counseling involves understanding and working with the individual to discover his/her unique needs, motivations and potentialities, and help to appreciate them.

   —*Bernard and Fullmer*

Characteristics of Counseling

1. Counseling is based on person-to-person relations.
2. It involves two individuals one seeking help and the other, a professionally trained who can help the first.
3. The main aim is to help the counselor to discover and solve client's personal problems independently.
4. In order to help and assist properly the counselor must establish a relationship of mutual respect, cooperation and friendliness between the two individuals.
5. The counselor will try to discover the problems and helps the client to set up goals and guide through difficulties and problems.
6. The main emphasis in the role of counseling process is laid on the counselor's self-direction and self-acceptance.
7. Counseling is democratic; the counselor sets up a democratic pattern and allows the counselee to do freely whatever client like while with the consultant not under the consultant.

Rules and Roles of Counseling (Fig. 26.6)

Remedial Role

1. Remedial role entails working with individuals or groups, to assist them in remedying problems of one kind or another.
2. As noted by Kagan et al (1988), remedial interventions may induce personal, social counseling or psychotherapy for an individual or couples (e.g. marital counseling).
3. Crisis intervention and various therapeutic services for students requiring assistance with unresolved life events are additional examples of work at the remedial level.

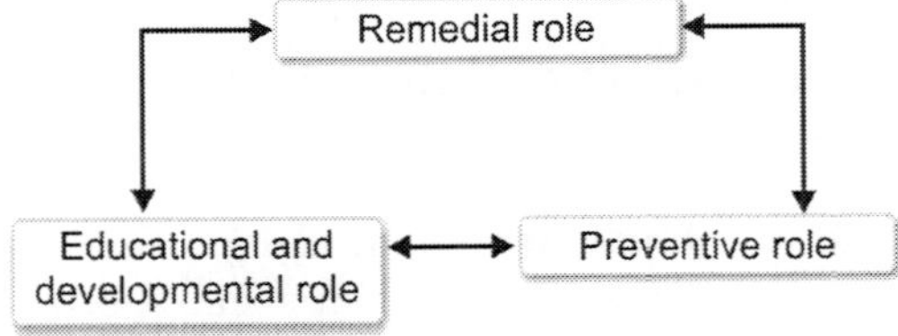

Figure 26.6: Rules and roles of counseling

Preventive Role

1. It is one in which the counseling psychologist seek to anticipate, circumvent and if possible, forestall, difficulties that may arise in the future.
2. Preventive interventions may focus on what are called 'psychoeducational program' aiming to forestall the development of problems or events.

   For example, drug prevention/awareness programs, suicide prevention programs for high risk and psychological adoption of orphan children, which gives them a feeling of belongingness.

Educational and Developmental Role

1. The purpose, which is to help individuals to plan, obtain and derive maximum benefits from the kinds of experiences, will enable them to discover and develop their potentialities.

   Examples of this would include various workshops or seminars. Another example might be a study skill class, where the college students aimed at making good students even more effective.
2. The key features of the developmental role are that when performing it one is going beyond prevention and is involved in enhancement.

Goals of Counseling

- Facilitating behavioral change
- Enhancing copying skills
- Promoting decision-making
- Improving relationships
- Facilitating client potential.

Comparison of Counseling with Other Terms

1. **Guidance and counseling:** These two are not synonyms. Counseling forms a part of guidance not all of it.
2. **Counseling and interview:** Usually interview is a part of counseling; it is only a technique, which is used in the process of counseling.
3. **Counseling and advising:** Counseling does not give advice; a wise counselor ever provides advice until it becomes absolutely essential.
4. **Counseling and teaching:** Counseling does not mean teaching. Teaching is related to academic and instinctual problems, whereas counseling is related to social and emotional problems.
5. **Counseling and psychotherapy:** Counseling is not considered as psychotherapy, although it is used by psychotherapist as one of the technique of treatment. Counselor does work in educational setting, while psychotherapist does work in medical setting.

Theories of Counseling

1. Williamson EG is the leading architect of this school of thought.
2. It is also called prescriptive or counselor-centered counseling.
3. It is considered to be problem centered and patient centered.
4. It is the counselor, who prepare plans and sees through the process.

Assumptions of Counseling

1. All the efforts should be done to tackle the problem of the counselee.
2. As counselor is more competent than the counselee, it means that the former plays a more active role than the client.
3. Counseling is more or less an intellectual rather than emotional process. Hence an intellectual aspect is assigned more weightage than emotional aspects.

Types of Counseling

There are three types of counseling:

- Directive counseling

- Non-directive counseling
- Eclectic counseling.

Directive Counseling

Steps

1. **Analysis:** Collection of data is carried out from a variety of sources by using a variety of tools and techniques.
2. **Synthesis:** Summarizing and organizing the data are to be carried out so as to reveal the client's assets, liabilities, adjustments and maladjustments.
3. **Diagnosis:** At this stage an attempt should be made to find out the root cause of the problem exhibited by the client.
4. **Prognosis:** At this stage the future development of the client's problems should be predicted.
5. **Treatment:** It includes establishing report, advice or plan programs.
6. **Follow-up:** Here the counselor makes an attempt to help the clients with new problem or with recurrences of the original problem and ascertains the effectiveness of counseling provided to them.

Advantages

1. It is more economical in time.
2. Its emphasis mainly lay on the problem, but not on the individual.
3. Directive counseling lays more emphasis on the intellectual rather than the emotional aspects of the personality of the individual, but not at the emotional level.
4. The directive counseling methods used have been direct, persuasive and are explanatory.

Limitations

1. The counselor would never become independent of the counselor.
2. Directive counseling is unable to keep the counselee away from making mistakes in future.

Non-directive Counseling

Carl Rogers is the chief architect of this school of thought:

1. It is also known as permissive counseling or client-centered counseling.
2. In this type of counseling, the counselor forms the pivot or the center. It is the counselee who plays the main role.
3. It is the counselee who actively participates in the process, gets insight into his/her problem by using the counselor and takes decisions to take action.

Assumption

1. Independence and integration of the client have been more important than the client.
2. Emotional aspects have been more significant than intellectual aspects.
3. Creating an atmosphere in which the clients can work out their understanding has been more important than cultivating self-understanding in the client.
4. Counseling results in a voluntary choice of goals and a conscious selection of courses of action.

Steps

1. The client is able to recognize the need of counseling and come for help. Help is sought and not given.
2. The counselor is able to define the situation and creates congenital atmosphere.
3. Attitude of the counselor has been friendship, sympathy and affection. Counselor is interested in the child and encourages free expression of feeling regarding the problem of individuals.
4. The counselor makes an attempt to understand the feelings of the individual.
5. The counselor accepts as well as recognizes the positive and negative feelings.
6. The counselor will pay attention to negatives self-feelings of the client or child and changes him/her from negative self-feelings to positive self-feelings, from emotional release to gradual insight.

7. The counselor makes the client to translate his/her insight to action.
8. A decreased need for help is desired and the client is the one who decides to the contact.
9. Positive steps towards the solution of the problem situation begin to start.

Advantages

1. It is a slow, but sure process, which makes the individual capable of making adjustments.
2. No tests are used in it and therefore avoid all that is laborious and difficult.
3. It is able to remove the emotional block and makes the individual to bring the repressed thoughts in conscious level, thereby reducing tension.

Limitations

1. It is quite slow and time-consuming process. In school it is not feasible as counselor has to attend many students.
2. The child, the client or the student, or the counselor is unable to make the decisions. Hence, we fail to rely upon their resources, judgment and wisdom.
3. There are many individuals who may lead from stages to stage. The counselor's passive attitude might be able to irritate the counselee so much that they might hesitate to express their feelings.

Eclectic Counseling

1. Eclectic counseling may be defined as the synthesis and combinations of directive and non-directive counseling.
2. In this counseling, the counselor has been neither too active as in directive counseling, nor too passive as in non-directive counseling.
3. In elective counseling, the counselor first of all consider the personality and needs of the counselee and then selects the directive or non-directive technique that would serve the purpose best.
4. Throne is the chief architect of eclectic counseling.

Steps

1. To diagnose the cause.
2. To analyze the problem.
3. To prepare a tentative plan for modifying factors.
4. To secure effective conditions for the counseling.
5. To interview and stimulate the clients to develop their own resources and to assume its responsibility for trying new models of adjustments.
6. To do proper handling of any related problems, which may be able to contribute to adjustments.

Generalizations

1. Generally passive methods should be used whenever possible.
2. Passive techniques are preferred in the early stages if the client is telling his/her story. This allows emotional release.
3. Active methods are to be used with specific indication.
4. Complicated methods should not be tried until simpler methods have failed.
5. All counseling should be client-centered.
6. Every child should be given an opportunity to resolve his/her problems non-directly.
7. Directive methods are generally involved in situational maladjustment where a solution cannot be achieved without involving cooperation of other persons.
8. Some degree of directiveness will be inevitable in all counseling even in reaching the decision to use passive methods.

Limitations

1. Eclectics are not possible because it is not possible to merge directive and non-directive concepts together.
2. According to some writers, eclectics are vague, superficial and opportunistic.

Basic Principles of Counseling

Acceptance: The client must be accepted as a whole person as a human being.

Respect for the individual: Importance is attached to respect for individual.

Permissiveness: All schools of counseling would accept relative permissiveness of counseling relationship.

Learning: All schools of counseling should accept the learning element in counseling.

Thinking in rather than for the client: It is another basic principle of counseling.

Functions or Duties of Counselor

1. Program of guidance and its organization, which includes such as vocational information service, self-inventory service and personal data collection service, counseling service, vocational preparatory service, placement and employment service, follow-up or adjustment service.
2. Orientation implies a sort of preparation, which includes collecting data about sources of jobs, disseminating information to pupils and planning activities.
3. Data collection should be done about the individual, administering the test and analyzing the same.
4. Interviews and individual counseling should be held.
5. Contact should be made outside agencies such as parents, guidance, bureaus and employment exchanges.
6. Placement and follow-up work should be done.

Characteristics or Qualifications of Counselor (Fig. 26.7)

Personality Traits

1. **Breadth of interest:** A counselor must be interested in various types of people, jobs and organization.
2. **Cooperation:** A counselor should cooperate with all the staff in a cheerful manner.

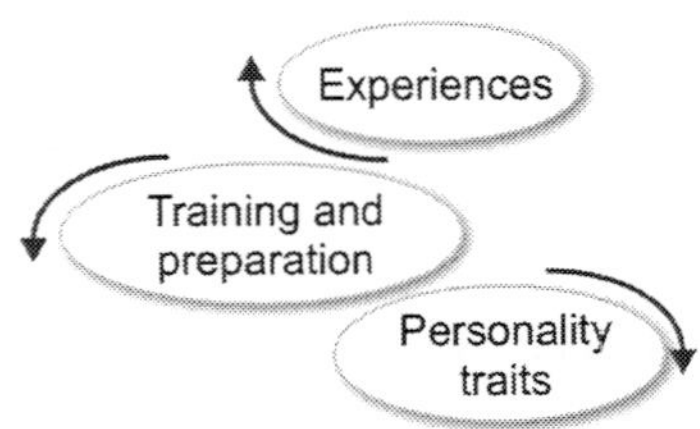

Figure 26.7: Characteristics or qualifications of counselor

3. **Refinement:** A counselor should not be overconfident, but should be modest and humble towards the pupils.
4. **Magnetism:** A counselor should create confidence in others and put other at ease.
5. **Considerateness:** A counselor should understand the difficulties of teachers, exhibit human understanding and possess real love for fellowmen.

Training and Preparation

Good education, which includes knowledge of humanities such as sociology, psychology, economics, history and geography, etc. It helps:

1. To know principles of guidance.
2. To know of objectives, curriculum and methods secondary schools.
3. To know vocational activities.
4. To know methods of imparting occupational information.
5. To know psychological tests in guidance services.
6. To know organization of guidance services.

Experiences

1. Competence as a leader in guidance programs.
2. Competence as a counselor.
3. Competence in interpreting and using information.
4. Competence in placement and follow-up services.

5. Competence in using community resources.
6. Competence in evaluating the counseling service itself.

CONCLUSION

Present day teachers have acquired some specialized knowledge regarding guidance and counseling in order to guide the students tactfully in this highly competitive world. Guidance services, which are aimed at bringing about desirable adjustment in any particular area of independence, must take into account the all-round development of the individual.

REVIEW QUESTIONS

Long Essays

1. Define guidance. Explain the concepts and elements of guidance.
2. Define counseling. Explain the meaning and characteristics of counseling.

Short Essays

3. Describe the principles of guidance.
4. List out the characteristics of guidance.
5. Discuss the types of guidance.
6. Stages of individual guidance services.
7. Enumerate the rules and roles in counseling.
8. Describe the various types of counseling.
9. Explain the functions and duties of counselor.

Short Answers

10. Purpose of guidance.
11. Aims of vocational guidance.
12. Objectives of educational guidance.
13. Individual guidance services.
14. Goals of counseling.
15. Eclectic counseling.
16. Basic principles of counseling.
17. Characteristics of counselor.

BIBLIOGRAPHY

1. Anthikad Jacob. Psychology for Graduate Nurses, 4th edition. New Delhi: Jaypee Brothers Medical Publisher (P) Ltd; 2007.
2. Bhatia BD, Craig Margaretta. Elements of Psychology and Mental Hygiene for Nurses in India. Chennai: Orient Longman (P) Ltd; 2005.
3. Bhatia BD, Craig Margaretta. Elements of Psychology and Mental Hygiene for Nurses in India. Chennai: Orient Longman; 2005.
4. Das G. Educational Psychology, New Delhi: Kind Books (P) Ltd.
5. Gabor D. First contact body language. In: How to Start a Conversation and Make Friends. Revised edition. Rockefeller center, New York: Fireside Publications; 2001.
6. Grant. Child development in India, 3rd edition. New Delhi: Ashish publishing house; 1992.
7. Gross Richard, Kinnison Nancy. Psychology for Nurses and Allied Health Professionals. London: Hodder Arnold; 2007.
8. Hilgard RE, Atkinson CR, Atkinson LR. Introduction to Psychology, 6th edition. New Delhi: Oxford & IBH Publishing Co (P) Ltd; 1975.
9. Hurlock B Elizabeth. Developmental Psychology: A Lifespan Approach, 5th edition. New Delhi: Tata McGraw-Hill Edition; 2002.
10. Khan MA. Psychology for Nurses. Delhi: Academa Publishers; 2004.
11. Kupuswamy B. An Introduction to Social Psychology. Bombay: Media Promoters and Publishers (P) Ltd; 1994.
12. Mangal SK. Advanced Educational Psychology, 6th edition. New Delhi: Prentice Hall of India (P) Ltd; 2007.
13. Mangal SK. General Psychology. New Delhi: Sterling Publishers (P) Ltd; 2006.
14. Matlin W, Margaret. Psychology, 3rd edition. Philadelphia: Harcourt Brace College Publishers; 1999.
15. Morgan CT. A Brief Introduction to Psycholog. New Delhi: Tata McGraw-Hill; 1975.
16. Morgan CT, King RA. Introduction to Psychology, 6th edition. New Delhi: Tata McGraw-Hill; 1982.

17. Morgan T Cifford, Kind A Richard, Weisz R John, et al. Introduction to Psychology, 7th Edition. New Delhi: Tata McGraw-Hill Publishing Company Limited; 2004.
18. Munn, Norman L. Introduction to Psychology. New Delhi: Oxford & IBH; 1973.
19. Myers G David. Social Psychology, 6th edition. Boston: Mc Craw-Hill College; 1991.
20. Nagaraja KR, Begum Shamshad B, Sudarshan CY. MCQs in Psychology for Nursing and Allied Sciences. New Delhi: Jaypee Brothers Medical Publishers (P) Ltd; 2006.
21. Ramnath Sharma. Psychology and Mental Hygiene for Nurses. Meerut: Kedarnath Ramnath & Co.
22. Robert S Feldman. Understanding Psychology, 6th edition. New Delhi: Tata McGraw-Hill Edition; 2004.
23. Robinson DN. An Intellectual History of Psychology. New York: Macmillan; 1976.
24. Santrock, JW Child Development, 7th edition. Sydney: Brown and Bench mark publishers; 1996.
25. Sinclair C Helen, Fawcett N Josephine. Altschul's Psychology for Nurses, 7th edition. London: Bailliere Tindall; 1991.
26. Skinner E Charles. Educational Psychology, 4th edition. New Delhi: Prentice-hall of India (P) Ltd; 1996.
27. Taylor E Shelley. Health Psychology, 6th edition. New York: Tata McGraw-Hill Edition; 2006.
28. Tendon BN. Management of severely malnourished children by village workers through ICDS in India. J Trop Pediatr. 1984;30(5):274-9.

CHAPTER 27

Psychological Assessment and Tests

■ INTRODUCTION

Psychological testing refers to the administration of psychological tests. A psychological test is 'an objective and standardized measure of a sample of behavior'. The term sample of behavior refers to an individual's performance on tasks that have usually been prescribed beforehand. The samples of behavior that make up a paper-and-pencil testing (PPT), the most common types of test are a series of items. Performance on these items produces a test score. A score on a well-constructed test is believed to reflect a psychological construct such as achievement in a school subject, cognitive ability, aptitude, emotional functioning, personality, etc. Differences in test scores are thought to reflect individual differences in constructing the test, which is supposed to measure. The technical term for the science behind psychological testing is psychometrics.

■ HISTORY OF PSYCHOLOGICAL TESTING

1. Circa 1000 BC, Chinese introduced written tests to help fill civil service positions.
2. In 1850, the United States begins civil service examinations.
3. In 1890, James Cattell developed a 'mental test' to assess college students. Test includes measures of strength, resistance to pain and reaction time.
4. In 1905, Binet-Simon scale of mental development used to classify mentally retarded children in France.
5. In 1914, World War I (WWI) produces need in US to quickly classify incoming recruits. Army Alpha test and Army Beta test developed.
6. In 1916, Terman developed Stanford-Binet test and develops the idea of intelligence quotient.
7. In between 1920 and 1940 factor analysis, projective tests and personality inventories first appear.
8. In 1941–1960, vocational interest measures developed.
9. In 1961–1980, item response theory and neuropsychological testing developed.
10. From 1980 till present, wide spread adaptation of computerized testing. 'Smart tests', which can give each individual different test items to develop.

■ DEFINITION

1. Psychological tests are written, visual or verbal evaluations administered to assess the cognitive and emotional functioning of children and adults.

2. Psychological testing means the use of one or more standardized measurements. Instruments, devices, or procedures including the use of computerized psychological tests, to observe or record human behavior and which require the application of appropriate normative data for interpretation or classification are used. It also includes the use of standardized instruments for the purpose of the diagnosis and treatment of mental and emotional disorders and disabilities, the evaluation or assessment of cognitive and intellectual abilities, personality or emotional states and traits, and neuropsychological functioning.

■ COMMON AREAS OF PSYCHOLOGICAL TESTING (Fig. 27.1)

Educational Testing

Intelligence tests and achievement tests are used from an early age in the US. From kindergarten, tests are used for placement and advancement.

Personnel Testing

Following World War I (WW I), business began taking an active interest in testing job applicants. Most government jobs require some civil service examination. At the Lally School of Management, the Myers-Briggs type indicator is used extensively to assess managerial potential. Type testing is used to hopefully match the right person with the job they are most suited for.

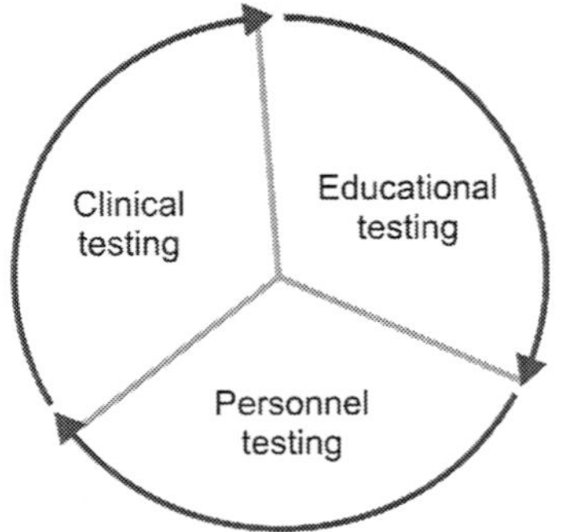

Figure 27.1: Common areas of psychological testing

Clinical Testing

Tests of psychological adjustment and tests, which can classify and/or diagnose patients are used extensively. Neuropsychological tests, which examine basic mental function, also fall into this category.

■ PURPOSES OF PSYCHOLOGICAL TEST

Psychological tests are used to assess a variety of mental abilities and attributes, including achievement and ability, personality and neurological functioning. For children, academic achievement, ability and intelligence tests may be used as tools in school placement, in determining the presence of a learning disability or a developmental delay, in identifying giftedness, or in tracking intellectual development. Intelligence testing may also be used with teens and young adults to determine vocational ability (e.g. in career counseling). Personality tests are administered for a wide variety of reasons, from diagnosing psychopathology (e.g. personality disorder, depressive disorder) to screening job candidates. They may be used in an educational setting to determine personality strengths and weaknesses.

Psychological tests are formalized measures of mental functioning. Most are objective and quantifiable; however, certain projective tests may involve some level of subjective interpretation. Also known as inventories, measurements, questionnaires and scales, psychological tests are administered in a variety of settings, including preschools, primary and secondary schools, colleges and universities, hospitals, outpatient healthcare settings, social agencies, prisons, and employment or human resource offices. They come in a variety of formats including written, verbal and computer administered.

■ MEANING OF PSYCHOLOGICAL TESTING

Psychological tests are used for assessment and evaluation of the test taker by a competent examiner. That is why it is also called psychological assessment. But of course, the tests can only be accurate and reliable, if you answer it carefully, honestly and seriously. A competent psychologist is generally the interpreter of these psychological tests. But it should be noted that psychological tests are advantageous only in certain situations. Free psychological tests circulated through the internet are usually bests for entertainment purposes.

Psychological testing, also called psychological assessment, is the foundation of how psychologists better understood a person and their behavior. It is a process of problem solving for many professionals to try and determine the core components of a person's psychological or mental health problems, personality, IQ, or some other component. It is also a process that helps to identify not only just weaknesses of a person but also their strengths. Psychological testing measures an individual's performance at a specific point in time—right now. Psychologists talk about a person's 'present functions functioning' in terms of their test data. Therefore psychological tests cannot predict future or innate potential.

Psychological testing is not a single test or even a single type of test. It encompasses a whole body of dozens of research-backed tests and procedures of assessing specific aspects of a person's psychological makeup. Some tests are used to determine IQ, others are used for personality and still others for something else. Since so many different tests are available, it is important to note that not all of them share the same research evidence for their use—some tests have a strong evidence base, while others do not.

Psychological assessment is something that typically done in a formal manner only by a licensed psychologist (the actual testing may sometimes be administered by a psychology intern or trainee studying to become a psychologist). Depending upon what kind of testing is being done, it can last anywhere from 1½ hours to a full day. Testing is usually done in a psychologist's office and consists largely of PPT (nowadays often administered on a computer for ease of use).

■ PRINCIPLES OF PSYCHOLOGICAL TESTS (Fig. 27.2)

Proper psychological testing is conducted after vigorous research and development in contrast to quick web-based or magazine questionnaires that say 'find out your personality color,' or 'what is your inner age?,' etc. Proper psychological testing consists of the following:

1. **Standardization:** All procedures and steps must be conducted with consistency and under the same environment to achieve the same testing performance from those being tested.
2. **Objectivity:** Scoring is free of subjective judgments or biases based on the fact that the same results are obtained from everyone.

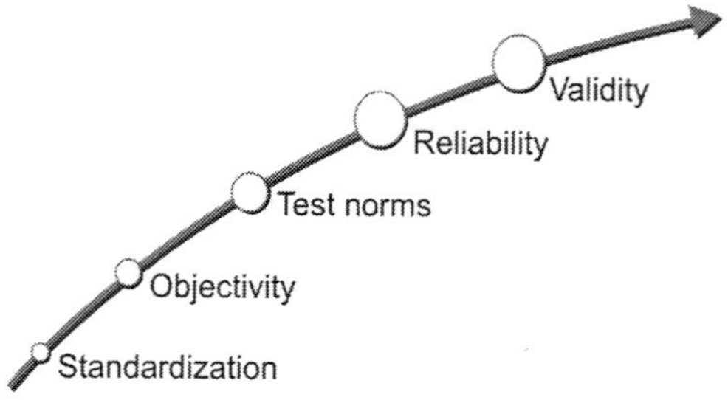

Figure 27.2: Principles of psychological testing

3. **Test norms:** The average test score within a large group of people where the performance of one individual can be compared to the results of others by establishing a point of comparison or frame of reference.
4. **Reliability:** Obtaining the same result after multiple testing.
5. **Validity:** The type of test being administered must measure what it is intended to measure.

CHARACTERISTICS OF PSYCHOLOGICAL TEST

1. **Reliability:** Test consistency or the ability to yield the same result under a variety of different circumstances.
2. **Validity:** Ability of a test to measure, what it is intended to measure.
3. **Percentile system:** Ranking of test scores that indicate the ratio of scores lower or higher than a given score.
4. **Norms:** Standard of comparison for test results developed by giving the test to large, well-defined groups of people.
5. **Intelligence:** Ability to acquire new ideas and behaviors, and adapt to new situations.
6. **Two-factor theory:** Proposes that two factors contribute to an individual's intelligence, first factor is 'G' for general intelligence and second is 'S' for specific mental abilities.
7. **Triarchic theory:** Proposes that it can be divided into three ways of processing information—analytical, creative, physical.
8. **Emotional intelligence:** It has four major aspects of interpersonal and intrapersonal intelligences.
9. **Intelligence quotient (IQ):** Standardized measure of intelligence based on a scale in which 100 is average.
10. **Heritability:** The degree to which a characteristic is related to genetic and inherited factors.
11. **Cultural bias:** An aspect of intelligence test in which the wording used in questions may be more familiar to people of one social group than the other group.
12. **Aptitude test:** Estimates the probability that a person will be successful in learning a specific new skill.
13. **Achievement test:** Measures how much a person has learned in a given subject or area.
14. **Interest test:** Measures a person's preferences, attitudes and interests in certain activities.
15. **Personality test:** Assesses personality characteristics and identifies problems.
16. **Objective test:** Forced-choice test in which a person must select one of several answers designed to study personal characteristics.
17. **Projective test:** Unstructured test, in which a person is asked to respond freely, giving his/her own interpretation of various ambiguous stimuli.

FUNCTIONS OF PSYCHOLOGICAL TESTS (Fig. 27.3)

1. **Detection of specific behavior:** Psychological test is used to measure and to detect the abilities of a person.
2. **Individual differences:** A psychological test is used to measure the individual differences, which are different between abilities of different persons and the performance of the same person at different time.

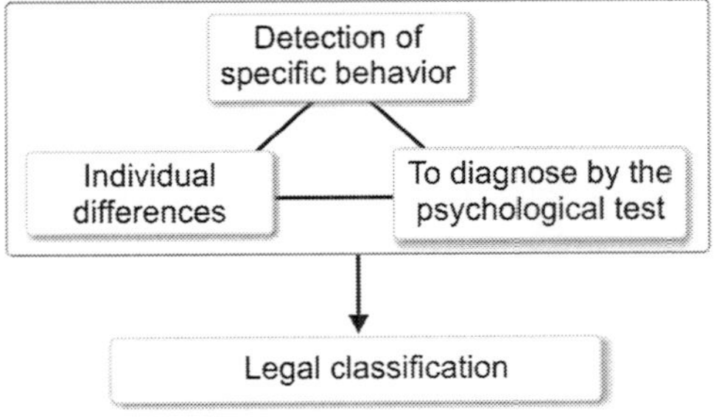

Figure 27.3: Functions of psychological testing

3. **To diagnose by the psychological test:** The psychological tests are usually used in clinical psychology. In clinical psychology a test's function is to diagnose mental disorders. So tests are used in mental hospitals and coaching, and guidance centers for the assessment and diagnose of mental disorders. Major tests are Minnesota Multiphase Personality Inventory (MMPI), Roteer Incomplete Sentences Blank (RISB), Bender-Gestalt Test, and Raven's Progressive Matrices (RPM), etc.
4. **Legal classification:** A psychological test helps in classifying a number of people into different categories, e.g. normal and abnormal, criminal and innocent, intellectual and mentally retarded, able and disable, etc.

■ METHODS OF LEGAL CLASSIFICATION

1. **Selection:** The people who express certain level of performance on a test are selected and others are rejected.
2. **Screening:** An ordinary test refers to a quick survey to located individuals who may need or be eligible for special treatment.
3. **Certification:** At the end of certain training program a test is used to recommend that the objectives of training program has been achieved and the person has acquired the desired skill to perform in the relevant field.
4. **Placement:** It is a sorting process that provides different level of serving for different persons.
5. **Promoting self-understanding:** A psychological test provide standardized information about the abilities, capabilities, aptitudes, potential competencies, interest, trait and states of a person, which helps in understanding one's personality and planning future prospective.
6. **Program evaluation:** An effectiveness of a particular program is assessed by the applications of some kind of test. This function is usually performed by an achievement test.
7. **Scientific inquiry or research:** Some experts use tests for research purpose, which provide information about the mental level and personality of the subject.
8. **Military selection:** A closely related application of psychological testing is to be found in the selection and classification of military personal. From simple beginnings in the WW I, the scope and variety of psychological tests employed in military situations underwent a phenomenal increase during WW II. Subsequently research on test development has been containing on a large scale in all brands of the normed services.
9. **Industry:** In industry and business tests are helpful in selection and classifying personal for placement in jobs that range from the simpler semiskilled to the highly skilled, from the selection of filling clerks and salesperson to top management for any of these position. However, test results are only one source of information though an important one industrial and organizational (IO) psychology (also known as IO psychology, work psychology, organizational psychology, work and organizational psychology, industrial psychology, occupational psychology, personnel psychology or talent assessment) applies psychology to organizations and the workplace.
10. **Education:** Psychological tests especially those of general intelligence and of specific aptitudes have very extensive use in educational classification, selection and planning from the 1st grade (and sometimes earlier) through the university. Prior to WW II schools and

colleges were the largest users of psychological tests.

11. **Mental hospitals:** In clinical or mental hospitals psychological tests are used primarily for individual diagnoses of factors associated with personal problems of learning, behavior attitudes or specific interpersonal relations.

■ IMPORTANCE OF PSYCHOLOGICAL TESTS

A psychological test is an instrument designed to measure unobserved constructs, also known as latent variables. Psychological tests are typically, but not necessarily, a series of tasks or problems that the respondent has to solve. Psychological tests can strongly resemble questionnaires, which are also designed to measure unobserved constructs, but differ in that psychological tests ask for a respondent's maximum performance whereas a questionnaire asks for the respondent's typical performance. A useful psychological test must be both valid (i.e. there is evidence to support the specified interpretation of the test results) and reliable (i.e. internally consistent or give consistent results over time, across raters, etc.).

It is important that people who are equal on the measured construct also have an equal probability of answering the test items correctly. For example, an item on a mathematics test could be 'in a soccer match two players get a red card; how many players are left in the end?' However, this item also requires knowledge of soccer to be answered correctly, not just mathematical ability. Group membership can also influence the chance of correctly answering items (differential item functioning). Often tests are constructed for a specific population and this should be taken into account when administering tests. If a test is invariant to some group difference (e.g. gender) in one population (e.g. England), it does not automatically mean that it is also invariant in another population.

Psychological assessment is similar to psychological testing, but usually involves a more comprehensive assessment of the individual. Psychological assessment is a process that involves checking the integration of information from multiple sources, such as tests of normal and abnormal personality, tests of ability or intelligence, tests of interests or attitudes, as well as information from personal interviews. Collateral information is also collected about personal, occupational, or medical history, such as from records or from interviews with parents, spouses, teachers, or previous therapists or physicians. A psychological test is one of the sources of data used within the process of assessment; usually more than one test is used. Many psychologists do some level of assessment when providing services to clients or patients and may use simple checklists used for treatment settings to assess a particular area of functioning or disability often for school settings, to help select type of treatment or to assess treatment outcomes, to help courts decide issues such as child custody or competency to stand trial, or to help assess job applicants or employees and provide career development counseling or training.

■ PSYCHOLOGICAL TEST AND ASSESSMENT

Tests and assessments are two separate, but related components of a psychological evaluation. Psychologists use both types of tools to help them arrive at a diagnosis and a treatment plan. Testing involves the use of formal tests such as questionnaires or checklists. These are often described as 'norm-referenced' tests. That simply means the tests have been standardized so that test-takers are evaluated in a similar way, no matter where they live or who administers the test. For example, a norm-referenced test of a child's reading abilities may rank that child's ability compared to other children of similar age or grade level. Norm-referenced tests have been developed and evaluated by researchers and proven to be effective for measuring a particular trait or disorder.

A psychological assessment can include numerous components such as norm-referenced psychological tests, informal tests and surveys, interview information, school or medical records, medical evaluation and observational data. A psychologist determines what information to use based on the specific questions being asked. For example, assessments can be used to determine if a person has a learning disorder, is competent to stand trial or has a traumatic brain injury. They can also be used to determine, if a person would be a good manager or how well they may work with a team.

One common assessment technique for instance is a clinical interview. When a psychologist speaks to a client about his/her concerns and history, they are able to observe how the client thinks, reasons and interacts with others. Assessments may also include interviewing other people who are close to the client, such as teachers, coworkers or family members (such interviews, however, would only be performed with written consent from the client). Together, testing and assessment allows a psychologist to see the full picture of a person's strengths and limitations.

■ PRECAUTIONS OF PSYCHOLOGICAL TEST

Psychological testing requires a clinically trained examiner. All psychological tests should be administered, scored and interpreted by a trained professional, preferably a psychologist or psychiatrist with expertise in the appropriate area. Psychological tests are only one element of a psychological assessment. They should never be used alone as the sole basis for a diagnosis. A detailed history of the test subject and a review of psychological, medical, educational, or other relevant records are required to lay the groundwork for interpreting the results of any psychological measurement. Cultural and language differences in the test subject may affect test performance and may result in inaccurate test results. The test administrator should be informed before psychological testing begins, if the test taker is not fluent in English and/or belongs to a minority culture. In addition, the subject's motivation and motives may also affect test results.

■ CLASSIFICATION OF PSYCHOLOGICAL TESTING

Psychological testing is divided into four primary types:

- Clinical interview
- Assessment of intellectual functioning
- Personality assessment
- Behavioral assessment.

Clinical Interview

The clinical interview is a core component of any psychological testing. Some people know the clinical interview as an 'intake interview,' 'admission interview' or 'diagnostic interview' (although technically these are often very different things). Clinical interviews typically last from 1 to 2 hours in length, and occur most often in a clinician's office. Many types of mental health professionals can conduct a clinical interview—psychologists, psychiatrists, clinical social workers, psychiatric nurses, amongst others. The clinical interview is an opportunity for the professional to gather important background and family data about the person. Think of it as an information gathering session for the professional's benefit (but ultimately for the benefit).

Assessment of Intellectual Functioning

Intellectual quotient is a theoretical construct of a measure of general intelligence. It is important to note that IQ tests do not measure actual intelligence—they measure what we believe might be important components of intelligence. There are two primary measures used to test a person's intellectual functions—intelligence tests and neuropsychological assessment. Intelligence tests are the more common type administered and include the Stanford-Binet and the Wechsler scales. Neuropsychological assessment, which can take up to 2 days to administer, is a far more extensive form of assessment. It is focused not only just on testing for intelligence but also on determining all of the cognitive strengths and deficits of the person. Neuropsychological assessment is most usually done with people who have suffered some sort of brain damage, dysfunction or some kind of organic brain problem, just as having a brain hemorrhage.

The most commonly administered IQ test is called the Wechsler Adult Intelligence Scale-Fourth Edition (WAIS-IV). It generally takes anywhere from hour to hour and a half to administer, and is appropriate for any individual aged 16 or older to take (children can be administered an IQ test especially designed for them called the Wechsler Intelligence Scale for Children–Fourth Edition, or the WISC-IV). The WAIS-IV is divided into four major scales to arrive at what is called 'full scale IQ'. Each scale is further divided into a number of mandatory and optional (also called supplemental) subtests. The mandatory subtests are necessary to arrive at a person's full scale IQ. The supplemental subtests provide additional, valuable information about a person's cognitive abilities.

■ TYPES OF PSYCHOLOGICAL TESTS

Achievement Tests

The IQ tests purport to be measures of intelligence, while achievement test are measures of the use and level of development of use of the ability. IQ (cognitive) tests and achievement test are common norm-referenced tests. In these types of tests, a series of tasks is presented to the person being evaluated, and the person's responses are graded according to carefully prescribed guidelines. After the test is completed, the results can be compiled and compared to the responses of a norm group, usually composed of people at the same age or grade level as the person being evaluated. IQ tests, which contain a series of tasks typically divide the tasks into verbal (relying on the use of language) and performance, or non-verbal (relying on eye–hand types of tasks, or use of symbols or objects). For example, verbal IQ test tasks are vocabulary and informative type (answering general knowledge questions). Non-verbal examples are timed completion of puzzles (object assembly) and identifying images, which fit a pattern (matrix reasoning).

Public Safety Employment Tests

Vocations within the public safety field (i.e. fire service, law enforcement, corrections, emergency medical services) often require industrial and organizational psychology tests for initial employment and advancement throughout the ranks. The National Firefighter Selection Inventory, the National Criminal Justice Officer Selection Inventory (NCJOSI) and the integrity inventory are prominent examples of these tests.

Attitude Tests

Attitude test assess an individual's feelings about an event, person, or object. Attitude scales are used in marketing to determine individual (and group) preferences for brands, or items. Typically attitude tests use either a Thurstone scale, or Likert scale to measure specific items.

Neuropsychological Tests

These tests consist of specifically designed tasks used to measure a psychological function known to be linked to a particular brain structure or pathway. Neuropsychological test can be used in a clinical context to assess impairment after an injury or illness known to affect neurocognitive functioning. When used in research, these tests can be used to contrast neuropsychological abilities across experimental groups. Although the content of individual neuropsychological evaluations may differ, the evaluation typically includes measures of intellectual functioning and some assessment of emotional/personality functioning. In addition, several domains of cognitive (thinking) ability are assessed.

Memory: The client will be asked to learn and remember new information (short stories, word lists, geometric designs and faces), and to recall them later. Ability to recall information learned in the past may also be assessed.

Language: Ability to name objects, comprehend and follow directions, speak, read, write and repeat may be assessed in different ways.

Spatial and perceptual: Ability to analyze visual designs, assemble puzzles or appreciate spatial relationships may be measured with specific tests.

Attention and concentration: Ability to pay attention for short or long periods of time may be assessed using tests of mental arithmetic, speeded writing or other abilities. Ability to concentrate, while distracted may also be accessed through tests requiring one to perform two tasks at once.

Problem solving: Real life or abstract problems to solve will be given. How these problems are analyzed and solved may be evaluated.

Motor and sensory abilities: One may be asked to perform some tasks in which fine motor coordination is assessed or to respond quickly to sensory input. Many neuropsychological examinations also contain measures that are designed to ensure that the patient is putting forth her best effort in performing the tasks.

Neuropsychological tests can be quite useful in defining cognitive and behavioral strengths and weaknesses as well as in diagnosis of specific medical conditions. If the results are abnormal, this does not necessarily mean that the person is cognitively impaired. Various emotional conditions (depression, anxiety, confusion and mental dullness) can impair neuropsychological test performance. Because of this, the neuropsychologist takes into account all reasonable explanations of the profile in interpreting the results. In most cases, the results will also lead to specific recommendations for treatment or management of the patient's problems.

Infant and Preschool Assessment

Due to the fact that infants and preschool aged children have limited capacities of communication, psychologists are unable to use traditional tests to assess them. Therefore, many tests have been designed just for children from birth to around 6 years of age. These tests usually vary with age respectively from assessments of reflexes and developmental milestones, to sensory and motor skills, language skills and simple cognitive skills. Common tests for this age group are split into categories such as infant ability, preschool intelligence and school readiness.

Common Infant Ability Tests

Gesell Developmental Schedules (GDS), which measures the developmental progress of infants, Neonatal Behavioral Assessment Scale (NBAS), which tests newborn behavior, reflexes and responses, modified-ordinal scales of psychological development (M-OS-PD), which assesses infant intellectual abilities, and Bayley-III, which tests mental ability and motor skills.

Personality Tests

Psychological measures of personality are often described as either objective test or projective tests. The terms 'objective test 'and 'projective test' have recently come under criticism in the Journal of Personality Assessment. The more descriptive 'rating scale or self-report measures' and 'free response measures' are suggested, rather than the terms 'objective tests' and 'projective tests,' respectively.

Objective Tests (Rating Scale or Self-report Measure)

Objective tests have a restricted response format such as allowing for true or false answers or rating using an ordinal scale. Prominent examples of objective personality tests include the MMPI, Millon Clinical Multiaxial Inventory, Child Behavior Checklist, Symptom Checklist 90, Beck Depression Inventory and objective personality tests can be designed for use in business for potential employees such as the NEO-PI, 16PF, and the occupational personality questionnaire, all of which are based on the big five taxonomy. The big five or five-factor model of normal personality has gained acceptance, since the early 1990s when some influential meta-analyses (e.g. Barrick and Mount, 1991) found consistent relationships between the big five personality factors and important criterion variables.

Projective Tests (Free Response Measures)

Projective tests allow for a freer type of response. For example, this would be the Rorschach test in which a person states what each of 10 inkblots might be. Projective testing became a growth industry in the first half of the 1900s, with doubts about the theoretical assumptions behind projective testing arising in the second half of the 1900s. Some projective tests are used less often today because they are more time consuming to administer and because the reliability and validity are controversial.

Direct Observation Tests

Although most psychological tests are 'rating scale' or 'free response' measures, psychological assessment may also involve the observation of people as they complete activities. This type of assessment is usually conducted with families in a laboratory, home or with children in a classroom. The purpose may be clinical, such as to establish a preintervention baseline of a child's hyperactive or aggressive classroom behaviors or to observe the nature of a parent-child interaction in order to understand a relational disorder. Direct observation procedures are also used in research, e.g. to study the relationship between intrapsychic variables and specific target behaviors, or to explore sequences of behavioral interaction.

Interest Tests

Psychological tests to assess a person's interests and preferences. These tests are used primarily for career counseling. Interest tests include items about daily activities among which applicants select their preferences. The rationale is that if a person exhibits the same pattern of interests and preferences as people who are successful in a given occupation, then the chances are high that the person taking the test will find satisfaction in that occupation.

Aptitude Tests

Psychological tests to measure specific abilities, such as mechanical or clerical skills. Sometimes these tests must be specially designed for a particular job, but there are also tests available that measure general clerical and mechanical aptitudes. For example, an aptitude test is the Minnesota Clerical test, which measures the perceptual speed and accuracy required to perform various clerical duties. Other widely used aptitude tests include the Differential Aptitude Tests (DATs), which assess verbal reasoning, numerical ability, abstract reasoning, clerical speed and accuracy, mechanical reasoning, space relations, spelling and language usage. Another widely used test of aptitudes is the Wonderlic test. These aptitudes are believed to be related to specific occupations and are used for career guidance as well as selection and recruitment.

Vocational Tests

Vocational tests also referred to as career tests or occupational tests are used to measure the interests, values, strengths and weaknesses. This information is then used in order to determine which careers or occupational settings are most suitable for. Career psychologists and counselors most commonly use vocational assessments to help their clients make decisions about their future educational goals and career choices.

■ PSYCHOLOGICAL TEST PREPARATION

Prior to the administration of any psychological test, the administrator should provide the test subject with information on the nature of the test and its intended use, complete standardized instructions for taking the test (including any time limits and penalties for incorrect responses), and information on the confidentiality of the results. After these disclosures are made, informed consent should be obtained from the test subject before testing begins (except in cases of legally mandated testing, where consent is not required for the subject). All psychological and neuropsychological assessments should be administered, scored and interpreted by a trained professional. When interpreting test results for test subjects, the test administrator will review with subjects—what the test evaluates, its precision in evaluation, any margins of error involved in scoring, and what the individual scores mean in the context of overall test norms and the background of the test subject.

Services that are described as 'psychological testing' shall only be administered and interpreted by persons credentialed by this board or who meet the formal academic training and experience qualifications described above, and who are otherwise exempt by statute:

1. Persons credentialed by this board, as well as other licensed or certified professionals, may also use tests of language, education and achievement, as well as tests of abilities, interests and aptitudes. With the exception of the test categories and psychological tests listed in Section 2 of this administrative regulation, the use of these other tests is not exclusively within the scope of this administrative regulation.
2. Members of other professions shall not train or supervise any person in performing psychological testing.
3. The practice of psychology shall be construed within the meaning of the definition contained in KRS 319.010(7) without regard to, if payment is received for services rendered.
4. Services that are described as 'psychological testing and treatment' shall be administered to minor children only upon the notification of and the granting of written permission by the parent or legal guardian, unless otherwise required by the courts subject to specific state or federal law.

■ ADVANTAGES OF PSYCHOLOGICAL TEST

Properly developed psychometric tests and questionnaires, when used by competent and appropriately qualified individuals have the following advantages:

1. They lead to judgments that are likely to be more valid than judgments made by other means. This is the most important advantage of psychometric assessment.
2. They are relatively cheap and easy to administer when compared to other approaches. For example, although it may seem relatively expensive for a company to pay for its staff to become qualified in psychometric assessment and then on top of this to pay for the cost of the testing itself, these costs pale into insignificance when one considers just how long it would take to obtain the same information about a person. At the risk of putting it simplistically, it could be argued that the information obtained from a good personality questionnaire might take several months of knowing and working with a person to obtain by other means.
3. They are likely to lead the considerable cost benefits in the long term. Whether it is for selection of new staff or development of existing staff, the expenses involved in psychometric assessment are minimal, when compared with the costs of high-turnover, under performance or misemployment of staff.

■ DISADVANTAGES OF PSYCHOLOGICAL TEST

1. There are numerous tests and questionnaires on the market, which purport to be 'psychometric instruments,' but which are not. Unfortunately, it is very difficult for untrained people to distinguish these from good psychometric instruments. In many cases, these tests and questionnaires have been put together by people with no background in psychometrics and they have very little actual utility and value for the purposes for which they are marketed.
2. Lack of correct training is also a significant danger in the use of psychometric testing. Although there exists in the UK, a training qualification system developed by the British Psychological Society, it is not uncommon for tests to be used by people who are not adequately trained to use them. Indeed, even attendance at a recognized training course is no guarantee that a person will at all times use tests and questionnaires correctly, since some instruments, particularly personality questionnaires, require considerable experience and the possibility of misinterpretation or inappropriate interpretation of results is ever present.
3. It is the use of personality questionnaires to try for assessing a person's ability or skill in a particular area. For example, if a person scores highly on a personality dimension called 'leadership,' this does not mean that he/she will actually possess a high level of leadership skill. Rather, it means that the person has the basic personality characteristics that are commonly found amongst effective leaders and with sufficient experience, and given the development of certain necessary skills, has the potential to become an effective leader. Unfortunately, however scores on scales such as this are often taken to imply that the person already has all the necessary skills and is already capable of performing at a high level in the area in question.

■ LIMITATIONS OF PSYCHOLOGICAL TEST (Fig. 27.4)

Psychological tests assess and evaluate information about an individual or group. Types of psychological tests include intelligence tests, neuropsychological tests, occupational tests, personality tests and specific clinical tests such as current level of anxiety

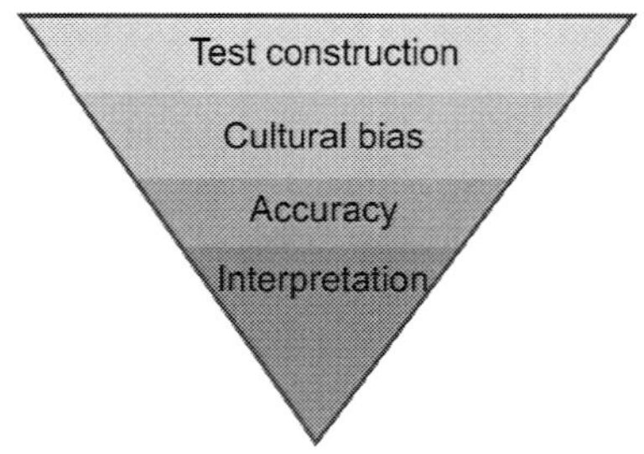

Figure 27.4: Limitations of psychological testing

or depression. Effective and accurate psychological tests are objective, reliable, valid, based on sound norms and standardized. Take the limitations of psychological testing into account, when evaluating results.

Test Construction

Some psychological tests are constructed in ways that make them unreliable and unscientific. The Enneagram and the Myers-Briggs Type Indicator tests are based on personality 'types' and not based on science. Another example is the Rorschach inkblot test, which involves presenting individuals with inkblots; they must then interpret for meaning. The reliability of this test is not high, as its interpretation depends on the psychologist and not objective results.

Cultural Bias

Many psychological tests, particularly intelligence tests can carry cultural biases. They assume all individuals have the same experiences and proficiency with the English language. Individuals from a ethnic minority may interpret items in a psychological test differently due to their culture and upbringing, which may result in a disproportionate and inaccurate result.

Accuracy

Psychological tests may be inaccurate for a number of reasons. Individuals taking the test may give false responses. They may fake or distort answers in a bid to portray themselves in a positive light. This issue becomes particularly salient during tests that involve employment suitability.

Interpretation

Even the most skilled in evaluating psychological test results can make errors, which becomes more likely when the test involves cognitive or emotional responses, which are more likely than behavioral responses to garner a subjective interpretation. The same response may receive different scores depending on who scores the test. This limitation may result in an inaccurate test result and compromise the validity of the test.

■ ROLE OF NURSES IN PSYCHOLOGICAL ASSESSMENT

Assessment of psychological conditions of patients is important for intervention. It is very important for the nurses to know what a psychological test is, how tests are constructed and used, what the uses of these tests are, and how to interpret the results of tests, etc. Then only she will be able to choose an appropriate test to suit particular purpose and particular person.

When a report of psychological testing is presented to a nurse, she must be in a position to understand and interpret these results. For example, when an X-ray along with report is presented to a nurse, she can definitely understand where the fracture is, what type of fracture and what precautions must be taken, etc. In the same way, when a report of intelligence test is presented, she should be in a position to know the level of mental retardation in a mentally challenged child. So, also a report about a neurotic case is presented, she should be in a position to understand the nature of the disease in that particular patient. For example, Eysenck's Personality Inventory (EPI) is administered to know the level of neuroticism, extraversion and introversion. Similarly MMPI is used to know psychoticism and other mental problems. Interests and aptitude tests are very useful in rehabilitation process of a patient. She can decide suitable recreational and occupational training for that patient. The nurses who go for higher studies and research in psychology definitely need this knowledge. In this way nurses have a major role to play in psychological assessment.

■ CONCLUSION

Psychological assessment is a process that involves the integration of information from multiple sources such as psychological tests and other information such as personal and medical history, description of current symptoms and problems by either self or others. Psychological test is one of the sources of data used within the process of assessment; usually more than one test is used. Psychological tests are standard measures devised to assess behavior objectively and used by psychologists to help people make decisions about their lives and understand more about themselves.

■ REVIEW QUESTIONS

Long Essays

1. Define psychological assessment. Explain the commonly used areas of psychological testing.
2. Describe the types of psychological tests in detail.

Short Essays

3. Describe the purpose of psychological testing.
4. Discuss the principles used in psychological testing.
5. Enumerate the functions and characteristics of psychological testing.
6. Enumerate the preparations needed for psychological testing.
7. List out the advantages, disadvantages and limitations of psychological testing.

Short Answers

8. Importance of psychological testing.
9. Clinical interview.
10. Achievement tests.
11. Interest tests.
12. Role of nurse in psychological assessment.

■ BIBLIOGRAPHY

1. American Educational Research Association, American Psychological Association, and National Council on Measurement in Education. Standards for Educational and Psychological Testing. Washington, DC: American Educational Research Association; 1999.
2. American Psychological Association. Standards for Educational and Psychological Testing. Washington DC: APA Press; 1999.
3. Braaten E, Felopulos G. Straight Talk About Psychological Testing for Kids. New York: Guilford Press; 2003.
4. Oscark. The Buros Institute of Mental Measurements at the University of Nebraska-Lincoln. In: Barbara S, Plake, James C, Lincoln I (Eds). The Fifteenth Mental Measurements Yearbook. NE: University of Nebraska-Lincoln Press; 2003.
5. Mellenbergh GJ. Item bias and item response theory. International Journal of Educational Research. 1989;13(2):127-43.

Appendices

APPENDIX I

Previous Years Psychology Questions

2015

■ LONG ESSAYS

1. a. Define thinking.
   b. Describe favorable elements in thinking.
2. a. Define personality.
   b. Explain in detail about psychoanalytical theory of personality.
3. a. Define psychology.
   b. Explain its factors and scope with special reference to nursing.

■ SHORT ESSAYS

4. Explain the sources of stress.
5. Factors affecting perception.
6. Attitudes during health and illness.
7. Methods of memorizing.
8. Describe the laws of learning.
9. Explain different types of defensive mechanism
10. Role of nurse in psychological assessment.
11. Grief and stages of grief.
12. Techniques of controlling emotions.

■ SHORT ANSWERS

13. Behavior.
14. Illusions.
15. Transfer of learning.
16. Reasoning.
17. Likert's attitude scale.
18. Superego.
19. Physical traits.
20. Competition.
21. Experimental psychology.
22. Incentives.

2014

■ LONG ESSAYS

1. Define psychology. Explain the methods of psychology.
2. Explain theories of emotion. What do you mean by emotional state?
3. How personality is assessed? What are the types of personality?

■ SHORT ESSAYS

4. What is the role of hereditary and environment in shaping behavior?
5. Distribution of intelligence.
6. Nature of factors influencing creativity.
7. What is thinking? Describe types of thinking.
8. Nature and biological causes of forgetting.
9. What is intelligence quotient? Discuss the present status of intelligence tests and its uses in nursing.
10. Role of nurse and attitude.
11. Explain the role of emotions in health and sickness.
12. Problem solving.

■ SHORT ANSWERS

13. Conflicts.
14. Extrasensory perception.
15. Span of attention.
16. Social motives.
17. Amnesia.
18. Self-actualization.
19. Genius.
20. Abstract thinking.
21. Genes.
22. Steps involved in creative thinking.

2013

LONG ESSAYS

1. Define intelligence. Explain the theories of intelligence.
2. Explain social motives.
3. Define emotion. Explain the theories of emotion.

SHORT ESSAYS

4. Explain the theories of forgetting.
5. Explain hereditary.
6. Explain body-mind relationship.
7. Explain factors that determine attention.
8. Explain principles of grouping and organization.
9. Explain types of thinking.
10. Physiological changes in emotion.
11. Explain trial and error method of learning.
12. Explain methods of improving memory.

SHORT ANSWERS

13. Psychology.
14. Attention.
15. Learning.
16. Memory.
17. Creative thinking.
18. Genius.
19. Hereditary.
20. Conflicts.
21. Attitude.
22. Interview.

2012

■ LONG ESSAYS

1. Define psychology. Explain experimental method with its merits and demerits.
2. Describe personality. Explain the types of personality.
3. What is learning? Explain Pavlov's classical conditioning theory of learning.

■ SHORT ESSAYS

4. Theory of intelligence.
5. Uses of psychology.
6. Types of memory.
7. Characteristics of mentally healthy person.
8. Types of thinking.
9. Hereditary environment.
10. Theories of forgetting.
11. James-Lange theory of emotions.
12. Types of conflicts.

■ SHORT ANSWERS

13. Case study.
14. Parapsychology.
15. Rationalization.
16. Attention.
17. Memory.
18. Motivation.
19. Sublimation.
20. Intelligence quotient.
21. Stress.
22. Introspection.

2011

■ LONG ESSAYS

1. Define defense mechanism. Explain any two with examples.
2. Explain the concepts and theories of motivation.
3. Define personality and theories of personality.

■ SHORT ESSAYS

4. Briefly explain the preventive strategies in mental health.
5. Explain trial and error method of learning.
6. Difference between learning by classical conditioning and operant conditioning.
7. What is reasoning? Explain errors of thinking.
8. Differentiate long- and short-term memory.
9. Describe the perceptual organization.
10. Elaborate effective way of memorizing.
11. Explain varieties of attention.
12. Explain two theories of emotion.

■ SHORT ANSWERS

13. Ego.
14. Biological motives.
15. Conflicts.
16. Motivational cycle.
17. Stress.
18. Principles of heredity.
19. Reasoning.
20. Tools of thinking.
21. Personal motives.
22. Aggression.

2010

LONG ESSAYS

1. Define conflicts. How it is related to motives?
2. Explain the importance of personality in nursing.
3. What emotions do patients usually experience? What provoke these emotions?

SHORT ESSAYS

4. What is perception?
5. Determinants of emotion.
6. Methods of psychology.
7. Individual differences.
8. Creativity.
9. Organization of perception.
10. Students' achievement tests.
11. Role of nurse and attitude.
12. Types of memory.

SHORT ANSWERS

13. Counseling.
14. Super ego.
15. Needs.
16. Rationalization.
17. Illusion.
18. Intelligent quotient (IQ).
19. Chromosomes.
20. Physical traits.
21. Introspection.
22. Reward and punishment.

2009

■ LONG ESSAYS

1. Define personality. Explain theories of personality.
2. Define perception. Explain the organization of perception.
3. Define intelligence. Explain the theories of intelligence.

■ SHORT ESSAYS

4. Briefly explain about the brain functions and behavior.
5. Illustrate factors affecting attention.
6. Write a note on classical conditioning.
7. Theories of intelligence.
8. Insightful learning.
9. Methods to improve learning.
10. Factors influencing attitude.
11. Write about abnormal behavior.
12. Role of nurse in mental health promotion.
13. Scope of psychology.
14. Theories of motivation.
15. Frustration.

■ SHORT ANSWERS

16. Applied psychology.
17. Heredity.
18. Aptitude.
19. Stress.
20. Mention the theories of emotions.
21. Types of motivation.
22. Thinking.
23. Learning.
24. Forgetting.
25. Types of psychological test.

2008

■ LONG ESSAYS

1. Explain the meaning and scope of educational psychology.
2. Define emotion and explain the theories of emotion.
3. Discuss the role of heredity and environment in causing individual differences.

■ SHORT ESSAYS

4. Explain Thorndike theory of trial and error learning, and their implications.
5. Describe introspection as a method of educational psychology with merits and demerits.
6. Write a short note on projective technique.
7. Explain the factors that influence the personality of a person.
8. Define intelligence. Explain different tests of intelligence.
9. Briefly explain Maslow's theory of hierarchy of needs.
10. Explain the causes of forgetting.
11. Briefly explain about teacher-learner relationship.
12. Write a note on formation of attitude.
13. Explain the factors influencing attention.

■ SHORT ANSWERS

14. Positive transference.
15. Extinction.
16. Schedules of reinforcement.
17. Define personality.
18. Branches of psychology.
19. Mnemonics.
20. Rationalization.
21. Drive and motive.
22. Body and mind relation.
23. Extrasensory perception.

2007

■ LONG ESSAYS

1. Distinguish between primary and secondary drives. Describe briefly the physiological drives that determine a person's daily behavior.
2. How would you define thinking? Describe the process by means of which concepts are formed.
3. Discuss various methods of psychology used to study the behavior.

■ SHORT ESSAYS

4. Describe the steps involved in scientific problem solving.
5. Describe the emotion that encourages health. List other emotions that hamper the healthy functioning of the body.
6. What is the general importance of psychology? Why should a student nurse study psychology?
7. What effect does acute illness have on personality?
8. What do you understand by adjustment mechanism? Do they serve any useful purpose?
9. Role of questionnaire in personality assessment.
10. Mention the meaning and nature of forgetting.
11. How attitude can be changed?
12. Discuss various traits composition necessary to have nurse-patient relationship.
13. Explain the role of environment in causing individual differences.

■ SHORT ANSWERS

14. Behavior.
15. Principles of heredity.
16. Integrated responses.
17. Hunger drive.
18. Distraction of attention.
19. Sensation.
20. Conflict.
21. Emotion as motives.
22. List the branches of psychology.
23. Creativity.

2006

LONG ESSAYS

1. Elucidate factors influencing the development of personality and its characteristics.
2. Discuss the laws of learning. Explain role of motivation and anxiety on learning process.
3. Define emotion. Describe various theories and state of emotion.

SHORT ESSAYS

4. Personality triats and an ideal nurse.
5. Factors influencing perception.
6. Explain the purposes of evaluation.
7. Explain the factors influencing memory.
8. Define frustration and its sources.
9. Role of nurse in change of attitude.
10. What are the types of memory? How can memory be improved?
11. Describe the factors that control and direct attention.
12. Explain the role of emotion in health and sickness.
13. Factors influencing the development of attributes.

SHORT ANSWERS

14. Conflict in motives.
15. Genius.
16. Maternal drive.
17. Chromosomes.
18. Amnesia.
19. Self-actualization.
20. Introverts.
21. Define concepts.
22. Insightful learning.
23. Interview method.

2005

■ LONG ESSAYS

1. Describe the scope of psychology. Explain it with reference to nursing.
2. What is ego defense mechanism? Explain any two with examples.
3. How are perceptions organized? Explain perceptual disturbances with examples.

■ SHORT ESSAYS

4. Distinguish between sensation and perception.
5. Define intelligence. How does it help in human adjustment?
6. Explain the factors influencing attention.
7. What is forgetting? List some factors affecting forgetting.
8. What is conflict of motives? Explain various types of conflicts.
9. What is a concept? How is it developed?
10. Explain experimental method in psychology?
11. What is transfer of learning? Describe some modern theories of transfer of learning.
12. Span of attention.
13. Explain the characteristics of an effective teacher.

■ SHORT ANSWERS

14. Levels of thinking.
15. Causes of individual differences.
16. Reasoning and types of reasoning.
17. Creativity.
18. Educational psychology and developmental psychology.
19. Integrated responses.
20. Habit interference.
21. Biological motives.
22. Emotion and health.
23. Types of intelligence.

2004

LONG ESSAYS

1. Define psychology. Explain its nature and scope with special reference to nursing.
2. How is personality assessed? What are different types of personality?
3. What are motives? Classify the different motives.

SHORT ESSAYS

4. What is forgetting? How can it be minimized?
5. Briefly describe the organization of personality.
6. Role of incentives and rewards in teaching.
7. Explain the importance of personality in nursing.
8. Name the verbal and performance tests of intelligence.
9. Describe the operant conditioning by skinner.
10. Elaborate theories of emotion.
11. Can attention be divided? Explain.
12. Differentiate long- and short-term memory.
13. What is thinking? Describe types of thinking.

SHORT ANSWERS

14. Biological motives.
15. Sensation and perception.
16. Creativity.
17. Extinction and spontaneous recovery.
18. Motivational cycle.
19. Conflicts.
20. Emotion as motives.
21. Observation method.
22. Steps of evaluation.
23. Reward and punishment.

2003

■ LONG ESSAYS

1. What is intelligence? Discuss the various intelligence tests and their use in nursing situation.
2. Discuss the various theories of emotion and bring the relationship between emotions and health.
3. Explain heredity and environment. Discuss their role in causing individual differences.

■ SHORT ESSAYS

4. Usefulness of questionnaires in education.
5. Role of heredity and environment on behavior.
6. Bring out the steps in creative thinking.
7. Elaborate effective ways of memorizing.
8. Explain educational implications of transfer of training.
9. Enumerate and explain determinants of attention.
10. Discuss the role of incentive and punishment in education.
11. What is forgetting? Explain the organic (biological) causes of forgetting.
12. Explain purpose of evaluation and their steps.
13. What are projective tests? Explain their role in personality assessment.

■ SHORT ANSWERS

14. Conflicts.
15. Motivational cycles.
16. 'Aha' effects in insight learning.
17. Short-term memory.
18. Span of attention.
19. Social motives.
20. Introspection.
21. Superego.
22. Stress.
23. Definition of psychology.

2002

LONG ESSAYS

1. Explain the various methods of psychology.
2. Define emotion. Explain how emotion can be a motive. What are the effects of emotion?
3. How do we resolve conflicts? Explain two ways of resolving conflicts.

SHORT ESSAYS

4. Role of endocrine glands on behavior.
5. What is extrasensory perception? Explain with examples.
6. Explain different principles of heredity.
7. What is operant conditioning? Explain with special references to skinner.
8. Explain the factors affecting memory. Describe various methods of memorizing.
9. Define learning. Explain the various types of learning.
10. Define attitudes. Explain its nature and characteristics.
11. Bring out the similarities and differences between introspection and observation.
12. Describe the present status of intelligence testing.
13. Explain Piaget and Bruner's contribution in concept formation.

SHORT ANSWERS

14. Factors affecting learning.
15. Effective teaching.
16. Definition of educational psychology.
17. Habit interference.
18. Distribution of intelligence.
19. Stress.
20. Conflicts.
21. Nursing and psychology.
22. Steps in evaluation.
23. Division of attention.

2001

■ LONG ESSAYS

1. Write an essay on the nature and scope of psychology. What is its relevance in the study of human behavior?
2. Give an account of the biological, personal and social motives. Classify motives.
3. Describe the scope and aims of educational psychology. Point out its significance in nursing profession.

■ SHORT ESSAYS

4. Definition of perception and attention.
5. Assessment of personality. What is its importance in nursing care?
6. Different tests of intelligence.
7. Heredity and environment.
8. What are the conditions for effective learning?
9. Problem-solving methods.
10. Meaning and nature of attributions.
11. Teacher-learner relationships.
12. Tools of evaluation.
13. Personal and social motives.

■ SHORT ANSWERS

14. Levels of functioning.
15. Span of attention.
16. Extrasensory perception.
17. Biological motives.
18. Types of personality.
19. Meaning of intelligence.
20. Behavior of an organism.
21. Principles of learning.
22. Types of thinking.
23. Evaluation.

2000

LONG ESSAYS

1. Explain the questionnaire and experimental methods of psychology.
2. Define personality. Explain the different theories of personality.
3. What is learning? Describe the concept of classical conditioning by Pavlov.

SHORT ESSAYS

4. What is extrasensory perception?
5. Enumerate theories of emotion.
6. Explain the trial and error learning.
7. What are the uses of intelligence tests?
8. Bring out the difference between biological and social motives.
9. Describe the types of conflicts.
10. Examine merits and demerits of introspection.
11. What are the determinants of attention?
12. Examine the influence of heredity and environment in human development.
13. Elucidate nature and factors influencing creativity.

SHORT ANSWERS

14. Division and distraction of attention.
15. Intelligence quotient (IQ).
16. Insight learning.
17. Mnemonics.
18. Emotions and health.
19. Transfer learning.
20. Factors influencing perception.
21. Definition of personality.
22. Reinforcement.
23. Errors in thinking.

1999

■ LONG ESSAYS

1. Explain the concept and theories of motivation. How could it facilitate in patient's quick recovery?
2. What is forgetting? Outline the factors responsible for forgetting.
3. Define personality. Mention any one classification.

■ SHORT ESSAYS

4. Application of psychology to nursing.
5. Determinants of attention.
6. General theories of emotion.
7. Importance of personality assessment in nursing.
8. Uses of intelligence tests.
9. Various methods of educational psychology.
10. Types of learning with illustrations.
11. Meaning and nature of thinking.
12. Attitude measurement and its implications in nursing.
13. Various tools of evaluation in educational psychology.

■ SHORT ANSWERS

14. Depth perception.
15. Define psychology and its application.
16. Needs and drives in human being.
17. States of emotion.
18. Personality types.
19. Chronological age (CA), mental age (MA) and intelligent quotient (IQ) concepts.
20. Hereditary studies for individual difference.
21. Trial and error learning methods.
22. Types of memory.
23. Incentive for effective teaching for teachers.

APPENDIX

II

Glossary

Abstract or general intelligence: It is the ability to respond to words, numbers and letters, etc. This type of intelligence is acquired by study of books and related literature. Mostly good teachers, lawyers, doctors and philosophers have this type of intelligence.

Abstract reasoning test: This test is intended as a verbal measure of the student's reasoning yielding ability. It has many picture tests yielding ambiguous scores because they require the student to discriminate between lines and areas, which differ, but slightly in size and shape. This test supplements the general intelligence aspects of the verbal and numerical tests.

Achievement testing: It is a systematic procedure for measuring a representative sample of learning tasks. Although the emphasis is usually on measuring a set of intended learning outcomes, as defined by the instructional objectives, it should not be implied that testing be limited.

Acute illness: Illness characterized by symptoms that are of relatively short duration, are usually severe and affect the functioning of the clients in all dimensions.

Adaptation: Process by which changes occur in any of a person's dimensions in response to stress.

Adjustment: An interaction between a person and his/her environment by which one adapts to depend upon the personal characteristics and circumstances of a situation producing a more harmonious relationship between himself/herself and the environment.

Aggression: A general term applied to behavior, aimed at hurting other people; also applies to feelings of anger or hostility. Aggression functions as a motive, often in response to threats, insults or frustrations.

Alarm reaction: The first stage of general adaptation syndrome that consists of prompt responses of the body; many of them mediated by the sympathetic system, which prepare the organism to cope with stressors.

Analytical intelligence: It is an academic problem-solving skill based on combined operations of execution, performance and knowledge. These three operations will enable us to encode stimuli, hold information in short-term memory, make calculations, perform mental calculations, mentally compare different stimuli and retrieve information from long-term memory.

Anxiety: These disorders range from feelings of uneasiness to immobilizing bouts of terror. Most people experience anxiety at some point in their lives and some nervousness in anticipation of a real situation. However, if a person cannot shake unwarranted worries or if the feelings are jarring to the point of avoiding everyday activities, the person most likely has an anxiety disorder. Anxiety can be associated with depression.

Appreciation learning: While conceptual learning is on the affective side, a child from the very beginning utilizes his/her inborn trait of esthetic sensibility and acquires concepts colored by appreciation.

Aptitude: It is a combination of characteristics indicative of an individual's capacity to acquire (with training) some specific knowledge, skill or set of organized responses such as the ability to speak a language, to become a musician and to do mechanical work.

Assimilation: In Piaget's theory of cognitive development, it refers to the modification of one's environment, so that it fits into already developed ways of thinking and behavior.

Associated areas: The regions of cerebral cortex involved in complex physiological functions such as understanding and production of language, thinking and imagery.

Associative learning: Conceptual learning is helped by associative learning in amassing a wealth of knowledge. New concepts are tagged with the past concepts through association.

Attitude: It is evaluation expressed by terms such as liking-disliking, pro-anti, favoring-not favoring and positive-negative. They are the feeling tone aroused by any attitude object. Attitude is thought to guide behavior, e.g. if a person is unfavorable towards smoking, he/she will show negative attitude towards smokers.

Attitude relevance: Because our world abounds with attitude issues, each of us can be concerned only with a limited number of issues those which are of special importance to us. It has been suggested recently that relevant attitudes are a better guide to subsequent behavior than are irrelevant attitude, i.e. for any given attitude issue, the link or correlation between attitudes and behavior should be much stronger for those individuals for whom the attitude is relevant than for those for whom it is not. This effect has been demonstrated for experimentally induced relevance.

Attitudinal learning: Attitudes are generalized dispositions for certain particular concepts, things, persons or activities. A child develops an attitude of affection towards his/her mother, an attitude of reverence towards the teacher and an attitude of belongingness towards the family. His/Her attitude towards play is most favorable. This entire child learns and adopts gradually.

Behavioral therapy: As the name implies, behavioral therapy focuses on behavior—changing unwanted behaviors through rewards, reinforcements and desensitization. Exposure therapy or desensitization is a process of confronting something that arouses anxiety, discomfort or fear and overcoming the unwanted responses. Behavioral therapy often involves the cooperation of others, especially family and close friends, to reinforce a desired behavior.

Behaviorism: The view that human and animal behavior can be understood predicted and controlled without recourse to explanations involving mental states.

Behaviorology: It is an independently organized discipline featuring the natural science of behavior. Behaviorologists study the functional relations between behavior and its independent variables in the behavior-determining environment. Behaviorological accounts are based on behavioral capacity of the species, the personal history of behaving organism, and the current physical and social environment in which behavior occurs. Behaviorologists discover the natural laws governing behavior.

Clairvoyance: It is the perception of objects or events not influencing the senses.

Clerical aptitude test: It is also a composite function; it involves several specific abilities such as perceptual ability, intellectual ability and motor ability.

Cloning: It is a technique of producing one or more individual plants or animals or human being, who are genetically identical to the original plant, animal or man. In short, it is the duplication process or carbon copy process.

Clouding of consciousness: It is a very mild form of altered mental status in which the patient has inattention and reduced wakefulness.

Cognitive dissonance: When two contradictory feelings, beliefs or behaviors exist, it creates a state of tension and the person tries to reduce tension by changing their feelings, beliefs or behaviors. For example, if a student nurse studies hard for a test, he/she expects to do well. But if studies hard and fails, dissonance is aroused.

Commitment: It is the extent to which a person feels reluctant to give up his/her initial position (attitude). Greater the strength of commitment to one's own attitude, it is harder for the individual to change his/her attitude.

Concepts: A concept is a symbol that stands for common properties of things. Concepts enable us to divide things into classes. Objects with common features are grouped under the same class. For example, we use the concept of flowers to refer to jasmine, lotus, etc. and with the concept of 'soft,' one can sort out objects into soft and hard. The concepts act as a tool and economize our efforts in thinking. For example, when we listen to the word 'elephant,' we are at once reminded not only about the nature and qualities of the elephants as a class but also our particular experiences and understanding about them emerges from our consciousness that stimulate the present thinking.

Conceptual learning: As concrete thinking leads to abstract thinking, perceptual learning is followed by conceptual learning. A concept is a general idea, which is universal in character. A child sees a particular cow and forms some ideas of a cow with some particular characteristics. Here the ideation is on the basis of one particular cow. This is the particular percept, but when the child sees a number of cows with some common characteristics, he/she locates certain general qualities in all the cows and on the basis of these, the child forms a conception of 'cow.' This is on the basis of percept, which is made general.

Conceptual or abstract thinking: Like perceptual thinking, it does not require the perception of actual objects or events. It is an abstract thinking where one makes use of concepts, the generalized ideas and language. It is regarded as a superior type of thinking to perceptual thinking, as it economizes efforts in understanding and problem solving.

Concrete intelligence: It is related to concrete materials. This type of intelligence is applicable when the individual is handling concrete objects or machines. The person uses this intelligence in the operation of tools and instruments. For example, engineers, mechanics generally have this type of intelligence.

Conditioning: It is a form of learning in which a reflex or some aspect of behavior is brought under the control of a stimulus; we will define conditioning in terms of the procedures used to bring it about. Although conditioning has been investigated in humans and animals, with generally similar findings, the majority of experiments on conditioning have employed animal subjects in which learning prior to the experiment can be more easily controlled.

Confusional state: It is a more profound deficit that includes disorientation, bewilderment and difficulty following commands. Lethargy consists of severe drowsiness in which the patient can be aroused by moderate stimuli and then drift back to sleep.

Consciousness: It is defined as the state of being mentally perceptive, alert and awake. For example, during some phases of deep sleep, the mind is active as it directs respiration, yet consciousness can be absent. So, consciousness is that bright spot of alertness within the much larger field of the mind. In this work, with the understanding that there are other uses of the word 'consciousness,' when it refers to that quality of alertness as an additional component within the mind, the word 'consciousness' will be capitalized.

Convergent thinking: The ability to produce responses that are based primarily on knowledge and logic.

Counseling: It is an accepting, trusting and safe relationship in which clients learn to discuss openly what worries and upsets them to define precise behavior goals to acquire essential social skills and to develop the courage and self-confidence to implement the desired new behaviors. Counseling is a process of enabling the individual to know oneself and his/her present and possible future situations in order that he/she may make substantial contributions to the society and to solve own problems through a face-to-face personal relationship with the counselor.

Creative intelligence: It involves insights, synthesis and the ability to react to novel situations and stimuli. It consists of ability, which allows people to adjust creatively and effectively to new situations. Novel tasks or situations are good measures of intellectual ability, because they assess an individual's ability to apply existing knowledge to new problems.

Creative process: It is referred to as any process by which something new is produced; an idea or an object including a new form or arrangement of old elements. The new creation must contribute to the solution of some problem.

Creative thinking: It means that the predictions and/or inferences for the individual are new, original, ingenious and unusual. The creative thinker is one who explores new areas and makes new observation, new predictions and new inferences. This type of thinking is chiefly aimed at creating something new. It is in search of new relationships and associations to describe and interpret the nature of things, events and situations. It is not bound by any pre-established rules. The individual himself/herself usually formulates the problem and is free to collect evidence and invent tools for its solution. The thinking of the scientists or inventors is an example of creative thinking.

Creativity: It is the capacity of a person to produce compositions, products or ideas, which are essentially new or novel and previously unknown to the producer.

Critical thinking: It is a higher order well-disciplined thought process, which involves the use of cognitive skills such as conceptualization, interpretation, analysis, synthesis and evaluation for arriving at an unbiased, valid and reliable judgment of the gathered or communicated information or data as a guide to one's belief and action.

Defense mechanism: It is a pattern of adjustment through which an individual relieves or decreases anxieties caused by an uncomfortable situation that threatens self-esteem. Ego defense mechanism is consciously or unconsciously operating device to keep confliction issues out of consciousness of the individual to bring some protective measures.

Delusional projection: Grossly frank delusions about external reality, usually of a persecutory nature. This defense mechanism is common feature of psychotic mental illnesses such as schizophrenia, delusional disorder, etc. These delusions are the false beliefs of the person which are not shared by race, age, educational background etc. Like, the person says that his family members are planning to kill him very soon.

Denial: It is protecting self from unpleasant reality by refusal to perceive it or face it. It is a defense mechanism in which a person is faced with a fact that is too painful to accept and reject it. The individual may deny the reality of the unpleasant fact altogether, admit the fact, but deny its seriousness or admit both the fact and seriousness, but denies responsibility. The concept of denial is particularly important to the study of addiction.

Differential aptitude test (DAT): It is developed by USA Psychological Corporation. It has proved more successful in predicting academic success, and found especially useful for providing educational and vocational guidance to secondary school children.

Distortion: A gross reshaping of external reality to meet internal needs. For example, mentally ill patients have no intact contact with reality. These patients are suffering with psychosis.

Drive: It is a tendency initiated by shifts in physiological balance, tissue tension, sensitivity to stimuli of a certain class and response in any of a variety of ways that are related to the attainment of a certain goals.

Echoic memory: A momentary sensory memory of auditory stimulus; if attention is elsewhere, sounds and words can still be recalled within 3–4 seconds. It would playback auditory information and gives time to recognize sounds as words.

Eclectic counseling: The strategy arises out of the appropriate knowledge of individual behavior and a combination of directive and other approaches. Irrespective of the differences, all approaches should have developmental, preventive and remedial values.

Educational guidance: This helps the students to get maximum benefit out of education and to solve their problems related to education. The emphasis is on providing assistance to students to perform satisfactorily in their academic work, choose the appropriate course of study, overcome learning difficulties, foster creativity, improve levels of motivation, utilize institutional resources optimally such as library, laboratory, etc.

Educational osychology: The branch of psychology used to study the behavior of learner in relation to educational environment. As a science of education, the subject matter of this branch helps in improving all the processes and products of education. The teachers can teach well and the students can learn well with the help of the knowledge and skills gained through the study of this subject. It also helps the teachers in gaining proper insight for bringing desirable modification in the behavior and seeking an all-round harmonious development of the personality of the students.

Emotion: A state of arousal involving facial and bodily changes, brain activation, cognitive appraisals, subjective feelings and tendencies toward action, all shaped by cultural rules.

Emotional intelligence: The ability to identify one's own and other people's emotions accurately, expresses emotions clearly and regulate emotions in oneself and others.

Emotionality: It has a powerful role to play in personality. The emotional stability and maturity is required for healthy personality.

Emotional quotient (EQ): The concept of EQ in understanding and measuring one's level of emotional intelligence in the same way and as we utilize the concept of intelligence quotient (IQ) in understanding, utilizing and measuring one's level of intelligence or intellectual potential. As a result, the term emotional quotient represents a relative measure of one's emotional intelligence potential in the same way as IQ does for the measurement of one's intellectual potential.

Environment: The totality of conditions within and surrounding the organism that serves to stimulate behavior or act to bring about change of behavior.

Environmental psychology: Field of psychology that focuses on the effects of environmental setting on an individual's feeling and behavior.

Episodic memory: It is concerned with information specific to a particular context, such as a time and place. It is used for more personal memories such as sensations, emotions and personal associations of a particular place.

Etiology: Identification of the cause of a problem. The cause may be direct or a contributing factor in the development of client problem or need.

Evaluation: It is determination of the worth or the value of an event, object or individual in terms of a specified criterion. Educators evaluate student progress by comparing student performance to the criteria of success based on instructional objectives. They evaluate a program in terms of how well children progress compared to how they might do in an alternative program.

Evolutionary psychology: The branch of psychology that seeks to identify behavior patterns that result from our genetic inheritance from our ancestors.

External environment: The environment after birth is more complex and powerful. It involves variety of physical and social contacts.

Extrinsic motivation: It comes from outside of the individual. Common extrinsic motivations are rewards such as money and grades, coercion and threat of punishment. Competition, in general, is extrinsic because it encourages the performer to win and beat others, not to enjoy the intrinsic rewards of the activity. A crowd cheering on the individual and trophies are also extrinsic incentives.

Fear: It is a basic survival mechanism or emotional response to a threat or specific stimuli. The stimuli or threat may be that of pain or danger of losing one's life. Fear is generally experienced by an individual with respect to a particular worsening situation.

General aptitude test: Battery developed by the Employment Service Bureau of USA has 12 tests, 8 of which are paper pencil tests, as for name comparison, computation, vocabulary, arithmetic, reasoning from matching, test matching, three-dimensional spaces, etc. The other 4 require the use of simple equipment in the shape of moving pegs on boards, assembling and dissembling rivets and washers.

General psychology: A field of psychology, which deals with fundamental rules, principles and theories of psychology to study the behavior of normal adult human being.

Genes: The parts of the chromosomes through which genetic information is transmitted.

Graphic art test: It requires the subject to produce sketches from given patterns of lines and figures. The created sketches of the subject are then evaluated according to the standards given by the author of this test.

Group counseling: This form of counseling is sometimes successful with clients, who have not responded well to individual counseling. This group interaction helps the individual to gain insight into his/her problems by listening to others discussing their difficulties. Group counseling often not only helps the individual to change but also enhances his/her desire and ability to help others faced with distressing life circumstances.

Guidance: It is the assistance made available by qualified and trained person to an individual of any age to help him/her manage his/her own life activities, develop own point of view, make own decision and carry on one's own burden. In educational context, guidance means assisting students to select courses of study appropriate to their needs and interests, achieve academic excellence to the best possible extent, derive maximum benefit of the institutional resources and facilities, inculcate proper study habits and satisfactorily participate in curricular and extracurricular activities.

Guilt: It is the emotional or cognitive experience, which succeeds the realization that one has violated a moral standard. The concept of remorse and guilt are closely related to each other.

Hallucinations: False sensory perceptions not associated with real external stimuli. Hallucinations may involve any of the five senses.

Health: Dynamic state in which an individual adapts to internal and external environments, so that there is a state of physical, emotional, intellectual, social and spiritual well-being.

Health behavior: Activities through which a person maintains, attains or regains behavior as an expression of personal health beliefs.

Health guidance: Health guidance implies the assistance rendered to students for maintaining sound health. Sound health is a prerequisite for participating in curricular and co-curricular activities. This type of guidance focuses on enabling students to appreciate conditions for good health and take steps necessary for ensuring good health, maintaining sound physical and mental health.

Health promoting behavior: Considered a third subcategory of health behavior and through assessment, reveal needs for vehicular safety, home safety, domestic violence recognition, recreational safety, occupational safety and health.

Health promotion: Activities directed toward maintaining or enhancing the health and well-being of clients.

Hereditary: Genetic transmission of characteristics from parents to their children or the totality of biologically transmitted factors that influence the structure of the body and thus, limit behavior.

Holistic health: A system of comprehensive or total care that considers the physical, emotional, social, economic and spiritual needs of the person, response to the illness, and the effect of illness on the person's ability to meet self-care needs.

Hormone: A secretion by a specific organ, often an endocrine gland, into the bloodstream, where it is carried to various organs of the body to have an effect; a chemical messenger.

Hypochondriasis: The transformation of negative feelings toward others into negative feelings toward self, pain, illness and anxiety. Hypochondriasis (or hypochondria), sometimes referred to as health phobia that refers to an excessive preoccupation or worry about having a serious illness. Often, hypochondria persist even after a physician has evaluated a person and reassured him/her that their concerns about symptoms do not have an underlying medical basis.

Iconic memory: A form of sensory memory that holds visual information for almost quarter of a second or more. It makes visual world appear smooth and continuous despite frequent blinks and an eye movements.

Identification test: It includes a wide variety of test situations representing various degree of realism. In some cases, a student may simply be asked to identify a tool or piece of equipment and to indicate its function. A more complex test situation might present the students with a particular performance task (e.g. locating a short in an electrical circuit) and ask them to identify the tools, equipment and procedures needed in performing the task.

Images: These, as mind pictures, consist of personal experiences of objects, persons or scenes once actually seen, heard or felt. These mind pictures symbolize the actual objects, experiences and activities. In thinking, we usually manipulate the images instead of actual objects, experiences or activities.

Individual counseling: This is a one-to-one helping relationship between the counselor and the counselee. It is focused upon the individual's need for growth and adjustment, problem solving and decision-making. This type of counseling requires counselors with the highest level of training and professional skills. In addition, it also requires that they have a certain personality type as well; counseling will be rendered ineffective unless counselors exhibit such personality traits as understanding, warmth, humaneness and positive attitudes toward the client.

Influencing ability: Most personality traits are not related to the ease with which someone is persuaded. A person's general personality profile will be of little use in predicting whether a given message will be persuasive. It is known, however, that some people are more easily influenced than others and that some people are downright gullible. The latter, bombarded with conflicting viewpoints, will believe the one they heard most recently. As might be expected, there are group differences in this trait. Obviously, children are more easily influenced than are adults, and poorly educated people are more easily influenced than are the well-educated.

Insight learning: In a typical insight situation, a problem is passed; a period follows during which no progress is made and then the solution comes suddenly. A learning curve of insight learning would show no evidence of learning for a time; and then suddenly learning would be almost complete.

Instinct: It is usually defined as a faculty of acting in such a way as to produce certain ends, without foresight of the ends and previous education in the performance.

Intelligence: It is the aggregate or global capacity of an individual to act purposefully, think rationally and deal effectively with his/her environment. Intelligence consists of an individual's those mental or cognitive abilities, which help him/her in solving the actual life problems and leading a happy and well-contented life. It is the capacity of an individual to learn and to solve problems and adjust to relatively new and changing conditions. There are individual differences, but it is desired from well-balanced personality in which intelligence is supplemented by healthy social being.

Intelligence quotient (IQ): It is a measure of intelligence obtained by dividing the individual's mental age as determined by his/her performance on standardized test items by his/her chronological age and multiplied by 100. It can be defined as the ratio between mental age and chronological age multiplied by 100.

Interest: It is a tendency to give selective attention to one activity or activities rather than to others in interest.

Internal environment: It refers to prenatal environment.

Intrinsic motivation: It refers to motivation that is driven by an interest or enjoyment in the task itself and exists within the individual rather than relying on any external pressure. Intrinsic motivation occurs when people are internally motivated to do something, because it either brings them pleasure, they think it is important or they feel that what they are learning is significant. It has been shown that intrinsic motivation for education drops from grades 3–9 though the exact cause cannot be ascertained.

Introspection: It means looking within or looking into the working of one's own mind and reporting what one finds there.

Language: It is the most efficient and developed vehicle used for carrying out the process of thinking. When one listens or read/writes words, phrases or sentences, or observes gestures in any language, the person is stimulated to think. Reading and writing of the written documents and literature also helps in stimulating and promoting the thinking process. The language broadens a person's thinking.

Learned motives: The motives those which are developed after birth. They are learned from the environment such as family and society. Learned motives include the need to be with others, to be approved by others, to be secure, to achieve success or social prestige.

Learning: It is the process by which an activity originates or is changed through reacting to an encountered situation, provided that the characteristics of the change in activity cannot be explained on the basis of native responses, tendencies, maturation or temporary states of the organism such as fatigue or effect of drugs.

Long-term memory (LTM): It has the unlimited capacity to store information for days, months, years and even lifetime. LTM codes information according to meaning, pattern and other characteristics. With the help of LTM, one can store, retain and remember most of the things in their life, at record notice, and thus make things quite easy.

Maturation: It is a developmental process within which a person, from time to time manifests different traits, the 'blueprints,' which have been carried in his/her cells from the time of conception. It produces an increase in competence, an ability to function at a higher level depending on the child's heredity. The changes in behavior of an organism resulting from physiological growth, the blueprints of which are provided by hereditary.

Mechanical aptitude: It is not a single unitary function; it is a combination of sensory and motor capacities and perception of spatial relations; the capacity to acquire information about the mechanical matters and the capacity to comprehend mechanical relationships.

Memory: The power to 'store' the experience and to bring them into the field of consciousness sometime after experiences have occurred, is termed memory.

Mental age: The average age of individuals who achieve a particular level of performance test.

Mental health: It refers to a sound, efficient mind and controlled emotions. It is the total and harmonious functioning of the whole personality of an individual for optimum functioning with maximum realization. A positive mental health shows an individual's ability to cope with the present and to adjust satisfactorily in future. A state of compromise and adaptation to a situation in a person's life leads to better adjustment. The individual fulfils his/her responsibilities, function effectively and is satisfied with the interpersonal relationships arid oneself.

Mental hygiene: It is an art and science, which includes application of scientific principles and practices for the promotion, preservation and maintenance of mental health, and prevention of mental disorders, enjoys healthy practices to lead productive, happy and contended life.

Mentally ill patients: They have no intact contact with reality. These patients are suffering with psychosis.

Mental retardation: It is defined as having significantly below-average intellectual functioning and limitations in at least two areas of adoptive functioning.

Motive: It is a state within the individual that under appropriate circumstances initiates or regulates behavior in relation to a goal.

Need: The lack of something which, if present, would tend to further welfare of the organism or of the species or to facilitate its usual behavior.

Neurobiology: The science of nervous system that includes neuroanatomy, neurophysiology, neurochemistry, neuropharmacology, neuroembryology, physiological psychology and other disciplines concerned with the structure, function and development of the nervous system.

Neurotransmitter: A chemical substance stored in vesicles and released into synaptic clefts or neuromuscular junction, to excite or inhibit neurons or muscle fibers.

Nursing: It is an art, science and profession by which one renders, serve human being to help regain or to keep a normal state of body and mind, and when it cannot accomplish this, it helps for the relief from physical pain, mental anxiety or spiritual discomfort.

Obtundation: It is a state similar to lethargy in which the patient has a lessened interest in the environment, slowed responses to stimulation and tends to sleep more than normal with drowsiness in between sleep states.

Operant conditioning: It refers to a kind of learning process whereby a response is made more probable or more frequently by reinforcement. It helps in the learning of operant behavior, the behavior that is not necessarily associated with known stimuli.

Panic attacks: The periods of intense anxiety, fear, physiological arousal, discomfort, stomach problems, etc. which occur suddenly and are discrete in nature are termed as panic attacks. They are associated with a variety of cognitive and somatic symptoms.

Paper-and-pencil performance: This test differs from the more traditional paper-and-pencil test by placing greater emphasis on the application of the knowledge and skill in a simulated setting. These paper-and-pencil applications might result in desired terminal learning outcomes or they might serve as an intermediate step to performance that involves a higher degree of realism (e.g. the actual use of equipment).

Perception: A process of organizing environmental stimuli into some meaningful patterns of wholes.

Perceptual learning: The child gets sensations through one's organs of sense and attaches meaning to each sensation. The earliest sensations of the infant are undifferentiated to the extent that he/she cannot differentiate between an object and another. In course of time, the child recognizes specific objects and perceives these separately.

Perceptual or concrete thinking: It is the simplest form of thinking. The basis of this type of thinking is perception, i.e. interpretation of sensation according to one's experience. It is also named as concrete thinking, as it is carried by the perception of actual or concrete objects and events. It is thinking of a lower order. Such type of thinking is present in animals and children.

Personal guidance: It refers to the guidance offered to students for enabling them to adjust themselves to their environment so that they become efficient citizens. Adolescent behavior to a great extent depends upon the moods and attitudes of the adolescent. Emotional instability is a characteristic of adolescents and this is often the cause of many of their personal problems. Personal guidance will help them to solve these problems.

Personality: The distinctive patterns of behavior, thought and emotions that characterize an individual's adaptation to the situations of his/her life. Personality is the individual's characteristic (and relatively enduring) organization (or integration), ways of behaving (or traits, interests, abilities, attitudes), and modes of adjustment to others and to the environment.

Personality disorders: These are psychological disorders characterized by lifelong maladaptive behavior patterns (refer antisocial personality disorder, schizotypal personality disorder, compulsive personality disorder and histrionic personality).

Personality dynamics:

a. The interactions among different characteristics (e.g. 'perro beauty'), especially motives.
b. The behavioral expression of personality characteristics in the process of adjusting to the environment.
c. In psychoanalysis, the management of the personality's energy system through the interactions of the id, ego and superego.

Personality structure: In general, the unique organization of traits, motives and ways of behaving that characterizes a particular person; in psychoanalytic theory, the conception of the personality in terms of id, ego, and superego (refer personality).

Personality tests: Tests to measure the characteristic ways a person behaves, thinks and feels, e.g. compatibility tests and the achievement tests.

Personalized system of instruction (PSI): An educational application of instrumental conditioning/operant conditioning in which the material in a course is divided into small units, each of which must be mastered at a high level of proficiency before the next unit is attempted.

Practical intelligence: It is the intelligence, which operates in the real world. People with this type of intelligence can adapt to or shape their environment. It is not only influenced by mental skills but also attitude and emotional factors.

Precognition: It is the perception of a future event. Precognition is a psychic knowledge of something in advance to its occurrence. In other words, it is the knowledge a person may have on another person's future thoughts.

Primary motives: These are those motives, which are necessary for survival; they are caused by the needs of our bodies. The main primary motives are hunger, thirst, avoidance of pain, need for air, sleep, elimination of wastes and regulation of body temperature.

Professional aptitude: The aptitude related to the activities of various professions and occupations are included in this category. These aptitudes are able to predict the future success of an individual in the field or profession related to these aptitudes.

Psi (pronounced 'sigh'): It is a term commonly used by parapsychologists to refer to both extrasensory perception (ESP) and kinesis taken together. The term was coined by Wiesner BP and recommended by Thouless RH.

Psychoanalysis: The method of psychotherapy based on Freud's psychoanalytic theory of personality; its basic premise is that the unconscious mind contains buried impulses and desires that must be brought to the surface, if anxiety is to disappear.

Psychoanalytic theory: Freud's theory states that all human behavior is dominated by instinctual biological urges that must be controlled. It is the conflict between the urges and efforts to control them that leads to emotional problems.

Psychodrama: A method of therapy in which one acts out scenes in order to bring out their emotional significance of behavior.

Psychokinesis (PK): Whereby a mental operation affects a material body or an energy system, e.g. wishing for a number affects what number comes up in the throw of dice.

Psychology: It is a systematic and scientific study of human and animal behavior. It has own special methods, which help us in gathering and organizing its subjective matter or the essential facts about it.

Psychometrics: Branch of psychology that deals with the development and application of statistical and other mathematical procedures to psychology.

Psychophysiological: It is pertaining to processes that have both bodily or material and psychological or mental aspects.

Psychosis: A severe mental disorder characterized by disorganization of the thought process, disturbances in emotionality, disorganization as to time, space and person, and in some other cases.

Psychosocial: It is pertaining to social relationships involving psychological factors.

Psychosocial development: Development of individual's interactions and understanding of each other and their knowledge, and understanding of themselves as the members of society.

Psychosomatic: A reference to the influence of mind or higher functions of brain (emotions, fears, desires, etc.) upon the functions of body; especially in relation to bodily disorders or disease.

Psychosomatic disorders: A disorder caused by a combination of organic and psychological factors. In psychosomatic disorders, there may be tissue changes as with peptic ulcers.

Psychotechniques: The practical application of psychological principles to control and manage the behavior.

Psychotherapy: The application of specialized techniques to the treatment of mental disorders or to the problems of everyday adjustment. The major techniques employed by psychotherapists include depth interviews, condition, suggestion and interpretation.

Psychotic: Characterizing a state of psychosis or resembling the behavior of an individual, who has a psychosis.

Puberty: The period, during which the capability for sexual reproduction is attained. It is marked by changes in both primary and secondary sexual characteristics, and is dated from menarche in girls and the emergence of pigmented pubic hair in boys.

Rational analysis: Involves the careful weighing of evidence for and against a particular attitude. The nurses giving health education in slums will influence their attitude for personal hygiene when informing about rationale of unhygienic conditions.

Reflective thinking or logical thinking: It aims at solving complex problems rather than simple problems. It requires reorganization of all the relevant experiences and finding new ways of reacting to a situation. Mental activity in reflective thinking does not undergo any mechanical trial and error type of effort. There is an insightful cognitive approach in reflective thinking. It takes logic into account in which all the relevant facts are arranged in a logical order, to get the solution of the problem in hand.

Registration: It is the short-term storage of the sensory input. Most of the information briefly held in the sensory register is lost. However, one pays special attention to some of the information in the sensory register. When a person does this, the attended information is passed onto the short-term store. The sensory register holds information for such a brief time that some psychologists prefer to discuss it as related to perception rather than memory.

Reinforcement: It is a collective term meaning either reward or punishment. It is often used when a principle is stated, which applies to both reward and punishment for instance, 'reinforcement is most effective when it occurs immediately after the response'.

Reliability: This is concerned with the consistency, stability and dependability of the results. In other words, a reliable result is one that shows similar performance at different times or under different conditions. For example, if a student takes a test several times and has not grown in area the test measures, he/she should earn a similar score each time.

Resistance to change/persuasion: Attitudes socialized early in life and to which the person is highly committed, do not change very much in adulthood. They are largely unaffected by mass communications or life changes such as aging, geographical mobility and social mobility.

Retention: It refers to a permanence of what was learnt. When active process of learning ceases, a comparatively passive process of retaining takes place. The material is retained when we are not thinking about it. People differ in their retentive capacity, which is largely due to genetic constitution.

Retrocognition: It is a type of clairvoyance involving knowledge of something after its occurrence through psychic menaces.

Selective attention and interpretation: Whether a message will influence a recipient or not depends upon how it is perceived and interpreted. Most important, it depends upon whether the message is attended to in the first place.

Semantic memory: It is the accumulation of facts and experiences gained over a lifetime. Semantic memory is used for remembering everyday types of facts and information. It is also called knowledge. Unlike other forms of memory, one usually does not remember where or when he/she has learnt the information in semantic memory.

Sensory defect: The defect in the function of one or more senses, resulting in visual, auditory or olfactory impairments.

Short-term memory (STM): It holds a relatively small amount of information about seven items, for a short period of (15–30 second) time, though not nearly as short-lived as the immediate memory.

Skill learning: Right from the birth, the child acquires skill. His/Her bodily organs learn to handle the things. He/She moves his/her legs and begins to crawl. In course of time, the child learns other motor skills, such as walking, speaking, drawing, writing, reading, playing music, cycling, swimming, etc.

Social guidance: This enables the student to make substantial contributions to the society, assume leadership, confirm to the social norms, work as team members, develop healthy and positive attitudes, appreciate the problems of society, respect the opinions and sentiments of fellow human beings, acquire traits of patience, perseverance and friendship. Its main purpose is to enable the student to become an efficient citizen.

Social intelligence: It is the ability of an individual to react to social situations in daily life. It includes the ability to understand people and act wisely in human relationships. Persons having this type of intelligence know the art of winning friends and influence them. For example, leaders, ministers, salesmen, diplomats are socially intelligent.

Social psychology: This branch of psychology studies the human behavior in relation to his/her social environment; one's behavior as a member of the group; the process of communication and interpersonal relationship, group dynamics and social relationship, etc. form the subject matter of this branch.

Space relations: It is the ability to visualize a constructed object from a picture of a pattern and an ability to imagine how an object would appear, if rotated in various ways for measurement of space perception. It means that these tests require mental manipulation of objects in three-dimensional spaces.

Stimulus: An occurrence or event that produces some effect on some organism. It is inborn, but not necessary for survival. It includes activity, curiosity, exploration, manipulation and physical contact.

Stress: It may be defined as an adjustive demand placed on the organism. The condition or force on object giving rise to this demand may be internal or external and is designated as the stressor.

Student performance: It emphasizes proper procedure. The student is typically expected to perform the same motions as those required in the actual performance of the task, but the conditions are simulated. In physical education, e.g. swinging a bat at an imaginary ball, shadow boxing and demonstrating various swimming strokes out of water are considered simulated performances.

Stupor: It means that only vigorous and repeated stimuli will arouse the individual and when left undisturbed, the patient will immediately lapse back to the unresponsive state.

Subconscious mind: Consciousness does not have access to the entire body/mind, thus the term subconscious. The subconscious mind refers to all parts of the body/mind that consciousness does not have access to. Because the body and mind cannot be separated, it is more accurate to call this the subconscious mind/body. This long phrase has been shorted in this work to simplify the subconscious.

Suggestion: Advertisers and propagandists often rely on suggestion, the uncritical acceptance of a statement. They design their messages in hopes that people will accept a belief, form an attitude or be incited to action by someone else say-so, without requiring facts.

Superego: According to Freud, the part of the personality that acquires the values and ideals of the parents and society, and imposes constraints on the id and ego, the conscience.

Telepathy: It is the perception of objects or events not influencing the senses.

Testing: A test is a set of specified, uniform tasks to be performed by students. These tasks are an appropriate sample from the knowledge or skills in a broader field of content. From the number of tasks performed correctly in the sample, the teacher makes an assumption of how the student is likely to perform in the total field. These delusions are the false beliefs of the person, which are not shared by race, age, educational background, etc. Similarly person says that his/her family members are planning to kill him/her very soon.

Thinking: It is a complex mental activity. It is symbolic in character; initiated by a problem, which the individual is facing, involves the response of the individual to this problem. Thinking is a problem-solving process in which we use ideas or symbols in places of overt activity.

Unconscious motivation: Some attitudes are held because they serve some unconscious function for an individual. For example, a person who is threatened by their homosexual feelings may employ the defense mechanism of reaction formation and become a crusader against homosexuals.

Verbal reasoning: It is a measure of ability to understand concepts framed in words. It is aimed at evaluation of the student's ability to abstract or generalize and to think constructively, rather than simple fluency or vocabulary recognition. The words used in these items may come from history, geography, literature, science or any other content area.

Visual memory: It is part of memory preserving some characteristics of our senses pertaining to visual experience. One is able to place in memory the information that resembles objects, places, animals or people in sort of a mental image.

Vocational guidance: It is the assistance provided for selection of a vocation and preparation for the same. It is concerned with enabling students to acquire information about career opportunities, career growth and training facilities.

Wernicke's area: An area in the temporal lobe of cerebrum, which is necessary for the recognition of speech sounds and therefore for the comprehension of language; also plays a part in the formulation of meaningful speech.

Index

A

D

E

F

G

H

I

N

Q

R

S

T

U